P9-BEE-263

a LANGE medical book

Evidence-Based Medicine

A Framework for Clinical Practice

NOTICE

Medicine is an ever-changing science. As new research and clinical experience broaden our knowledge, changes in treatment and drug therapy are required. The authors and the publisher of this work have checked with sources believed to be reliable in their efforts to provide information that is completely and generally in accord with the standards accepted at the time of publication. However, in view of the possibility of human error or changes in medical sciences, neither the authors nor the publisher nor any other party who has been involved in the preparation or publication of this work warrants that the information contained herein is in every respect accurate or complete, and they disclaim all responsibility for any errors or omissions or for the results obtained from use of the information contained in this work. Readers are encouraged to confirm the information contained herein with other sources. For example and in particular, readers are advised to check the product information sheet included in the package of each drug they plan to administer to be certain that the information contained in this work is accurate and that changes have not been made in the recommended dose or in the contraindications for administration. This recommendation is of particular importance in connection with new or infrequently used drugs.

a LANGE medical book

Evidence-Based Medicine

A Framework for Clinical Practice

Edited by
Daniel J. Friedland, MD
Assistant Clinical Professor
Department of Medicine
University of California, San Francisco

Lange Medical Books/McGraw-Hill
Medical Publishing Division

New York St. Louis San Francisco Auckland Bogotá Caracas Lisbon London
Madrid Mexico City Milan Montreal New Delhi San Juan
Singapore Sydney Tokyo Toronto

McGraw-Hill

A Division of The **McGraw·Hill** Companies

Evidenced-Based Medicine: A Framework for Clinical Practice

Copyright © 1998 by Appleton & Lange. All rights reserved. Printed in the United States of America. Except as permitted under the United States Copyright Act of 1976, no part of this publication may be reproduced or distributed in any form or by any means, or stored in a data base or retrieval system, without the prior written permission of the publisher.

6 7 8 9 10 QSR/QSR 0 9 8 7 6 5 4 3

ISBN: 0-8385-2476-1 (domestic)
ISSN: 1098-0059

Acquisitions Editor: Shelley Reinhardt
Development Editor: Cara Lyn Coffey
Production Editor: Elizabeth C. Ryan
Art Coordinator: Eve Siegel
Illustrations: Wendy Beth Jackelow
Interior Design: Janice Barsevich Bielawa

I dedicate this book to my loving and supportive parents, Yvonne and Bernard Friedland, and my love, Susan Hunt.

—Daniel J. Friedland, MD

CONTENTS

CONTRIBUTORS

Peter E. Alperin, MD
Assistant Clinical Instructor, Department of Medicine, University of California, San Francisco
Application of the Guide to Study Examples of Diagnostic Tests, Intervention & Prognosis

Stephen W. Bent, MD
Clinical Research Fellow, Department of Internal Medicine, University of California, San Francisco
Internet: steve_bent@quickmail.ucsf.edu
Treatment and Testing Thresholds; Evaluating Integrative Literature

J. Ben Davoren, MD, PhD
Assistant Clinical Professor of Medicine, University of California, San Francisco; Assistant Chief, Medical Service, Department of Veterans Affairs Medical Center, San Francisco
Internet: davoren@itsa.ucsf.edu
Searching MEDLINE; Searching the Internet

Daniel J. Friedland, MD
Assistant Clinical Professor, Department of Medicine, University of California, San Francisco
Internet: djf@itsa.ucsf.edu
Treatment and Testing Thresholds; Guide for Assessing the Validity of a Study; Application of the Guide to Study Examples of Diagnostic Tests, Intervention, & Prognosis; Evaluating Integrative Literature

Alan S. Go, MD
Clinical Epidemiology Fellow, General Internal Medicine Section, Department of Veterans Affairs Medical Center, San Francisco
Internet: alan_go@quickmail.ucsf.edu
Refining Probability

Terrie Mendelson, MD
Associate Professor of Medicine & Director, Housestaff Education, University of California, San Francisco; Program Director, Internal Medicine/Evidence Based Medicine Residency (PRIME), Department of Veterans Affairs Medical Center, San Francisco, & University of California, San Francisco
Internet: tmend@itsa.ucsf.edu
Keeping Up With the Medical Literature; Evaluating Integrative Literature

Michael G. Shlipak, MD, MPH
Senior Resident, Department of Internal Medicine, University of California, San Francisco
Internet: shlip@itsa.ucsf.edu
Decision Analysis; Evaluating Integrative Literature

Leslee L. Subak, MD
Adjunct Assistant Professor, Department of Obstetrics, Gynecology, & Reproductive Science, University of California, San Francisco
Internet: leslee_subak@quickmail.ucsf.edu
Cost-Effectiveness Analysis; Evaluating Integrative Literature

Philippe O. Szapary, MD
Senior Resident, Department of Internal Medicine, University of California, San Francisco
Internet: szapary@mail.med.upenn.edu
Application of the Guide to Study Examples of Diagnostic Tests, Intervention, & Prognosis

Jeffrey A. Tice, MD
Fellow, General Internal Medicine, University of California, San Francisco
Internet: jeffrey_tice@ucsfdgim.ucsf.edu
Application of the Guide to Study Examples of Diagnostic Tests, Intervention, & Prognosis

FOREWORD

Medical knowledge is expanding rapidly. Learning to access, interpret, and apply this knowledge appropriately is a daunting but crucial task for all clinicians. In *Evidence-Based Medicine: A Framework for Clinical Practice,* common clinical examples serve to illustrate a practical, logical, and efficient approach to making medical decisions on the basis of sound evidence.

The authors present an approach to finding relevant literature and present uniform guides for evaluating studies and integrative literature. Key issues, such as the validity of measurements and the representativeness of subjects, are developed in detail, so that users of this book can become independent readers of the medical literature. The book provides tools in the section on medical decision-making techniques to help readers further decide whether and how the results of a study apply to their patients.

If you have ever faced the problem of deciding which, if any, articles to read when a journal arrives or of finding the most relevant study when confronted with a specific clinical question, the advice in this book will be helpful. Whether you are considering the recommendations of a particular clinical practice guideline or how to interpret and apply the results of a case-control study, decision analysis, or other types of medical literature, the practical approaches contained within these pages will be invaluable.

Deborah Grady, MD, MPH
Associate Professor of Epidemiology
and Medicine, University of
California, San Francisco

Warren S. Browner, MD, MPH
Professor of Medicine, Epidemiology
and Biostatistics, University of
California, San Francisco
Chief, General Internal Medicine,
Department of Veterans Affairs Medical Center,
San Francisco

PREFACE

Evidence-Based Medicine: A Framework for Clinical Practice provides an introduction to the most important components of evidence-based decision making:

- Medical decision-making techniques
- Accessing medical information
- Evaluating the validity of medical information

AUDIENCE

This book can improve evidence-based decision making at all levels of experience, from students to clinicians in training, to clinicians in practice. The principles of evidence-based medicine can be applied in all fields of medicine and will be useful to any type of health care provider in the privileged position of helping a patient make a diagnostic or therapeutic decision. In addition, this text may be invaluable to those involved in making policies or to anyone who critically evaluates medical literature.

OBJECTIVES

After reading this book, the reader will be able to:

- Estimate the probability that a particular diagnosis is present
- Understand the fundamental components of decision analysis
- Estimate the treatment and testing thresholds for various medical conditions
- Understand the fundamental components of cost-effectiveness analysis
- Use a systematic approach to search MEDLINE
- Understand the key components of the Internet and how the Internet is used to search for medical information
- Keep up to date with the mass of medical information
- Use a systematic approach to critically evaluate studies
- Use a systematic approach to critically evaluate integrative literature (ie, overviews, meta-analyses, practice guidelines, and decision and cost-effectiveness analyses)

OUTSTANDING FEATURES

- The Introduction presents the significance, definition, and components of evidence-based medicine and outlines the organization of the book.
- The text is divided into three sections covering the three major components of evidence-based medicine.
- An organizational algorithm of the book's structure provides a context at the beginning of each chapter.

- Each chapter is outlined.
- Topical clinical vignettes and examples are used extensively throughout.
- A problem-solving approach to refining probability and estimating treatment and testing thresholds is used.
- Evidence-based medicine terms are provided for searching MEDLINE.
- Examples of premiere medical Internet sites are included.
- Includes examples of premiere publications for keeping up to date with medical information.
- Contains a study guide that is a novel five-step approach to evaluating studies based on epidemiologic and clinical research principles.
- Examples are provided of how the study guide is applied to a published study of an intervention, diagnostic test, and prognosis ("reprints" of the articles evaluated are included).
- Contains a novel five-step approach to evaluate integrative literature.
- Chapters are summarized.
- The text is readable—and possibly even fun!

ACKNOWLEDGMENTS

The contributors and I are indebted to the following persons for providing their precious time to review the manuscript and for offering invaluable comments: Dr. Warren Browner, Dr. Deborah Grady, Dr. Stephen Hulley, Dr. Thomas Newman, Dr. Karla Kerlikowske, Dr. Peter Salzmann, Dr. Steven Cummings, Dr. Joel Simon, Dr. Andrew Avins, Dr. Shanta Suryaraman, Dr. Craig Frances, Gail Sorrough, and Gloria Won.

I am indebted to Dr. Keith Marton, Dr. Merlynn Bergen, Dr. Lawrence Tierney, Jr., and Dr. Stephen McPhee for providing encouragement and constructive advice during the formative stages of this project.

I am grateful to Sylvia Miles for her patient grammatical review of parts of the text and the tireless effort of Diane Bartholomew in taking care of numerous administrative details.

I also owe gratitude to the Department of Epidemiology and Biostatistics at the University of California, San Francisco, for supporting my fellowship, during which time much of this project evolved.

Finally, we have had the good fortune of working with a truly gracious and consummately professional team at Appleton & Lange: Cara Coffey, who was meticulous and an absolute pleasure to work with during her development and copy edit of the text; Elizabeth Ryan for production; Janice Bielawa for design; Eve Siegel for her artwork; and Shelley Reinhardt, who supervised the development and production of the book.

DISCLAIMER

Although we have endeavored to ensure the accuracy and validity of all information in this book, we acknowledge the possibility of unforeseen errors. In the spirit of evidence-based medicine, the individual clinician should ensure that any information provided to the patient is valid and accurate and that a reasonable decision-making process has been used. Medicine is not an exact science but a science of probabilities. Medicine involves uncertainty. Ultimately, persons involved in making decisions must assume responsibility. The authors and publisher disclaim all responsibility for any liability, loss, injury, or damage incurred as a consequence, directly or indirectly, of the use or application of any contents of this book.

Daniel J. Friedland, MD
San Francisco, California
May 1998

Please send comments, suggestions, or corrections to Dr. Daniel J. Friedland, c/o Appleton & Lange, 107 Elm St, PO Box 120041, Stamford, CT 06912-0041.

INTRODUCTION

Daniel J. Friedland, MD

The goal of this book is to provide an introductory framework for evidence-based medicine. In this introduction, we first address the importance of evidence-based medicine and provide its definition. Next we discuss the individual components of evidence-based medicine that serve as the basis for the structure of the book.

IMPORTANCE OF EVIDENCE-BASED MEDICINE

Consider these two scenarios:

> Your patient has just had a Q-wave myocardial infarction that resulted in moderate congestive heart failure. You are considering administering a beta-blocker in the patient, but a professor in the Division of Cardiology advises against this, stating that instituting such medication will further decrease cardiac function.

What should you do?

> You are a fresh-out-of-residency surgeon caring for a patient with 70% occlusion of the left carotid artery. The patient has had no neurologic symptoms and was referred to you after his primary care physician noted a left carotid artery bruit. You are being asked to consider the patient for carotid endarterectomy. You discuss the case with a former attending physician, who states that the intervention makes good sense and is supported by recent medical literature. The attending physician also states, "This is now what we always do."

What should you do?

Evidence-based medicine is a movement that has developed to help us make such decisions with our patients *systematically*. This movement is represented by a recent profusion of literature and course work in evidence-based medicine and, as described below, has been characterized as a paradigm shift.[1]

The **traditional medical paradigm** comprises four assumptions:

1. Individual clinical experience provides the foundation for diagnosis, treatment, and prognosis. The measure of authority is proportional to the weight of individual experience.
2. Pathophysiology provides the foundation for clinical practice.
3. Traditional medical training and common sense are sufficient to enable a physician to evaluate new tests and treatments.
4. Clinical experience and expertise in a given subject area are a sufficient foundation to enable the physician to develop clinical practice guidelines.

The new **evidence-based medicine paradigm** comprises a different set of assumptions:

1. When possible, clinicians use information derived from systematic, reproducible, and unbiased studies to increase their confidence in the true prognosis, efficacy of therapy, and usefulness of diagnostic tests.
2. An understanding of pathophysiology is necessary but insufficient for the practice of clinical medicine.
3. An understanding of certain rules of evidence is necessary to evaluate and apply the medical literature effectively.

If we use the traditional paradigm to make decisions in the first scenario, we would avoid the use of a beta-blocker in a patient who has just had a myocardial infarction that resulted in moderate congestive heart failure. According to pathophysiologic principles, a negative inotropic agent could decrease cardiac pump function and therefore should not be used in a patient with moderate congestive heart failure. Furthermore, the stature and experience of the consultant contributes considerable weight to our decision.

In the new evidence-based medicine paradigm, decisions are based primarily on certain rules of evidence that are applied to systematic studies. In this paradigm, we are more likely to recommend a beta-blocker on the basis of results of the Beta-Blocker Heart Attack Trial,[2,3] which showed a mortality benefit of beta-blockers after Q-wave myocardial infarction. With the application of a simple calculation, we note that the number of patients who were treated to prevent a single death was smaller in the group who had their infarct complicated by congestive heart failure than it was in the asymptomatic subset. In other words, the mortality benefit of the medication after myocardial infarction is expected to be greater in patients with congestive heart failure than in those who are asymptomatic.

If we were following the traditional paradigm in the second scenario, we would undoubtedly recommend the surgical intervention. Our recommendation would be strongly influenced by the counsel of an experienced surgeon, as well as the biological plausibility that if our patient has narrowing in the internal carotid artery, removal of this narrowing should decrease subsequent risk of cerebrovascular events. Although the new evidence-based medicine paradigm does not always provide a definitive answer, it does provide an explicit framework that helps us evaluate the validity of the relevant literature[4] and, with application of certain key concepts and calculations, better estimate the net benefit of this intervention for our patient. In Chapter 9, we demonstrate how to assess the validity of the information relevant to this scenario and how to determine its net benefit for the patient. With this framework, we are able to counsel our patients more effectively.

Although evidence-based medicine has been beneficial in providing a new systematic approach to medical decision making, its characterization as a paradigm shift has met with some resistance. This resistance may be due to the presumption that before the development of evidence-based medicine, medical decisions were not made on the basis of any evidence at all. A letter recently published in *The Lancet*[5] states that the new evidence-based medicine paradigm presumes ". . . the practice of medicine was previously based on a direct communication with God or by tossing a coin." An alternative and possibly more palatable way of characterizing evidence-based medicine is *not as a paradigm shift* but rather as an *evolution of the tools used to practice scientific medicine*. The paradigm shift to practice scientific medicine probably dates to 1910, when Abraham Flexner reported on the quality of education at approximately 130 US medical schools.[6] Medicine was no longer practiced and taught as a trade. Its new foundation rested on *biomedical science*, which at that time served as the best available evidence on which medical decisions were made. Medical decision-making tools of the time thus relied on a thorough knowledge of pathophysiology and clinical judgment. As an evolution of these tools, evidence-based medicine by no means substitutes for clinical judgment or pathophysiology, but rather incorporates them within a more explicit and rigorous framework.

Our assumption is that evidence-based medicine will lead to an improvement in patient outcomes and teaching and result in more cost-effective medical care by providing an explicit framework to make medical decisions in following rules of evidence applied to systematically obtained information. With further development, evidence-based medicine itself will need to be systematically evaluated to provide supporting evidence for its role in medical practice.

So, then, what is this term, evidence-based medicine?

DEFINITION OF EVIDENCE-BASED MEDICINE

Evidence-based medicine is the practice of making medical decisions through the judicious identification, evaluation, and application of the most relevant information.

COMPONENTS OF EVIDENCE-BASED MEDICINE

The definition makes reference to a number of components of evidence-based medicine. First, we frame a given medical problem to identify the specific information we need. When this information is identified, we retrieve it and then evaluate it to ensure that it is valid. Finally, if we believe the information, we need to know how to apply it to the care of our patient.

The care of our patients usually involves making diagnoses and providing effective counseling to help them make choices that will either cure disease, prolong life, prevent disease or disease progression, or facilitate quality of life. Framing a medical problem thus entails the application of strategies to make diagnoses and choices. Although there are many ways to frame a clinical problem, the one that is most rigorous involves medical decision-making techniques. These techniques not only help you identify the information you need but—once you assess the validity of this information—also assist you in applying this information to patient care. In this book, we thus focus on three primary components of evidence-based medicine, discussed below (Figure I–1).

Medical decision-making techniques

These techniques are **quantitative methods** that we may apply to medical decision making. However, the methods are often used **qualitatively** as well. These techniques may be divided into those that help us make diagnoses and those that help us make choices.

For a given medical problem, we generate a differential diagnosis. Before any test is performed, we assign each diagnosis in the differential a probability of being present (ie, pretest probability). We then perform a test that may change the probability of the diagnosis being present (ie, posttest probability). This process, the technique of **refining probability,** helps us determine the likelihood of each given disease process in the differential, thereby assisting us in making a diagnosis.

Refining probability in isolation, however, does not enable us to make choices (eg, to perform another diagnostic test or to observe or treat the patient). When our refined probabilities are applied to **treatment and testing thresholds,** however, the appropriate choice may become apparent.

Decision analysis helps us choose between any number of strategies by providing an accounting method that takes into consideration the probabilities of multiple outcomes as well as the relative value of each outcome. As you will see later in this book, decision analysis is also integral to determine the treatment threshold.

Another technique to help us make choices is **cost-effectiveness analysis.** This technique helps us place the medical decision within a larger context: the finite resources of society. This type of analysis enables us to choose the best intervention on the basis of an evaluation of the costs and efficacy of therapy.

Finally, when we apply the relevant information to make decisions with our patients, we do so within the context of the patient's preferences. To that end, techniques that help us make choices with our patients incorporate the relative values patients assign to the possible outcomes.

Access to medical information

Access to the vast body of medical information presents two major challenges: (1) finding the relevant information for a given problem and (2) keeping up with the literature.

Our options for finding the relevant reference material include asking experts, searching our personal library of textbooks and articles, and performing a computer-assisted literature search. The latter is the most effective method for finding a relevant article, because it enables us to search vast medical databases of published journal articles (eg, MEDLINE). In recent years, much medical information has become available via the Internet.

Keeping up with the medical literature in our precious spare time dictates a need for efficiency. One approach may be to target specific journals, continuing medical education (CME) updates, and publications that provide summaries of key articles from many journals.

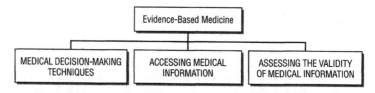

Figure I–1. The three principal components of evidence-based medicine.

Assessment of the validity of medical information

When we are presented with medical information, it is critical that we assess its validity. This may involve a determination of the credibility of the source or, optimally, an evaluation of the literature. Structured approaches are available to evaluate the literature and have been applied to articles addressing prognosis, diagnostic tests, efficacy and risk of therapy, as well as overviews, practice guidelines, decision analysis, and economic analysis.[7-20] Assessing validity of information derived from the Internet is more difficult, especially because of the lack of peer review in this medium.[21]

STRUCTURE OF THIS BOOK

(See Figure I–2.)
This book consists of three sections in a modular format that is intended to provide a framework for the practice or study of evidence-based medicine. The practitioner of evidence-based medicine may use the medical decision-making techniques presented in Section 1 to frame the medical problem. The first chapter, "Refining Probability," helps us make diagnoses. The next three chapters, "Decision Analysis," "Treatment & Testing Thresholds," and "Cost-Effectiveness Analysis," help us make choices with our patients. Framing the particular problem helps us identify information that we need to retrieve. The chapters in Section 2, "Accessing Medical Information," enable us to locate the relevant information by searching MEDLINE and the Internet. In addition, Section 2 also includes a chapter to help you keep up to date with the medical literature. After retrieving the relevant information, we evaluate it critically. Section 3 of the book, "Assessing the Validity of Medical Information," is dedicated to this process. A systematic five-step approach is presented in Chapter 8, "Guide for Assessing the Validity of a Study." The next chapter provides examples of the guide applied to studies of an intervention, diagnostic test, and prognosis. Once we have retrieved and critically appraised the relevant information, we apply the information to the care of our patient, again turning to the principles described in Section 1 and Chapter 8. In this way, we use the best evidence to make diagnoses, facilitate patients' choices, and provide patients with appropriate counseling.

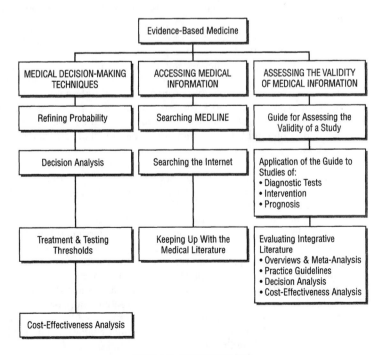

Figure I–2. Structure of the book.

The book's modular format may facilitate the teaching of evidence-based medicine. Consider the structure of a month-long course for fourth-year medical students in preparation for their residency. The first week of the course would be dedicated to learning the different medical decision-making techniques, including the use of computer software such as decision analysis programs. The student would then use a particular technique to frame an important clinical scenario that they might encounter in their chosen specialty. A student entering medicine might choose to determine the treatment and testing thresholds for pulmonary embolism (as in Chapter 3). A prospective surgical intern, on the other hand, might be interested in these thresholds for appendicitis (also in Chapter 3). Alternatively, either student might be interested in using a decision analysis to determine whether they should use immunosuppressive therapy or surgery in the patient with ulcerative colitis in whom administration of corticosteroids has failed (see Chapter 2).

By the end of the first week, the student will have used a particular technique to frame the clinical problem at hand, thereby identifying the information they need to retrieve. For example, the student tackling the thresholds for pulmonary embolism will discover that it is imperative to retrieve specific information regarding the natural history of untreated pulmonary embolism, the risks and benefits of anticoagulation, and the test characteristics of the ventilation-perfusion lung scan. The second week of the course would be dedicated to learning MEDLINE and Internet search techniques to find these needles of information in the haystack of medical literature.

During the third week, students would learn the skills to evaluate medical information critically. These skills would then be applied to the systematic evaluation of the key articles they have retrieved (possibly using a journal club format). During the final week, the students would present to their colleagues their evidence-based approach for their selected scenarios.

What is the proper context of this book? To answer this, we need to consider many issues regarding evidence-based medicine. Does the practice of evidence-based medicine mean that we no longer exercise clinical judgment, rather becoming quantitative automatons? What do we do when faced with time constraints and lack of data in daily practice? Can you imagine performing a decision or threshold analysis every time you wanted to determine the best therapeutic option? You would not have time to see your patients—for that matter, you would have no free time at all! Although many of this book's principles are presented quantitatively, the limits of data and time will more likely lead to these principles being used qualitatively. For example, use of the principles of decision analysis reminds us to at least consider the probabilities of the possible outcomes as well as the patient's preferences for those outcomes. Similarly, application of the principles of threshold analysis helps us to explicitly weigh the risks and benefits of a therapy that may better clarify whether we should have a high or low threshold for treating the patient. Furthermore, if evidence is lacking, we do not need to forestall decision making; the principles of evidence-based medicine highlight areas of uncertainty and provide us with an explicit framework for discussion and planning. As such, evidence-based medicine principles do not substitute for clinical judgment but rather help improve it by more explicitly highlighting the individual factors that contribute to our decision-making process.

For common clinical questions, the practitioner may feel unable to find the time to identify, retrieve, evaluate, and apply the most relevant information. However, a clinician who has invested time to develop an evidence-based approach to a commonly seen medical problem may subsequently save time by decreasing the use of unnecessary tests and treatment or the numbers of referrals made for patients.

The physician may save even more time by referring to literature that synthesizes and integrates information obtained from individual studies into a summary finding or recommendation. This type of information is known as integrative literature and comprises overviews, meta-analyses, practice guidelines, decision analyses, and cost-effectiveness analyses. In the growing mass of published studies and the increased pressure to see more patients in less time, clinicians will likely become more dependent on integrative literature to guide their practice. Clinicians will therefore need to become more facile in critically evaluating this literature. To that end, the final chapter of this book instructs the reader in how to assess the validity of integrative literature.

REFERENCES

1. Evidence-based medicine: A new approach to teaching the practice of medicine. Evidence-Based Medicine Working Group. JAMA 1992;268:2420.
2. Beta-Blocker Heart Attack Trial Research Group: A randomized trial of propranolol in patients with acute myocardial infarction. JAMA 1982;247:1707.
3. Furberg CD et al: Effect of propranolol in postinfarction patients with mechanical or electrical complications. Circulation 1984;69:761.
4. Executive Committee for the Asymptomatic Carotid Atherosclerosis Study: Endarterectomy for asymptomatic carotid artery stenosis. JAMA 1995;273:1421.
5. Fowler PBS: Letter to the editor. Lancet 1995;346:838.
6. Flexner A: *Medical Education in the United States and Canada: A Report of the Carnegie Foundation for the Advancement of Teaching.* Institution: Carnegie Foundation, 1910.
7. Oxman AD et al: Users' guides to the medical literature. I. How to get started. Evidence-Based Medicine Working Group. JAMA 1993;270:2093.
8. Guyatt GH et al: Users' guides to the medical literature. II. How to use an article about therapy or prevention. A. Are the results of the study valid? Evidence-Based Medicine Working Group. JAMA 1993;270:2598.
9. Guyatt GH et al: Users' guides to the medical literature. II. How to use an article about therapy or prevention. B. What were the results and will they help me in caring for my patients? Evidence-Based Medicine Working Group. JAMA 1994;271:59.
10. Jaeschke R et al: Users' guides to the medical literature. III. How to use an article about a diagnostic test. A. Are the results of the study valid? Evidence-Based Medicine Working Group. JAMA 1994;271:389.
11. Jaeschke R et al: Users' guides to the medical literature. III. How to use an article about a diagnostic test. B. What are the results and will they help me in caring for my patients? The Evidence-Based Medicine Working Group. JAMA 1994;271:703.
12. Levine M et al: Users' guides to the medical literature. IV. How to use an article about harm. Evidence-Based Medicine Working Group. JAMA 1994;271:1615.
13. Laupacis A et al: Users' guides to the medical literature. V. How to use an article about prognosis. Evidence-Based Medicine Working Group. JAMA 1994;272:234.
14. Oxman AD et al: Users' guides to the medical literature. VI. How to use an overview. Evidence-Based Medicine Working Group. JAMA 1994;272:1367.
15. Richardson WS, Detsky AS: Users' guides to the medical literature. VII. How to use a clinical decision analysis. A. Are the results of the study valid? Evidence-Based Medicine Working Group. JAMA 1995;273:1292.
16. Richardson WS, Detsky AS: Users' guides to the medical literature. VII. How to use a clinical decision analysis. B. What are the results and will they help me in caring for my patients? Evidence Based Medicine Working Group. JAMA 1995;273:1610.
17. Hayward RSA et al: Users' guides to the medical literature. VIII. How to use clinical practice guidelines. A. Are the recommendations valid? Evidence-Based Medicine Working Group. JAMA 1996;274:570.
18. Hayward RSA et al: Users' guides to the medical literature. VIII. How to use clinical practice guidelines. B. What are the recommendations and will they help you in caring for your patients? Evidence-Based Medicine Working Group. JAMA 1996;274:1630.
19. Drummond MF et al: Users' guides to the medical literature. XIII. How to use an article on economic analysis of clinical practice. A. Are the results of the study valid? Evidence-Based Medicine Working Group. JAMA 1997;277:1552.
20. Drummond MF et al: Users' guides to the medical literature. XIII. How to use an article on economic analysis of clinical practice. B. What are the results and will they help me in caring for my patients? Evidence-Based Medicine Working Group. JAMA 1997;277:1802.
21. Kassirer JP, Angell M: The Internet and the journal. N Engl J Med 1995;332:1709.

SUGGESTED READING

Gelbach SH: *Interpreting the Medical Literature,* 3rd ed. Macmillan, 1992.
 This text provides an understanding of the medical literature through discussion of different study designs and measurements and interpretation of important concepts such as distributions, averages, statistical significance, diagnostic test characteristics, risk, and causation.

Hulley SB, Cummings SR: *Designing Clinical Research: An Epidemiologic Approach.* Williams & Wilkins, 1988.
 This is the classic text on how to design clinical research. An understanding of the important issues of study design facilitates an ability to appraise a published study critically. The basic principles in

Hulley and Cummings' book serve as the foundation of the study guide presented in Chapter 8 of our text.

Panzer RJ et al: *Diagnostic Strategies for Common Medical Problems.* American College of Physicians Press, 1991.

This book provides instruction on how you can refine probability using likelihood ratios. It presents data that help you estimate the pretest probability of disease as well as the characteristics of diagnostic tests, thereby facilitating diagnoses. Diagnostic strategies for many medical problems are presented.

Sackett DL et al: *Clinical Epidemiology: A Basic Science for Clinical Medicine,* 2nd ed. Little, Brown, 1991.

In many ways, this is a forerunner to Sackett and coauthors' 1996 text. It presents an epidemiologic approach to diagnosis and management, including an approach to evaluate studies and how to apply them to patient care. The book presents information to help you review your performance in patient care, search for relevant information, keep up to date with medical information, read reviews and economic analyses, and derive benefit from continuing medical information.

Sackett DL et al: *Evidence-Based Medicine: How to Practice and Teach EPBM.* Churchill Livingstone, 1996.

This pioneering text provides a clinically practical approach to frame the clinical question, search for the information, appraise the information's validity, and apply the information to patient care. In addition, an approach to evaluating the effect of your decisions is included. The text devotes individual attention to diagnosis, prognosis, treatment, and harm.

Sox HC Jr et al: *Medical Decision Making.* Butterworth-Heinemann, 1988.

This text presents key concepts in medical decision making. It has chapters on differential diagnosis, quantifying uncertainty in terms of probability, using Bayes' theorem to apply new information, measuring the accuracy of clinical data, selecting and interpreting diagnostic tests, as well as decision, cost-effectiveness, and cost-benefit analyses.

Weinstein MC: *Clinical Decision Analysis.* Saunders, 1980.

This is an early classic text in decision analysis.

1

MEDICAL DECISION- MAKING TECHNIQUES

REFINING PROBABILITY: AN INTRODUCTION TO THE USE OF DIAGNOSTIC TESTS

Alan S. Go, MD

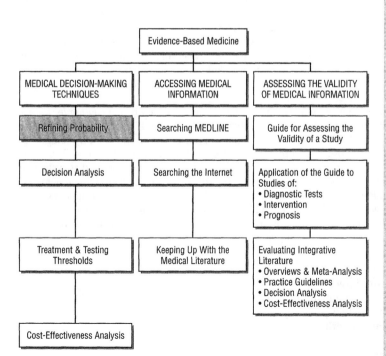

Evidence-Based Medicine

MEDICAL DECISION-MAKING TECHNIQUES
- Refining Probability
- Decision Analysis
- Treatment & Testing Thresholds
- Cost-Effectiveness Analysis

ACCESSING MEDICAL INFORMATION
- Searching MEDLINE
- Searching the Internet
- Keeping Up With the Medical Literature

ASSESSING THE VALIDITY OF MEDICAL INFORMATION
- Guide for Assessing the Validity of a Study
- Application of the Guide to Studies of:
  • Diagnostic Tests
  • Intervention
  • Prognosis
- Evaluating Integrative Literature
  • Overviews & Meta-Analysis
  • Practice Guidelines
  • Decision Analysis
  • Cost-Effectiveness Analysis

INTRODUCTION: AN APPROACH TO THE ART OF MEDICAL DIAGNOSIS

A 6-month-old baby girl is brought to your pediatric office by a worried mother. The baby has been having poor feeding, tactile fever, rhinorrhea, and a progressive cough for 1 week. *What are the possible causes of these symptoms and signs, and how would you refine the probability of each of them?*

A 28-year-old woman who is in her third trimester of pregnancy comes to your obstetrics office for a routine visit. She reports mild headaches over the last couple of weeks and intermittent epigastric pain not associated with meals. She heard about a pregnancy-related complication called preeclampsia and was concerned that she may have it. *What are other possible causes of her symptoms, and how would you refine the probability of preeclampsia and the rest of the possible etiologies?*

A 63-year-old man with a history of hypertension presents to the local emergency department complaining of progressive headache and neck pain. *What are the possible causes, and how would you refine the probability of each of them?*

As you can see, when a person presents with a medical complaint, the physician is often faced with a daunting diagnostic dilemma. As physicians in this situation, we generate a **differential diagnosis** that includes the most important possible causes, and then we use various pieces of information (eg, history, physical examination, clinical laboratory tests, and radiographic studies) to help us **refine the probability of disease** for *each* significant diagnostic prospect.

The first step in the art of medical diagnosis is learning to generate a differential diagnosis. This is simply assembling a list of all the possible causes that may explain your patient's symptoms and signs. How do we generate this list? Many clinicians develop a short list of specific diseases in a random or haphazard fashion, but this approach often leaves out important considerations of the underlying cause because it is not systematic. A method commonly taught early in medical training is the use of a strict *anatomic* approach, which can be effective for certain types of diseases. For example, a young man presents with the acute onset of periumbilical abdominal pain that moves to the right lower quadrant and is accompanied by nausea and vomiting. What is on your differential diagnosis list? A strict anatomic approach to abdominal pain in the right lower quadrant might move from the outward structures inward. In this case, one can start at the skin (eg, herpes zoster) and muscle wall (eg, inguinal hernia) and move to the peritoneal lining (eg, peritonitis), right ascending colon (eg, diverticulitis), terminal ileum (eg, inflammatory bowel disease), and, finally, the appendix (eg, appendicitis). In certain cases, the strict anatomic approach may also result in inclusion of the ureter (eg, kidney stone) and bladder (eg, cystitis), depending on other symptoms and signs. Unfortunately, there is not always a strong correlation between anatomy and the true underlying cause.

Another approach that is commonly taught focuses primarily on *pathophysiologic* processes (eg, inflammation, infection, and ischemia) to guide thinking about the imaginable list of diagnoses. As with use of only the anatomic approach, use of only the physiologic approach can lead to omissions of potentially important and more likely diagnoses. Therefore, although there are different approaches one can use, a very helpful mnemonic that systematically includes most of the major categories is "**VINDICATE.**" To remember this mnemonic, keep in mind that after we've generated a differential diagnosis and used the techniques of refining probability, we will feel "**VINDICATE**d" by obtaining the most likely diagnosis! This mnemonic combines anatomic, pathophysiologic, and systems approaches and can be applied successfully to almost any patient complaint, as described below:

V ascular
I nflammatory/infectious
N eoplastic/neurologic and psychiatric
D egenerative/dietary
I ntoxication/idiopathic/iatrogenic
C ongenital
A llergic/autoimmune
T rauma
E ndocrine and metabolic

Now let's see how the VINDICATE approach works practically. Let's go back to the example of the 63-year-old man with a history of hypertension who complained of progressive headache and neck pain. Using the mnemonic VINDICATE, the following differential diagnosis can be generated:

Vascular: subarachnoid hemorrhage, stroke/transient ischemic attack, vertebrobasilar insufficiency, temporal arteritis, subdural hematoma

Inflammatory/infectious: bacterial, fungal, or mycobacterial meningitis or brain abscess; sinusitis

Neoplastic/neurologic and psychiatric: brain tumor, carcinomatous meningitis, migraine, tension headache, cluster headache, anxiety reaction, somatization, panic attack

Degenerative/dietary: cervical osteoarthritis

Intoxication/idiopathic/iatrogenic: cocaine ingestion, ethanol withdrawal, idiopathic or iatrogenic causes

Congenital: none

Allergic/autoimmune: hay fever, ankylosing spondylitis, lupus cerebritis

Trauma: cervical musculoskeletal strain, vertebral fracture, cerebral contusion

Endocrine and metabolic: pheochromocytoma, carcinoid syndrome, hypercalcemia

And so we have an example of one approach—VINDICATE—to generating a differential diagnosis list. There are many resources available to assist in problem-based or symptom-specific differential diagnoses.[1,2] Now that we have a method to systematically develop a list of possible causes for our patient, we now need a way to determine which cause is the *most likely*. Typically, the list is long—but on the basis of the history and physical examination, along with other more formal diagnostic tests, we can narrow the possibilities to end up with a much shorter list. In other words, we refine the probability of *each* possible choice to ultimately arrive at the most likely diagnosis.

Unfortunately, many of us don't understand how the results of diagnostic tests change the likelihood of a particular diagnosis. Therefore, the primary goal of this chapter is to help you improve your use of diagnostic tests by applying the evidence-based medicine techniques of **refining probability**. As you'll see, this chapter is an interactive one, and completion of its exercises will enable you to sequentially expand your diagnostic armamentarium. It may be helpful to keep a calculator nearby.

AN EQUATION FOR THE USE OF DIAGNOSTIC TESTS:
"WHAT WE THOUGHT BEFORE" + "TEST INFORMATION" = "WHAT WE THINK AFTER"

Let's illustrate the process of refining probability with an example from internal medicine. Below is a hypothetical patient who you may see on a typical clinic day.

It's 5:30 PM and near the end of your medical clinic shift. Ms Venus Klott, a 50-year-old executive who is an 60-pack-year cigarette smoker, drops in complaining of an acute onset of shortness of breath and a vague pleuritic chest pain starting 30 minutes after eating a large chicken burrito.

Based on this information, what are the top five possible diagnoses on your **differential diagnosis list**?

1. _____
2. _____
3. _____
4. _____
5. _____

Although we could easily produce a laundry list of possible causes, a reasonable list of the most likely five candidates includes pulmonary embolism, acute myocardial infarction, gastroesophageal reflux disease or peptic ulcer disease, esophageal obstruction, and airway foreign body obstruction.

In actual clinical practice, we will often attempt to "rule in" or "rule out" *each* of these significant possibilities, but for simplicity, let's concentrate only on the possibility of *pulmonary embolism* (ie, a blood clot that has traveled from the deep venous system in the legs or pelvis into one or both of the pulmonary arteries). However, the principles demonstrated in refining the probability of pulmonary embolism can easily be used for *any* diagnostic possibility.

For each situation, write in your estimate of the probability (0–100%) that Ms Venus Klott is experiencing a pulmonary embolus (PE):

Based on her history alone, what is her probability of having a PE? _____ %

An arterial blood gas (ABG) measurement obtained with the patient breathing room air showed the PaO_2 (partial pressure of oxygen) to be 70 mm Hg (normal, 80–100 mm Hg).

With the added information from the ABG measurement, what is her cumulative probability of having a PE? _____ %

An electrocardiogram (ECG) obtained in the office showed atrial fibrillation with an $S_1Q_3T_3$ pattern and a right bundle branch morphology (ie, suggestive of right ventricular strain).

With the added information from the ECG, what is her cumulative probability of having a PE? _____ %

You obtain a ventilation-perfusion (V/Q) lung scan that was notable for multiple segmental, unmatched defects in the left upper lobe, right upper lobe, and right apex (ie, a "high-probability" scan).

Given all of this diagnostic test information, what is her final probability of having a PE? _____ %

We'll return to this example throughout our discussion to see how accurate we were and how we can improve our estimation of probability!

As physicians, we routinely order diagnostic tests—but why? Some of the reasons often stated for ordering diagnostic tests include

- "It's what we always do." (*Tradition*)
- "The hospital has to make money somehow." (*Economic Gain*)
- "I just wanted to know the ceruloplasmin level." (*Curiosity*)
- "(Fill a name in the blank) told me to do it." (*Hierarchy*)
- "We have to learn how to perform procedures somehow." (*Practice*)

Although these reasons are frequently cited, ultimately, the most important reason we order diagnostic tests is to **refine probability,** which is defined here:

Refining probability = modifying our estimate of the likelihood of a disease through the application of diagnostic tests

This is another way of stating a mathematical principle called **Bayes' theorem.** Bayes' theorem simply says that the probability of an event depends on new information applied to what is previously known about the event. Regarding diagnostic tests, this simplifies to the following equation:

What we thought before + Test information = What we think after

Pretty easy, right? New diagnostic test information is applied to what we thought before the test to yield what we think after the test. By the end of this chapter, we'll convert this equation into one that we can apply practically in the care of our patients:

What we thought before + Test information = What we think after
⇓   ⇓   ⇓
Pretest probability + Likelihood ratios = Posttest probability

When we think about disease in our patients, "What we thought before" and "What we think after" from the above equation are merely estimates of the likelihood of a disease. These estimates lie along the same scale of **probability** that ranges from 0% (disease ruled out) to 100% (disease ruled in).

Over the next several sections, let's work our way through each component of the above equation. Then we'll put the whole equation back together. Let's start with "What we thought before."

What we thought before + Test information = What we think after

⇕

Prestest Probability + Likelihood Ratios = Posttest Probability

MAXIMIZING YOUR PRETEST PROBABILITY ESTIMATES: "WHAT WE THOUGHT BEFORE"

In all arenas, especially sports, the probability of winning is an important topic of discussion for many people. In many cities across the country, a major issue weighing on the hearts and minds of many fans and bookmakers is, What is the preseason probability that their major league sports teams will win the national championship?

Well, the mention of "probabilities" is heard not only in sports bar chatter, but it is also ubiquitous in the halls of medicine. Probabilities are indispensable in describing the likelihood of a disease in a particular patient. As you'll see, determining the probability of a disease *before* you order a diagnostic test (ie, pretest probability) will help you more effectively arrive at your final estimate of disease (ie, posttest probability). We've been using the term probability frequently, so let's define it explicitly:

Probability = a number between 0 and 1 (or 0% and 100%) that expresses the likelihood of something happening or being true

Therefore, the following definitions logically follow:

Pretest (or prior) probability = the probability that a patient has the disease *before* undergoing a test

Posttest (or posterior) probability = the probability that a patient has the disease, *given* the result of a test

In other words, we start with a certain **pretest probability,** and after the application of a diagnostic test, we finish with a **post-test probability** of disease. Armed with these definitions, let's start the process of refining probability.

From the above discussion, it is clear that we must start with learning how to determine the pretest probability. A key concept about pretest probability is the importance of assigning a number to our qualitative descriptions of pretest probability while using general rules to help us generate a more accurate estimate.

Many of us have learned only to *qualitatively* estimate our patient's pretest probability of disease. For example, it is quite common to hear colleagues (or ourselves) describe a patient's likelihood of disease as "possible," "probable," or "ruled in." Note, however, that although we are comfortable with these qualitative terms, it is important to learn to put a *number* on the estimated pretest probability. By assigning a number to our qualitative descriptions, we improve our precision and more clearly convey to other physicians what we actually mean. One physician's conversion of verbal descriptions to numerical probabilities is shown in Figure 1–1. Would your assigned probabilities be exactly the same? Probably not.

In fact, when posed to a group of physicians, ranges of answers were obtained (Figure 1–2). Given the wide range of numerical estimates for the *same* verbal description, it's no surprise that people get confused when they try to communicate using only qualitative, verbal expressions of pretest probability.

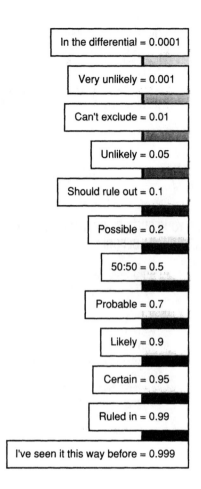

Figure 1–1. Numerical probabilities of disease assigned to qualitative estimates.

Besides understanding the need to communicate in quantitative terms, what methods do we use to generate our estimates of pretest probability? There are generally two methods:

1. Personal experience
2. Published data

Personal experience: the pinnacles & the pitfalls

Personal experience is a critical part of determining pretest probability and is part of the reason why the most skilled diagnosticians who have had many years of clinical experience seeing patients and diseases arrive at more accurate estimates. When physicians are confronted with any diagnostic dilemma, they often fall back on personal experience through the application of a process psychologists call *heuristics*.[4] Heuristics are often referred to as diagnostic *rules of thumb* that are used to help one generate a differential diagnosis and then refine probability. In other words, heuristics are cognitive processes used to learn, remember, or understand knowledge that are assembled through personal experience as a set of approaches to problems. Unfortunately, although heuristics can be helpful in estimating pretest probability, physicians' experiences are not comprehensive, and this shortcoming can lead to significant errors in our estimates. Understanding the potential errors that can be made will reduce your likelihood of making mistakes in overestimating or underestimating pretest probability.[4,5] The three most common heuristical errors occur in **sampling, saliency,** and **simple weighting of clinical characteristics.**

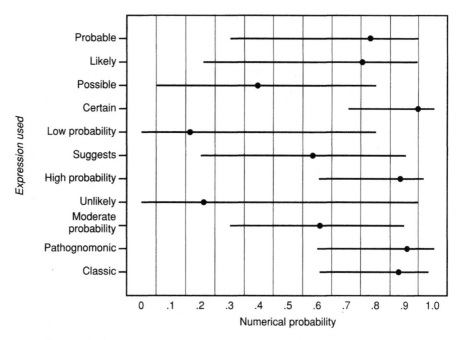

Figure 1–2. Probability estimates of disease associated with various qualitative verbal expressions. Mean values are indicated by a dot and ranges by a horizontal line. (Reprinted by permission of *The New England Journal of Medicine*. Modified from Bryant GD, Norman GR: Expressions of probability words and numbers. N Engl J Med 302:411. Copyright (1980]), Massachusetts Medical Society).[3]

Sampling. Sampling bias can lead to either an underestimation or overestimation of disease pretest probability secondary to overall clinical inexperience or an unrepresentative experience. An example of sampling bias:

> You are a medical student in the first month of your internal medicine ward rotation at a tertiary care hospital. You've seen a total of five patients with shortness of breath and wheezing, and because you're at a tertiary care center, three of the five were referred patients who turned out to have Wegener's granulomatosis (a rare disease). You're now on-call and go down to see a patient in the emergency department complaining of shortness of breath and wheezing.

Because of sampling bias from both a small overall clinical experience and an unrepresentative experience, you may make mistakes in your pretest probability estimates. Because you've only been at a tertiary care center, you may greatly overestimate the pretest probability of Wegener's granulomatosis because of the five previous cases you've seen. Similarly, you may underestimate the pretest probability of reactive airway disease (ie, asthma or exacerbation of chronic obstructive pulmonary disease), which is far more likely in this patient given how common this illness is in the general population.

Saliency. Webster's defines saliency as "a striking point or feature, or highlight."[6] Therefore, saliency bias occurs in medicine when a particular "highlight" of a disease makes it much easier to remember compared with other more likely diagnoses in a given patient. Specifically, these memory highlights may be based on the *recency* of a case of the disease, the *rarity* of the illness, its *novel clinical features,* or a past experience of being *"burned" by missing a case* of the disease. Any one of these highlights may bias you to overestimate the pretest probability of a particular disease in the next patient you evaluate. For example, the last patient with neck pain whom you assessed turned out to have an atypical presentation of a dissecting aortic aneurysm that was missed and that later required emergent surgery, which led to a long, complicated hospital course. Saliency bias (ie, recency, rarity, novelty, or being "burned") may lead to the next five patients complaining of neck pain receiving unnecessary computed tomographic scans of the chest because of an overestimation of the pretest probability of aortic dissection. Similarly, this experience would lead to a compensatory underestimation of more likely diseases such as musculoskeletal strain, tension headaches, or even meningitis.

Simple weighting of clinical characteristics. A final class of heuristics that can lead to an overestimation of the pretest probability of a disease is the problem of simple weighting of clinical characteristics in a patient. A simple weighting system assigns *equal* weights to the presence or absence of the different clinical characteristics being considered in making a particular diagnosis. Let's look at an example.

> A 60-year-old man with a strong family history of early coronary artery disease and multiple other cardiac risk factors comes to your office complaining of the acute onset of crushing, substernal chest pressure for the last 30 minutes. The chest pressure was accompanied by shortness of breath, diaphoresis, mild nausea, intermittent palpitations, and minimal lightheadedness.

The main concern is whether this patient is experiencing acute myocardial infarction (AMI). A simple weighting system would assign equal value to each of the clinical characteristics (eg, family history, other cardiac risk factors, chest pain, shortness of breath) in determining a pretest probability of AMI. Therefore, most clinicians would estimate that this patient has a very high pretest probability of AMI based solely on the presence of eight clinical characteristics consistent with this disease. How would your estimate change if the patient had only a family history of early coronary disease and had acute onset of crushing, substernal chest pressure for the last 30 minutes? It may surprise some readers that the pretest probability of AMI when you have only these two clinical characteristics is almost the *same* as when you have all eight, since family history and typical angina carry much more weight in the diagnosis of AMI than all of the other features combined. In fact, the remaining six characteristics contributed very little because they either are not strong, independent predictors of AMI (eg, lightheadedness or palpitations) or provide redundant information of the same underlying physiologic process (eg, diaphoresis and mild nausea from increased vagal tone). As you can see, it is very important to consider the appropriate weights of each individual clinical feature when evaluating a patient for a specific illness.

In thinking about all of these issues, you will gain insight into how you mentally assign estimates of pretest probability on the basis of your own experience. By remembering the potential biases of sampling, saliency, and simple weighting, you should decrease the number of gross errors you make in either overestimation or underestimation of the probability of disease in your patient.

PUBLISHED STUDIES: SIFTING THE WHEAT FROM THE CHAFF

Published studies in the medical literature can be invaluable in determining pretest probability when the studies are well-designed and have clinically useful results. Given this caveat, there are two main ways that we can use published data in our estimates of pretest probability, ways that are presumably more objective than personal experience (although this may be debated):

1. Estimating pretest probability using the *prevalence* of a disease associated with a certain **clinical symptom or sign** (eg, the prevalence of pulmonary embolism in outpatients who complain of the acute onset of dyspnea or the prevalence of hemachromatosis in white men with an abnormally high serum ferritin level)
2. Estimating pretest probability using **discriminant score clinical prediction rules** (eg, to determine the likelihood of myocardial infarction in patients presenting to an emergency department with chest pain)

It is important to remember that there are limitations of published data, including bias and lack of generalizability (see Chapter 8). But often, the main problem is the sheer lack of information that is needed to answer the desired question.

So what's the bottom line for estimating pretest probability? Skilled clinicians maximize the use of both **personal experience** and **published data** (while recognizing their limitations) to more accurately predict pretest probability in an individual patient. Another important characteristic of skilled diagnosticians is their ability to recognize that whenever considering the probabilities of different diseases in a specific patient, all of the probabilities must add up to 100%. For example, 60% chance of pneumonia + 20% chance of asthma + 15% chance of viral upper respiratory tract infection + 5% chance of pneumothorax = 100% total probability of disease.

Having just reviewed ways to estimate pretest probability, let's return to the case of Ms Klott. Again, for simplicity, we are considering only one diagnosis, pulmonary embolism, whereas in actual clinical practice, we would use the same techniques for all significant possibilities in the differential diagnosis list. Remember, the first question we need to answer is:

> For a 50-year-old woman with acute onset of dyspnea and pleuritic chest pain who presents to an outpatient primary care clinic, what is the pretest probability of a pulmonary embolus?
> - Using personal experience *alone,* the pretest probability is _____ (only you can determine this).
> - After an extensive search for the published prevalence of pulmonary embolism in patients presenting to an outpatient clinic with dyspnea and pleuritic chest pain, you find that no actual studies have been published from 1966 to 1997. However, published data on the prevalence of pulmonary embolism in patients admitted to the hospital with acute shortness of breath provide a reasonable estimate of the pretest probability that ranges between **5% and 15%**.[7-9]
> - Putting these two values together, what is your combined pretest probability? _____

Starting with this estimate of "What we thought before" (or pretest probability), we're now ready to use "Test information" to finally arrive at "What we think after" (or posttest probability).

What we thought before + *Test information* = What we think after

SENSITIVITY, SPECIFICITY, PREDICTIVE VALUE, & LIKELIHOOD RATIOS EXPLAINED: "TEST INFORMATION"

Test information (ie, diagnostic test characteristics) has traditionally been reported in terms of **sensitivity, specificity,** or **predictive value** throughout the bulk of the medical literature. However, we will quickly see that only when test information is presented as **likelihood ratios** can we easily refine the estimated probability of disease in our patients. Sensitivity, specificity, and predictive value have significant limitations that prevent us from extracting the most information from diagnostic tests. However, it is important to gain an understanding of these concepts before fully appreciating the advantages of using likelihood ratios.

Let's start with sensitivity and specificity.

Sensitivity & specificity re-examined

One of the key prerequisites to breaking down the concepts of sensitivity and specificity is to understand the (in)famous 2 × 2 table shown in Figure 1–3. Remember, sensitivity and specificity can be used primarily for diagnostic tests that have only two outcomes (ie, dichotomous tests). Also, as with all diagnostic tests reported in the medical literature, sensitivity and specificity are meaningful only when the studied population underwent an acceptable "gold standard" that was used to "rule in" or "rule out" the disease of interest (eg, evaluating the diagnostic capabilities of serum ferritin level for iron deficiency anemia in patients with microcytic anemia who all underwent bone marrow biopsy to determine actual marrow iron stores).

The table in this figure shows us that there are only four possible outcomes of a dichotomous test:

Disease

		Present	Absent	
Test result	Positive	a TP = True-positives	b FP = False-positives	a + b
	Negative	c FN = False-negatives	d TN = True-negatives	c + d
		a + c	b + d	a + b + c + d

Figure 1–3. 2 × 2 table for a dichotomous test.

1. A positive test result in persons with the disease = **a** = **true-positive**
2. A positive test result in persons without the disease = **b** = **false-positive**
3. A negative test result in persons with the disease = **c** = **false-negative**
4. A negative test result in persons without the disease = **d** = **true-negative**

Using this 2 × 2 table and these definitions, sensitivity and specificity are easily derived by thinking *vertically.* Let's start with the concept of sensitivity as shown in Figure 1–4.

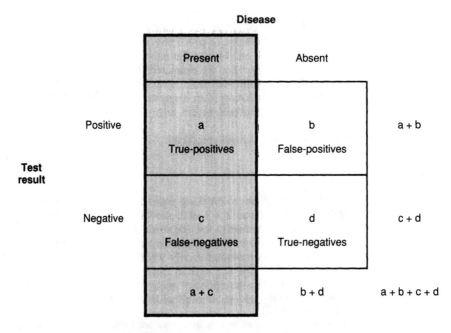

Figure 1–4. Sensitivity presented vertically in a 2 × 2 table for a dichotomous test.

Sensitivity = the proportion of patients *with* the disease who have a
positive test result. In Figure 1–4, this is represented by a/(a + c) =
true positives/(true positives + false negatives)

Some people like mnemonic devices to help them remember. For sensitivity, one can use **PID,** which stands for **positive in disease,** because sensitivity tells us how often the test result is **positive in** people who are already known to have the **disease.**[10]

The complementary term to sensitivity is **specificity,** which is shown in Figure 1–5.

Specificity = the proportion of patients *without* the disease who have a
negative test result. In Figure 1–5, this is represented by d/(b + d) =
true negatives/false positives + true negatives)

A complementary mnemonic for specificity is **NIH,** which stands for **negative in health,** because specificity tells us how often a test result is **negative in** people who are known not to have the disease (ie, in good **health**).[10]

Note that sensitivity and specificity describe the proportion of positive and negative test results in a population in whom we *already know* who has the disease or not. This, therefore, gives us insight into the major clinical limitation of sensitivity and specificity in the use of diagnostic tests—*we don't know who has the disease before the test!* Otherwise, we wouldn't need to order the diagnostic test.

Instead, what we really want to know is, What is the meaning of a positive or negative test result? In other words, we want to know a test's **predictive value.**

The usefulness of predictive value

The predictive value of a diagnostic test is based on both its sensitivity and specificity as well as the prevalence of the target disease in the population being evaluated. Thus, the predictive value of a diagnostic test includes information about both the test itself and the tested population to give a more useful clinical measure.

Because we care more about how "good" a test is at "predicting" who has the disease and who doesn't, we will now think *horizontally* across in the 2 × 2 table instead of vertically (as we did for sensitivity and specificity).

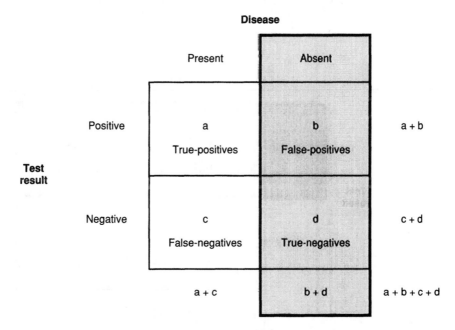

Figure 1–5. Specificity presented vertically in a 2 × 2 table for a dichotomous test.

We'll start with **positive predictive value (PPV),** which is used to help us predict the likelihood of having the disease if you have a *positive* test result (Figure 1–6).

Positive predictive value (PPV) = the proportion of patients with a
positive test result who *have* the disease. In Figure 1–6, this is
represented by a/(a + b) = true positives/(true positives + false positives)

Key synonyms for PPV that you may encounter in the medical literature include **posttest probability** and **posterior probability of having the disease.** These synonyms arose because of the assumption that the pretest probability is the prevalence of the disease in the studied population and that a positive test result will yield a "posttest" or "posterior" = "after the test" probability of having the disease.

As you would expect, the complementary term of PPV is **negative predictive value (NPV),** which helps us predict the likelihood of *not* having the disease in the setting of a *negative* test result (Figure 1–7).

Negative predictive value (NPV) = the proportion of patients with a
negative test result who do *not have* the disease. In Figure 1–7, this is
represented by d/(c + d) = true negatives/(false negatives + true negatives)

Key synonyms for NPV that you may encounter in the medical literature include **posttest probability** and **posterior probability of not having the disease.** Similar to the explanation for PPV above, these names arose because of the assumption that the pretest probability of not having the disease is (1-prevalence) in the studied population and that a negative test result will yield a "posttest" or "posterior" probability of *not* having the disease.

Does this all sound confusing? With one test result, you get the probability of *having* the disease, whereas with the other, you get the probability of *not having* the disease! This added complexity is one reason why predictive value is not very useful.

Furthermore, since predictive value is dependent on the fixed prevalence/pretest probability of disease in the studied population, predictive value is limited in helping us to refine probability in our particular patient population—composed of patients who usually have a different prevalence/pretest probability of disease.

By using diagnostic test information in the form of likelihood ratios, we are freed from the constraints of the 2 × 2 table and the fixed prevalence/pretest probability of disease in our patient. Two additional advantages of likelihood ratios are that:

Disease

		Present	Absent	
Test result	**Positive**	a True-positives	b False-positives	a + b
	Negative	c False-negatives	d True-negatives	c + d
		a + c	b + d	a + b + c + d

Figure 1–6. Positive predictive value presented horizontally in a 2 × 2 table for a dichotomous test.

Disease

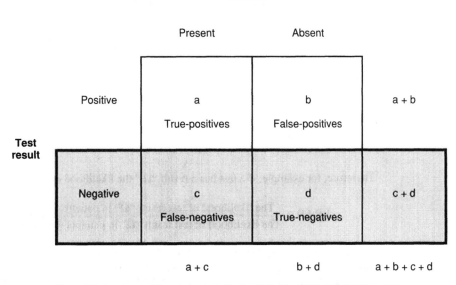

Figure 1–7. Negative predictive value presented horizontally in a 2 × 2 table for a dichotomous test.

1. they can be derived for diagnostic tests that have multiple levels/categories of results.
2. likelihood ratios from different, *independent* tests can be used together sequentially to easily calculate a single estimate of a patient's posttest probability of disease.

Likelihood ratios: the final frontier

As we've said before, we order diagnostic tests to help us refine probability. Let's briefly review the basic equation of diagnostic tests:

What we thought before + *Test information* = What we think after
⇕
Pretest probability + *Likelihood ratios* = Posttest probability

Since we don't usually have truly perfect tests (ie, a "gold standard"), test results can only *increase* or *decrease* our likelihood (probability) of disease. What's more, diagnostic tests that have different levels or categories of results can give us more information than tests that have just a positive or negative result, because with the former we will be able to change our probability of disease with greater accuracy and precision. So how do we best express test information? **Likelihood ratios.**

As you can imagine from the above equation, the magnitude of the likelihood ratio, when applied to the pretest probability, directly affects the magnitude of the posttest probability. Also, since diagnostic tests can have multiple levels/categories of results, each possible level/category has its own likelihood ratio with a value ranging from 0 to +∞. The generalized effect of likelihood ratios on the posttest probability of disease is provided in Table 1–1.

By now, I'm sure you're wondering, "Okay, likelihood ratios sound really good, but what exactly are they?" Simply put, **a likelihood ratio (LR) is a ratio of likelihoods.** Sound easy? It is! The easiest way to remember the correct ratio is with the mnemonic **WOWO**, which stands for **W**ith **O**ver **W**ith**O**ut. This gives you the proper placement of likelihoods that comprise the ratio as shown below:

$$LR = \frac{\text{Likelihood of a particular test result in someone } \textit{\textbf{with}} \text{ disease}}{\text{Likelihood of the same test result in someone } \textit{\textbf{without}} \text{ the disease}}$$

TABLE 1–1. EFFECT OF THE VALUE OF A LIKELIHOOD RATIO
ON THE POSTTEST PROBABILITY OF DISEASE

Likelihood Ratio	Posttest Probability of Disease
0	No disease
0.1	Lower
1	Unchanged
10	Higher
$+\infty$	Disease certain

Therefore, for example, if a test has a result "Ω," the likelihood ratio for that result is

$$LR(\Omega) = \frac{\text{The likelihood of test result "}\Omega\text{" in patients with the disease}}{\text{The likelihood of test result "}\Omega\text{" in patients without the disease}}$$

Before getting back to the example of Ms Klott, let's calculate our likelihood ratios for the pulmonary ventilation-perfusion (V/Q) scan that was used as the final diagnostic test in our example. Using data from the Prospective Investigation of Pulmonary Embolism Diagnosis (PIOPED) study, which evaluated the value of the V/Q scan in the diagnosis of pulmonary embolism, investigators obtained the numbers in Figure 1–8 from a multicenter sample of patients.[11] For this part of the example, we will make the results dichotomous, with a (+) V/Q scan including high probability and intermediate probability results and a (−) V/Q scan including low probability and normal results (Figure 1–8).

This test has only two types of results, positive and negative, so we can calculate a likelihood ratio for a positive test result (**LR[+]**) and a likelihood ratio for a negative test result (**LR[−]**):

$$LR(+) = \frac{\text{The likelihood of a positive test result in patients with PE}}{\text{The likelihood of a positive test result in patients without PE}} = \frac{a/a + c}{b/b + d}$$

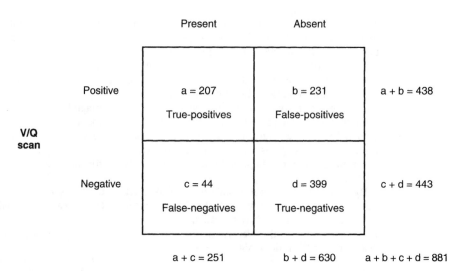

Pulmonary embolism

		Present	Absent	
V/Q scan	Positive	a = 207 True-positives	b = 231 False-positives	a + b = 438
	Negative	c = 44 False-negatives	d = 399 True-negatives	c + d = 443
		a + c = 251	b + d = 630	a + b + c + d = 881

Figure 1–8. Results for the ventilation-perfusion (V/Q) scan in the diagnosis of pulmonary embolism using pulmonary angiography as the "gold standard."[11]

Do the numerator and denominator look familiar? Of course they do! The numerator, **a/a + c,** is the equation for our old friend sensitivity, and the denominator, **b/b + d,** is the equation for 1-specificity. Therefore, the equation for **LR(+)** reduces to:

$$LR(+) = \frac{sensitivity}{1 - specificity}$$

Consequently, for dichotomous tests in which only sensitivity and specificity values are reported, LR(+) can be effortlessly calculated using the above equation.

Just as we calculated an LR(+), we can also generate an **LR(−):**

$$LR(-) = \frac{\text{The likelihood of a negative test result in patients with PE}}{\text{The likelihood of a negative test result in patients without PE}} = \frac{c/a + c}{d/b + d}$$

In this case, the numerator, **c/a + c,** is the equation for 1-sensitivity, whereas the denominator, **d/b + d,** is our familiar friend, specificity. Therefore, the equation for LR(−) reduces to:

$$LR(-) = \frac{1 - sensitivity}{specificity}$$

Similar to LR(+), for dichotomous tests in which sensitivity and specificity values are known, LR(−) can also be easily calculated using the above equation.

Using these equations, let's make some calculations based on the PIOPED data in Figure 1–8.

1. What is the LR(+) for a V/Q scan using the PIOPED data in Figure 1–8? _____

2. What is the LR(−) for a V/Q scan using the same data? _____

Answers for these and subsequent questions can be found in the Appendix at the end of this chapter.

If you only remember:

$$LR(+) = \frac{sensitivity}{1 - specificity} \qquad \& \qquad LR(-) = \frac{1 - sensitivity}{specificity}$$

it will be easy to calculate values for LR(+) and LR(−) for any diagnostic test reported in the literature that describes only sensitivity and specificity—and you can do so without necessarily having to construct your own 2 × 2 table.

Calculating the LR(+) and LR(−) is helpful, but have we maximized the amount of information from the V/Q scan results? Of course not. V/Q scan results do not have just a positive or negative result; rather, they have different levels or categories of results (eg, high probability, intermediate probability, etc). When we consider these categories, we can generate more beneficial likelihood ratios.

Let's take the previous PIOPED data and present them according to scan category results (Table 1–2).

TABLE 1–2. COMPARISON OF V/Q SCAN CATEGORY TO THE PRESENCE OR ABSENCE OF PULMONARY EMBOLISM (PE).[11]

Scan Category	PE	No PE
High probability	102	14
Intermediate probability	105	217
Low probability	39	273
Near normal/normal	5	126
Totals	**251**	**630**

Using the generic equation for a likelihood ratio presented above, calculate the likelihood ratios for the V/Q scan test results (check the Appendix to this chapter to see if your answer is right). Remember, a likelihood ratio is a ratio of likelihoods in the following format (WOWO = with over without):

$$LR(\Omega) = \frac{\text{The likelihood of test result “}\Omega\text{” in patients with the disease}}{\text{The likelihood of test result “}\Omega\text{” in patients without the disease}}$$

Calculation of V/Q Scan Likelihood Ratios

V/Q Scan Likelihood Ratios

LR (high probability)	$\frac{102/251}{14/630}$	=	18.3
LR (intermediate probability)	_____	=	_____
LR (low probability)	_____	=	_____
LR (normal probability)	_____	=	_____

Congratulations! You now know how to calculate likelihood ratios for tests with *any* number of results!

PUTTING THE EQUATION BACK TOGETHER USING LIKELIHOOD RATIOS: "WHAT WE THINK AFTER"

We are finally ready to use likelihood ratios in the basic equation to arrive at posttest probability:

What we thought before + Test information = *What we think after*
⇕
Pretest probability + Likelihood ratios = *Posttest probability*

There are two methods by which we apply likelihood ratios to refine probability: using likelihood ratios with a nomogram and using likelihood ratios with simple math.

Using likelihood ratios with a nomogram

Figure 1–9 is a nomogram that, when used with a straight edge, determines posttest probabilities of disease in your patients. Pretest probabilities are lined up along the *left* column, likelihood ratios are lined up in the *center* column, and posttest probabilities are lined up along the *right* column. Look familiar? This is simply the basic equation in nomogram form!

What we thought before + Test information = What we think after
⇕ ⇕ ⇕
Pretest probability + Likelihood ratios = Posttest probability

To use the nomogram, you need follow only three steps:

1. Choose your pretest probability on the left and anchor a straight edge on that point.
2. Take the likelihood ratio for the test result and line up the straight edge through that value in the middle.
3. The straight edge will land on a value on the far right that represents the posttest probability.

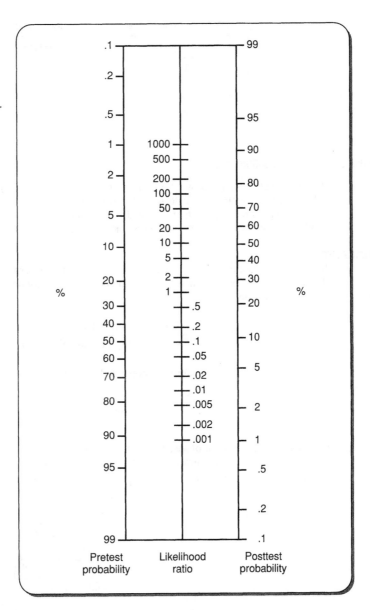

Figure 1–9. Nomogram for likelihood ratios. (Reprinted by permission of *The New England Journal of Medicine*. Adapted from Fagan TJ: Nomogram for Bayes' theorem. N Engl J Med 293;257. Copyright (1975), Massachusetts Medical Society).[12]

Using this process, let's now refine our probability for Ms Klott using likelihood ratios from the V/Q scan (Table 1–3) and the nomogram (Figure 1–9).

Ms Klott's pretest probability could be estimated at **10%** (this can be argued), and she had a high probability V/Q scan. Using the three-step approach,

1. What is her posttest probability of having a pulmonary embolus? _____
2. What is her posttest probability if she had an intermediate-probability V/Q scan? _____
3. What is her posttest probability if she had a normal V/Q scan? _____

TABLE 1–3. Calculated likelihood ratios for each V/Q scan category.[11]

Scan Category	Likelihood Ratio
High probability	18.3
Intermediate probability	1.2
Low probability	0.4
Near normal/normal	0.1

Using likelihood ratios with simple math

It's often inconvenient to carry a nomogram around. Also, many physicians prefer being able to directly calculate a posttest probability. Such calculation turns out to be another relatively simple process, but first we need to talk about the concept of **odds**, which are just another way of expressing the likelihood or probability of an event.

Getting odds straight

In medicine, we aren't used to dealing with odds, but they turn out to be fairly easy to understand and are powerful when used in the context of likelihood ratios. Simply, odds are a ratio of proportions:

$$\text{Odds} = \frac{\text{The probability of something happening}}{\text{The probability of something not happening}}$$

If we rewrite this, with probability represented as **p,** the ratio becomes

$$\text{Odds} = \frac{p}{1-p}$$

Odds can also be thought of visually. Suppose you and your friend are splitting a warm apple pie after a delicious dinner. You, of course, decide to take the smaller piece and your friend takes the rest of the pie.

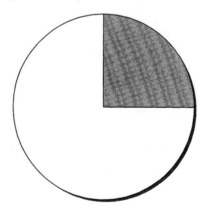

What proportion of the pie did you take? _____ = **p**
What proportion of the pie is left? _____ = **1 – p**
What is the ratio of your portion to your friend's? _____ = **p/(1 – p)**

Congratulations! In calculating this final ratio, you converted a probability into an odds.

Comparing probability & odds

There are different ways of thinking about converting probability to odds and vice versa that are helpful in becoming adept at moving between these two concepts. Below is one way of understanding this conversion process:

$$\text{Probability} = \frac{\text{Odds}}{\text{Odds} + 1} \qquad \& \qquad \text{Odds} = \frac{\text{Probability}}{1 - \text{Probability}} = \frac{p}{1 - p}$$

Therefore, suppose the probability of your winning the state lottery is 20%, or 0.2. The odds of your winning, then, are:

$$\text{Odds} = \frac{p}{1 - p} = \frac{0.2}{1 - 0.2} = \frac{0.2}{0.8} = \frac{1}{4} = 0.25$$

Likewise, if the odds of enjoying these exercises are 9, then the probability that you like doing this is:

$$\text{Probability} = \frac{\text{Odds}}{\text{Odds} + 1} = \frac{9}{9 + 1} = \frac{9}{10} = 0.9$$

Let's do a few more examples to assist you in becoming skilled at converting between probability and odds (Table 1–4).

After filling in this table (and reviewing the Appendix to ensure you are correct), several features about probability and odds become clear:

- When either the probability or odds is low (ie, <0.1), they are essentially interchangeable values.
- When the probability is 0.5, the odds are 1.
- Probability is limited to values between 0 and 1, whereas odds range from 0 to $+\infty$.

Putting it all together

If we now combine all these concepts we've discussed, they simplify to the following equation:

Pretest probability   Posttest probability
$\downarrow$ $\uparrow$

Pretest odds $\times$ Likelihood ratio $=$ Posttest odds

Here again, similar to using the nomogram, it takes only a few steps to generate a more quantitative estimate of posttest probability:

1. Estimate the pretest probability.
2. Convert pretest probability to pretest odds.
3. Multiply the pretest odds by the likelihood ratio to get posttest odds.
4. Convert the posttest odds to a posttest probability.

Let's reassure ourselves that the simple mathematical method for determining Ms Klott's posttest probability of a pulmonary embolus generates the same result as when we used the nomogram. Remember that our estimated pretest probability was **10%** and the LR for a high probability scan was about **18.** We have all the tools, so let's get to work:

TABLE 1–4. CONVERSIONS BETWEEN PROBABILITIES AND ODDS.

Probability	Odds
0.01	
0.1	
0.5	
	3
	5
	19

If pretest probability = 10% (or 0.1), then pretest odds = P/1 – P = ___

Pretest odds	×	Likelihood ratio	=	Posttest odds
_____	×	_____	=	_____

If posttest odds = ___, then posttest probability = odds/odds + 1 = ___

Congratulations! You now have two ways (nomogram and simple math) that you can use likelihood ratios to help you more precisely and accurately estimate the posttest probability of a disease in your patients.

Using likelihood ratios in sequence

One useful and interesting mathematical property of likelihood ratios is that they can be used in sequence, so that you can keep modifying your posttest probability on the basis of a series of test results.

The posttest probability of one test result becomes the pretest probability for the next test result and so on and so on for each additional test result. Instead of performing each calculation separately, however, you can use the following mathematical approach to combine *all* the likelihood ratios from separate tests into a *single* equation:

$$\text{Pretest probability} \qquad\qquad\qquad \text{Posttest probability}$$
$$\downarrow \qquad\qquad\qquad\qquad\qquad\qquad\qquad \uparrow$$
$$\text{Pretest odds} \ \times \ LR_1 \ \times \ LR_2 \ \times \ LR_3 \ = \ \text{Posttest odds}$$

Let's use three different test results to produce the most refined probability of Ms Klott having a pulmonary embolus. We have her arterial blood gas measurement, electrocardiographic findings, and V/Q scan.

It turns out that the likelihood ratios for the results of Ms Klott's tests are:

Test	LR
PaO_2 < 90 mm Hg on arterial blood gas	~2
New $S_1Q_3T_3$ pattern and RBBB on ECG	~1
High probability V/Q scan	~18

Using the equation above, what is a reasonable cumulative estimate of Ms Klott's posttest probability of having a pulmonary embolus on the basis of the above test results?

$$\text{Pretest probability} \ \_\_\_ \qquad\qquad\qquad \_\_\_\text{Posttest probability}$$
$$\downarrow \qquad\qquad\qquad\qquad\qquad\qquad\qquad \uparrow$$
$$\text{Pretest odds} \ \_\_\_ \ \times \ \underset{LR_1}{\_\_\_} \ \times \ \underset{LR_2}{\_\_\_} \ \times \ \underset{LR_3}{\_\_\_} \ = \ \_\_\_ \ \text{Posttest odds}$$

Congratulations again! You now have the ability to combine results from multiple tests to generate a final posttest probability. An important caveat to remember when combining LRs is that you can combine only *unadjusted* likelihood ratios when they are results of independent tests. Tests are independent when they measure different aspects of a given condition and when the chance of obtaining a particular test result is not influenced by the result of a different test in the sequence. A more in-depth discussion of this important limitation can be found elsewhere.[10]

As you can see, the effect of the high probability V/Q scan's likelihood ratio on the posttest probability far outweighed the combined effect of the arterial blood gas measurement or electrocardiographic findings. Therefore, the V/Q scanning result is the more useful diagnostic test result for the evaluation of pulmonary embolism when it is actually obtained.

Now that we finally have our most refined posttest probability for a disease in our patient, what do we do next?

Depending on how much our diagnostic test result affects our estimate of the probability of disease, we make choices about whether to treat or not treat by considering whether we have crossed a **treatment threshold.** This concept and its practical use will be extensively discussed in Chapter 3.

Computers, the internet, & refining probability

Finally, in this era of increasingly improved computer capabilities and access to the Internet, several types of medical diagnostic support programs have become available. These programs assist in both generating a differential diagnosis list and refining the probability of disease for patients seen in the office or at the bedside. Some of the more popular programs use Bayesian logic (eg, ILIAD, Dxplain), whereas others use primarily case-based reasoning (eg, Quick Medical Reference [QMR], HELP). In addition to references that include lists of published likelihood ratios,[13] many Internet access sites are being rapidly developed to provide on-line diagnostic support and up-to-date information on likelihood ratios for various diagnostic tests.

SUMMARY

We have transformed the theoretical perspective of Bayes' theorem into a practical application for diagnostic tests by converting the basic equation into an efficient, effective tool that we can use in the first step toward better medical decision making.

$$\text{What we thought before} + \text{Test information} = \text{What we think after}$$
$$\Downarrow$$
$$\text{Pretest probability} + \text{Likelihood ratios} = \text{Posttest probability}$$

As you leave this chapter armed with the skills to improve medical diagnosis, remember the following important points:

1. The mnemonic VINDICATE can be used to systematically generate a differential diagnosis list, which is the first step in refining probability.
2. Pretest probability is determined by two things:
   - Personal experience: Avoid sample bias, saliency bias, and simple weighting of clinical characteristics.
   - Published data: Use prevalence data for clinical symptoms and signs, and use clinical prediction rules.
3. Convert diagnostic test information into likelihood ratios:

$$\bullet \quad LR(W) = \frac{\text{The likelihood of test result ``}\Omega\text{'' in patients with the disease}}{\text{The likelihood of test result ``}\Omega\text{'' in patients without the disease}}$$

If you have only sensitivity and specificity, use

$$LR(+) = \text{sensitivity}/(1 - \text{specificity}) \text{ and } LR(-) = (1 - \text{sensitivity})/\text{specificity}$$

4. Using either a nomogram or simple math, combine pretest probability and likelihood ratios to arrive at the final posttest probability of disease.

REFERENCES

1. Saint S, Frances C: *Saint-Frances Guide to Inpatient Medicine.* Williams & Wilkins, 1997.
2. Collins RD: *Differential Diagnosis in Primary Care,* 2nd ed. Lippincott, 1987.
3. Bryant GD, Norman GR: Expressions of probability: Words and numbers. N Engl J Med 1980;302:411.
4. Tversky A, Kahneman D: Judgment under uncertainty: Heuristics and biases. Science 1974;185:1124.
5. Detmer DE et al: Heuristics and biases in medical decision making. J Med Ed 1978;53:682.
6. *Webster's New Collegiate Dictionary.* Merriam, 1979, p 1012.

7. Stein PD, Henry JW: Prevalence of acute pulmonary embolism among patients in a general hospital and at autopsy. Chest 1995;108:978.
8. Leeper KJ et al: Clinical manifestations of acute pulmonary embolism: Henry Ford Hospital experience, a five-year review. Henry Ford Hosp Med J 1988;36:29.
9. Stein PD et al: Clinical characteristics of patients with acute pulmonary embolism. Am J Cardiol 1991;68:1723.
10. Sackett DL et al: *Clinical Epidemiology: A Basic Science for Clinical Medicine,* 2nd ed. Little, Brown and Company, 1991.
11. The PIOPED Investigators: Value of the ventilation/perfusion scan in acute pulmonary embolism. Results of the prospective investigation of pulmonary embolism diagnosis (PIOPED). JAMA 1990;263:2753.
12. Fagan TJ: Nomogram for Bayes' formula. N Engl J Med 1975;293:257.
13. Sox HC Jr et al: *Medical Decision Making.* Butterworths, 1988. (Appendix contains a list of published likelihood ratios.)

APPENDIX: ANSWERS TO CHAPTER EXERCISES

Page 25

1. What is the LR(+) for a V/Q scan using the PIOPED data in Figure 1–8?

$$\frac{207/251}{231/630} = 2.2$$

2. What is the LR(−) for a V/Q scan using the same data?

$$\frac{44/251}{399/630} = 0.3$$

Page 26

Calculation of V/Q Scan Likelihood Ratios

LR (high probability)	$\dfrac{102/251}{14/630}$ =	18.3
LR (intermediate probability)	$\dfrac{105/251}{217/630}$ =	1.2
LR (low probability)	$\dfrac{39/251}{273/630}$ =	0.4
LR (near normal/normal)	$\dfrac{5/251}{126/630}$ =	0.1

Page 27

1. What is her posttest probability of having a pulmonary embolus? ~**70%**
2. What is her posttest probability if she had an intermediate-probability V/Q scan? ~**10%**
3. What is her posttest probability if she had a normal V/Q scan? ~**1%**

Page 28

What proportion of the pie did you take? $^1/_4 = \mathbf{p}$

What proportion of the pie is left? $^3/_4 = \mathbf{1 - p}$

What is the ratio of your portion to your friends'? $\dfrac{^1/_4}{^3/_4} = {}^1/_3 = \mathbf{p/(1 - p)}$

Page 29

TABLE 1–4. CONVERSIONS BETWEEN PROBABILITIES AND ODDS.

Probability	Odds
0.01	0.01/0.00 = 0.01
0.1	0.1/0.9 = 0.11
0.5	0.5/0.5 = 1
3/(3 + 1) = 0.75	3
5/(5 + 1) = 0.83	5
19/(19 + 1) = 0.95	19

Page 30

If pretest probability = 10% (or 0.1), then pretest odds = p/1 − p = **0.1/0.9**

Pretest odds   ×   Likelihood ratio   =   Posttest odds
  0.11   ×   18.3   =   2.0

If posttest odds = 2.0 , then posttest probability = odds/odds + 1 = 2.0/3.0 **= 0.67**

Page 30

Pretest probability   0.1   0.80 Posttest probability
      ↓   ↑
  Pretest odds   0.11   × $\dfrac{2}{LR_1}$ × $\dfrac{1}{LR_2}$ × $\dfrac{18}{LR_3}$ =   4.0 Posttest odds

DECISION

ANALYSIS

Michael G. Shlipak, MD, MPH

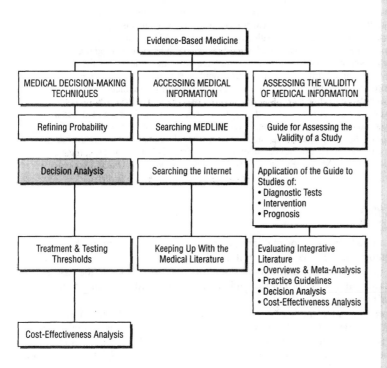

Evidence-Based Medicine

MEDICAL DECISION-MAKING TECHNIQUES

Refining Probability

Decision Analysis

Treatment & Testing Thresholds

Cost-Effectiveness Analysis

ACCESSING MEDICAL INFORMATION

Searching MEDLINE

Searching the Internet

Keeping Up With the Medical Literature

ASSESSING THE VALIDITY OF MEDICAL INFORMATION

Guide for Assessing the Validity of a Study

Application of the Guide to Studies of:
- Diagnostic Tests
- Intervention
- Prognosis

Evaluating Integrative Literature
- Overviews & Meta-Analysis
- Practice Guidelines
- Decision Analysis
- Cost-Effectiveness Analysis

You are discussing treatment options in your office with your patient, SM, a 40-year-old man who has persistent exacerbation of chronic ulcerative colitis. He continues to experience severe abdominal pain, poor appetite, and diarrhea despite taking high doses of oral corticosteroids. In his 20 years of living with ulcerative colitis, during which he has experienced frequent severe flares of the disease, SM has never seemed so distraught. "Doc, you've got to do something. You've got to make me better! I just can't take this any longer!" As his primary care physician for the past decade, you reflect on his long-term battle with ulcerative colitis—the hospitalizations, the occasional bouts of fecal incontinence, and the constant fear of colorectal cancer. You realize that SM is at a crossroads concerning his disease and that the two of you must make a decision.

Unfortunately, your consultants are in disagreement about a decision. The general surgeon recommends total colectomy, using a relatively new technique—**ileal pouchanal anastomosis.** This two-stage procedure involves total colectomy, but the ileum is anastomosed to the anus so that ileostomy is usually avoided. Because a "pouch" is created from the ileum to serve as a rectum, continence is usually maintained; however, many patients experience daily soiling of stool that requires them to wear diapers. On the basis of her experience, the surgeon assures you that the operation is *safe,* that ileostomy is a *rare complication,* and that the *vast majority* of patients are continent after the procedure. You think this sounds too good to be true. Moreover, what do "safe," "rare," and the "vast majority" really mean? SM has told you many times during the years how fearful he is of spending the rest of his life attached to an ileostomy bag. Can this outcome really be avoided?

The gastroenterology service, on the other hand, is furious at the surgeon for wanting to "rush" your patient to the operating room. The consultant recommends starting **immunosuppressive therapy with 6-mercaptopurine,** which he claims is highly effective both to stem the current exacerbation, allowing you to taper SM off the corticosteroids, and to prevent further episodes that would require surgery. You have never used this drug, and you worry about its associated toxicities. You have heard that it increases the subsequent risk of lymphoma. Furthermore, if this treatment works only in the short term, will SM still require surgery in the near future or can proctocolectomy be avoided forever?

As you discuss these treatment options with SM, you realize that you do not have a practical framework for weighing the risks and benefits. Not only do you lack the evidence to evaluate the potential outcomes, but you feel overwhelmed by your inability to characterize the decision. Nonetheless, since the consultants have offered contradictory recommendations and have refused to speak with one another, the decision is left to you and your patient. How will you and SM decide? *Can you make an evidence-based decision?*

INTRODUCTION TO DECISION ANALYSIS

In Chapter 1 we refined our skills of making diagnoses by addressing the probabilities of each possible diagnosis. In this chapter, we will develop a method for determining a course of action to make the *right* decision. In critical situations, such as the one in the case example above, physicians often rely on clinical judgment—their ability to make tough decisions in the face of uncertainty.

Many approaches to making medical decisions are commonly used by physicians; some of these are listed in Table 2–1. Skilled physicians intuitively make decisions on the basis of consideration of the likelihood of the possible results and the patient's preferences for each outcome. Although experienced clinicians have well-developed intuition, the

TABLE 2–1. EMPIRICAL METHODS FOR CLINICAL DECISION MAKING[1]

Dogmatism	This is the best way to do it.
Policy	This is the way we do it around here.
Experience	This way worked the last few times.
Whim	This way might work.
Nihilism	It doesn't really matter what we do.
Rule of least chagrin	Do what you'll regret least.
Defer to experts	How would you do it?
Defer to patients	How would you like us to proceed?

complexity of some decisions involves the integration of more information than the mind could possibly handle.

Optimal decision making requires that physicians identify each possible strategy, accurately predict the probability of future events, and balance the risks and benefits of each possible action, all while tailoring to the values of the individual patient. To this end, a technique called **decision analysis** was developed to assist clinicians in making rational decisions that reflect the best available evidence and the patient's individual needs.[2]

Described as a "systematic articulation of common sense"[2] **decision analysis is a formalization of the medical decision-making process.** The method of decision analysis can be thought of as a scale to weigh the risks and benefits of each potential strategy (Figure 2–1). The process is developed using a **decision tree,** a type of flow diagram that outlines the outcomes that could follow each potential decision and calculates the probability and the value of each possible event.[3]

By demanding that the clinician consider all possible consequences for the decision in question and by placing a value on the desirability of each result, the decision tree helps to diagram and structure uncertainty. Uncertainty surrounds clinical medicine: We constantly are unsure about the presence or absence of disease in a patient or about the probabilities of various outcomes of a particular treatment. In the absence of a crystal ball, decision analysis offers a technique for making a definitive choice despite the inherent conditions of uncertainty. In this chapter, we will develop a decision analysis model using a decision tree to represent our uncertainty regarding our patient SM, and we will use the results to direct our therapeutic decision.

Now that we have introduced decision analysis, when should we use this technique? Certain types of problems are best handled by decision analysis, in either a clinical situation involving an individual patient or a policy dilemma involving a population of similar patients. The following situations may benefit from the structure of a decision tree:

- **Complicated, high-stakes situations:** The presence of multiple competing risks and benefits requires a formal, quantitative method to evaluate the optimal strategy.
- **When important data are not known with certainty:** Decision analysis may reveal that a critical parameter is not well defined in the literature, rendering a single "best answer" unobtainable. Focusing the uncertainty on the missing variable rather than on the entire decision may permit a more informed choice by explicitly describing the effect of this variable on the outcome over a range of possible values.

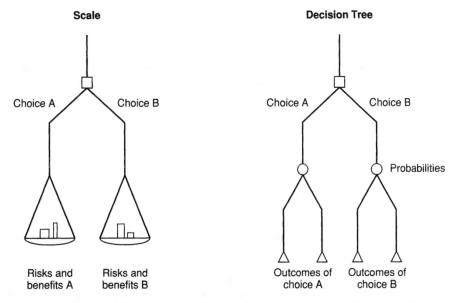

Figure 2–1. A decision tree (right) is analogous to a scale (left) that weighs the relative risks and benefits of each possible strategy.

- **When patient input is critical:** The best decision may depend heavily on how an individual patient values life with a particular disability. For our patient SM choosing between surgery and medicine, the "right" decision may be critically dependent on his personal values for the potential health outcomes he faces.
- **When important events occur at different points in time:** Many patients value the present much more than they value the future; this time preference is easily forgotten when making decisions implicitly. How do we compare death resulting from surgery today with death resulting from cancer in the distant future?

The major advantages of decision analysis arise from dividing a problem into its component parts. The method is explicit and quantitative, forcing the physician to identify all possible treatment alternatives and outcomes, to determine which data are necessary to make an educated decision, and to evaluate precisely the relative preference for each possible outcome. By providing an absolute best alternative, decision analysis is prescriptive. The decision tree does not merely represent an overview of the problem; rather, it tells us what we should do. The final product of a decision analysis model should be a rational decision made on the basis of a complete understanding of the clinical situation.[2,4]

THE FIVE STEPS OF DECISION ANALYSIS

Let's now discuss the steps to using the decision analytic technique as a tool for solving difficult problems in clinical medicine. As we outline each step, the case of SM will be used as an example of the method's application to an individual patient. These are the five steps of decision analysis:

1. Formulate an explicit question.
2. Structure the decision and make the tree.
3. Fill in the data (probabilities and outcomes).
4. Determine the value of each competing strategy.
5. Perform sensitivity analyses

Formulate an explicit question

Although this seems like an obvious step for any type of decision making, the exercise of transforming a difficult clinical situation into the form of an explicit question can be enlightening. The physician must clearly delineate all the reasonable courses of action that are available and the time frame during which the outcomes would occur. When an exhaustive list of the clinical alternatives has been made, the mechanics of structuring the decision tree can begin.

In the case of SM, the status quo is not reasonable because the situation demands an intervention. The two rational treatment interventions are surgery to cure colitis (proctocolectomy) and immunosuppressive therapy in an attempt to induce and maintain remission of ulcerative colitis (thus avoiding surgery). We will formulate our clinical question simply and explicitly:

Choose medicine or choose surgery?

Structure the decision and make the tree

The structuring step in decision analysis begins with listing the possible outcomes that could result from either strategy and ends with a completed decision tree. As a flow diagram, the decision tree should represent the logical sequence of events over time. Each therapeutic strategy may require further interventions, depending on the patient's clinical course, which should be reflected in the decision tree. For example, if immunosuppressive therapy does not improve the condition of our patient, the decision tree should indicate that he requires surgical intervention. Of course, in clinical medicine there is no limit to the potential complexity of most case scenarios; nonetheless, part of the art of decision analysis is reducing a complex decision into a finite number of straightforward components. Each aspect of the clinical scenario will eventually be defined by a choice, probability, and outcome.[3]

The drawing of the decision tree may seem unnatural for readers who are new to the concept, but with practice the tree can be as easy to use as an outline or a flow chart. We recommend that tree-building begin with envisioning the possible outcomes or health states that could result from each therapeutic strategy. When a complete list has been made of these outcomes, the outcomes should be arranged temporally to provide a representation of the time course of the clinical situation. The outcomes can then be separated into branches to represent the probability of each outcome occurring. These branches may be simply dichotomous—yes or no—outcomes (eg, "lymphoma develops" or "no lymphoma"), but the branches can also contain any number of possible outcomes. The final decision tree will result from the arrangement of these multiple branches, as we will now illustrate.

We will begin structuring our patient's decision tree by identifying the most likely outcome states of each strategy, which happen to be included in the clinical scenario. Because we are interested mostly in the long-term quality of life for SM, we will include only those outcomes that have long-term consequences. Outcomes that cause only short-term discomfort and no long-term sequelae are deliberately left out. The long-term consequences of *surgery* could be **intra-operative mortality, permanent ileostomy, permanent incontinence** (defined as daily soiling of stool), or **surgical success** to end colitis. *Medical therapy* with immunosuppressive agents may **induce remission or it may fail** because of toxicity or treatment inadequacy; thus, SM would still **need surgery.** Despite an initial period of remission, SM may experience a **severe relapse** of ulcerative colitis, forcing him to **undergo surgery at a later time.** The medicine could continue to control the ulcerative colitis, but either **colorectal cancer** or **lymphoma** may develop; SM could **survive** either of these malignant processes or he could **die.** Finally, SM may avoid surgery, experiencing **chronic ulcerative colitis,** which entails a normal life-expectancy,[5] and eventually dying of unrelated causes. A list of these final outcomes, arranged temporally, thus includes

Surgery: immediate death, ileostomy, incontinence, surgical success
Medicine: initial treatment failure requiring surgery, disease relapse requiring surgery, death resulting from lymphoma, death resulting from colorectal cancer, chronic ulcerative colitis

Having delineated the two treatment strategies and defined all the major possible outcomes, we are ready to construct our decision tree. Typically drawn from left to right—the decision is on the left and the outcomes are on the right—the decision tree is composed of decision nodes, chance nodes, and health outcomes. A **decision node,** represented on the tree as a square (Figure 2–2), is a crossroads in clinical medicine at which the physician must choose an action or strategy. As SM's doctor, you currently stand at a decision node until you decide on a treatment strategy.

Chance nodes, which appear as circles on the decision tree, represent events that are beyond our control; they are the uncertainty in clinical medicine. Although we cannot predict with accuracy which outcome will occur, we define the probability of each and assign these values to the chance node. The chance nodes are arranged left to right based on the temporal sequence in which the uncertainty is expected to occur. Finally, all branches of the tree must eventually reach a **terminal state,** representing one of the final outcomes. These are usually represented by a triangle in the decision tree.

Having drawn the initial decision node, dividing the tree into "Choose surgery" or "Choose medicine," let's translate our description of the surgical strategy into a decision tree format (Figure 2–3). A chance node will represent the possibility of surviving surgery or dying, death being a terminal state of the tree. Surviving surgery is followed by another chance node to identify the likelihood of the pouch procedure remaining viable ("Pouch succeeds") or resulting in an eventual ileostomy. Because the ileostomy would be permanent,

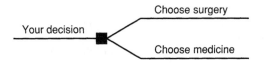

Figure 2–2. A decision node, represented by a square, indicates a clinical crossroads where the clinician must make a decision. Here, the decision must be made between medical and surgical strategies.

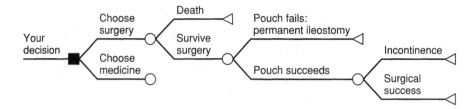

Figure 2–3 The surgery branch of the tree. The circles in the tree are called chance nodes; they represent the uncertainty in clinical medicine. In this tree, chance nodes represent the possibility of dying as a result of the surgical procedure, of being left with a permanent ileostomy, of having chronic incontinence, and of having a completely successful surgical outcome.

this branch is represented with a terminal state. The " Pouch succeeds" branch then separates into two final outcome states, surgical success and incontinence.

Although the medicine strategy appears more complicated, we can transform its possible outcomes into a decision tree by representing each possible outcome as a yes or no possibility (Figure 2–4). Thus, our first chance node is a dichotomous yes or no representing initial treatment success or failure (because of actual treatment failure or adverse effects of treatment). Treatment failure would require surgery, so we can label this outcome as "Need surgery" for now. The second chance node similarly represents the future success or failure of medical therapy to prevent a severe relapse that would require surgery.

As shown in Figure 2–4, the following chance nodes are similarly dichotomous: lymphoma develops (yes or no); if lymphoma develops, survive (yes or no). If no lymphoma occurs, colorectal carcinoma may develop (yes or no); if colorectal carcinoma develops, survive (yes or no). If treatment succeeds and malignancy does not develop (or the patient survives lymphoma), then the patient will reach the terminal state of chronic ulcerative colitis. The astute reader will notice in our tree that we have assumed that no patient will be so unfortunate as to have both lymphoma and colorectal carcinoma develop. Although possible, this occurrence is so unlikely that it is not worth including in the model.

The outcome "Need surgery" encountered in the medical tree is essentially equivalent to the "Choose surgery" subtree in Figure 2–3. Therefore, we can copy this subtree onto each "Need surgery" terminal node in Figure 2–4, except for the final one, which follows colorectal cancer. A patient with colorectal cancer will not be a candidate for ileal pouch anastomosis but will instead undergo traditional proctocolectomy, which results in a permanent ileostomy. Thus, a patient who survives colorectal cancer will have the terminal state of permanent ileostomy. Having replaced the "Need surgery" outcomes in Figure 2–4, we now have our final tree represented in Figure 2–5.

Fill in the data

Thus our decision tree is drawn. We are now ready for step 3, filling in the data. Each chance node has a probability associated with each branch that follows, and each terminal health state has a relative preference, or utility. In this step, we quantify the probability of events and the values of outcomes and insert these numbers into the decision tree.

Probability

A **probability** is a prediction of the *future*. But we must estimate the frequency of the events in our tree using evidence from the *past*. To arrive at an evidence-based solution to a clinical problem, we must derive these probabilities using the best possible information available. Major sources of probability that we can incorporate into a decision analysis include

- Clinical studies
- Clinical databases
- Expert opinions and educated guesses

Clinical studies. Medical literature probably provides the most reliable source of evidence because the data are quantitative and the studies presumably peer-reviewed.[2] The methods for evaluating the medical literature described in Section 3 of this book will help you determine

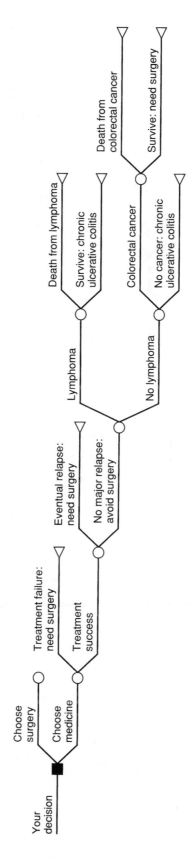

Figure 2–4. The medicine branch of the tree.

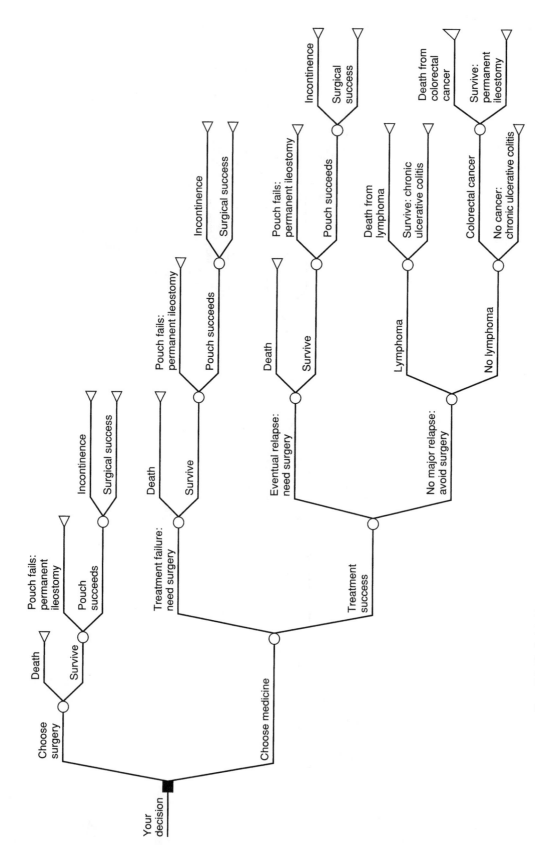

Figure 2-5 The final decision tree. Although this tree appears complex, it simply combines the surgery and medicine trees drawn in Figures 2–3 and 2–4.

the validity of these sources of data. Even if published information is valid, however, it may not be applicable to your patient. The study population may be different, the treatment may have changed, a new test may be available, or a surgical technique may have been improved. As in applying any source of published literature to an individual patient, care must be taken in constructing a decision tree to ensure that the published probability applies to the clinical situation at that chance node. Using a poor source of evidence can be less valid than having no data at all.

Clinical database. Local patterns of disease or outcomes of treatment are often more relevant than published clinical studies. For example, the complication rate of patients undergoing ileal pouch anastomosis for the particular surgeon at your hospital is more applicable to your patient than the rate published in a peer-reviewed journal. For our hypothetical patient and for the purpose of generalization, the surgical complication rate for this procedure will be taken from published literature.

Expert opinions/educated guesses. Often we cannot find adequate data to provide an evidenced-based estimate for a chance node. Rather than incorporate data that are not truly applicable to the clinical situation, it is preferable to seek the opinion of one or more experts—the "educated guess." In the absence of an evidence-based approach, this intuitive method would be the entire basis for decision making. But by structuring the problem with decision analysis, we can limit the "guess" to the probabilities of one or two specific events. The accuracy of the subjective probability is of course dependent on the experience of the individual making the estimate; however, the ability to derive probabilities is a teachable skill that is crucial to the practice of evidence-based medicine (see Chapter 1, discussion of heuristics). The importance of the "educated guess" to the overall decision can be determined via sensitivity analysis, as discussed in step 5 on page 48.

We will now address the probabilities in our decision tree using available evidence. We learned in Chapter 1 that the sum of all probabilities must add up to 1.0 and that we can revise probabilities to adjust for added information. The probabilities in Table 2–2 were obtained by a thorough review of the literature, using the techniques described in Chapter 5 on searching MEDLINE. The notation p[outcome] in this table stands for the probability of that outcome occurring. You will note that the sum of the probabilities placed around each chance node equals 1.0.

Note that no increase in the risk of lymphoma was found among patients with ulcerative colitis who received 6-mercaptopurine. Although the risk of lymphoma is not zero, as suggested in Table 2–2, this branch can be eliminated from the decision tree because the risk is

TABLE 2–2. PROBABILITY ESTIMATES FOR EACH CHANCE NODE IN THE DECISION TREE.*

Probability Variable	Estimate	Reference No.
p[death]	0.002	6
p[survive]	0.998	
p[pouch succeeds]	0.93	
p[ileostomy]	0.07	6
p[incontinence]	0.18	7
p[surgical success]	0.82	6,7
p[initial medical treatment failure]	0.37	8,9
p[initial medical treatment success]	0.63	9
p[eventual relapse requiring surgery]	0.20	10
p[permanent medical treatment]	0.80	10
p[lymphoma]	0.0	9
p[no lymphoma]	1.0	9
p[colorectal cancer]	0.09	11,12,13
p[no colorectal cancer]	0.91	11,12,13
p[colon cancer mortality]	0.30	13
p[colon cancer survival]	0.70	13

* p[event] = the probability of the event occurring.

the same whether the patient receives surgical or medical therapy. The incidence and survival rates of colorectal cancer are based on patients who received active surveillance with colonoscopy, as documented in the reference. The only probability that is not explicitly derived from clinical literature is the probability of eventual relapse requiring surgery. The long-term efficacy of chronic immunosuppressives in avoiding surgery has not been extensively studied. We therefore consulted an "expert" gastroenterologist for an educated estimate of this probability. A similar estimate was found in the referenced article.

Valued outcomes

As our clinical scenario has demonstrated, the range of possible outcomes for an important clinical decision may be broader than just life or death. To compare the results of clinical strategies, a method for ranking outcomes must be devised. How would levels of disability, discomfort, or inconvenience be ranked? These values must be considered as rigorously and quantitatively as our sources of probability if our analysis is to be valid. The most commonly used method of ranking health states in medical decision making is called utility assessment.

Utility = a quantitative measure of the strength of a
patient's preference for a particular state of health or outcome

Utilities are the currency used to trade among possible outcomes. Because the individual patient determines utility, utilities are appropriately and necessarily subjective and are essential to the decision tree.[3] Alternative outcomes to utilities could include life expectancy,[14] functional status, or satisfaction. We, however, will focus on utility.

The first step in assigning a quantitative utility to an outcome state is to rank the outcomes from most desirable to least desirable. Our patient SM states that the most desirable outcome would be a cure of his ulcerative colitis to avoid all medications and worry, yet avoiding the surgical complications of incontinence or ileostomy; in other words, **surgical success** is his best outcome. Next best would be prolonged remission resulting in asymptomatic **chronic ulcerative colitis** that avoids surgery and does not result in colorectal cancer. The third best option is surgical cure of ulcerative colitis that leaves him with the nuisance of being somewhat **incontinent** but without an ileostomy. The fourth best option is surgical cure that results in a **permanent ileostomy.** The outcome of **colorectal cancer–related death** is almost the worst option. The worst possible outcome, though, is immediate **surgery-related death.** Remember, these are the rankings of one individual patient. They reflect his values alone.

Let's now list these ranked outcomes from 1 to 6:

1. Surgical success
2. Chronic ulcerative colitis
3. Postsurgical incontinence
4. Permanent ileostomy
5. Colorectal cancer–related death
6. Surgery-related death

Ranking the outcomes from 1 to 6 helps us understand SM's preferences for the possible outcomes of our decision, but for decision analysis this is insufficient. Where does ileostomy fall on a continuum of death to perfect health? Would future death resulting from colorectal cancer be valued akin to immediate death or be closer to permanent ileostomy? We need to quantify the patient's preference for each of these outcomes if we are to continue with decision analysis.

Because utilities are quantitative measures, they require a scale, which is determined arbitrarily. For convenience the scale usually is 0–1.0, with 0 being the worst possible outcome (eg, immediate death) and 1.0 being a state of perfect health relative to the particular patient. All other outcomes are valued with a utility somewhere between these two extremes, depending on the patient's preference. The techniques for deriving an individual's personal utilities arise from basic economic theory. The fundamental assumption is that individuals will behave rationally in order to maximize their personal satisfaction or utility.

The methods for determining an individual's utilities, described below, are tools for forcing the patient to reveal his or her preferences for potential outcomes; thus, the decision analysis is tailored to fit the patient's own values.

We will focus on three common methods for calculating personal utilities:

- Visual analog scale
- Time trade-off
- Standard gamble

Visual analog scale (interval scaling). This method for determining utilities relies on the patient's ranking of health states using a linear scale. The scale (basically a ruler) is presented to the patient with a health state at either end. The patient demonstrates his or her relative preference for an intermediate outcome, relative to the health states at either end, by marking the line at the desired point. Using this example, we might ask our patient SM to mark the line where he would value an ileostomy, if surgery-related death = 0 and surgical success = 1.0.

$$\text{Incontinence}$$
$$(0) - \text{Surgery-related death} \text{———} X \text{———} \text{Surgical success} - (1)$$

If he chose a point three-fourths of the distance between 0 and 1.0, as shown in the example above, his utility for incontinence would be 0.75. Similarly, the value of another intermediate outcome (eg, ileostomy) may be scaled by repeating this technique.

$$\text{Ileostomy}$$
$$(0) - \text{Surgery-related death} \text{———} X \text{———} \text{Surgical success} - (1)$$

The primary problem with this method is that it may bias results toward the middle of the scale, so utilities may be scored inappropriately low. Rarely would an X be placed at 0.98, for example, because persons tend to avoid marking the extremes of a scale.

Time trade-off. This technique involves presenting the patient with a trade-off between the quality of his or her life and the length of life in time. The assumption is simply represented for health states A and B, where A is perfect health and B is a less desirable health state:

$$\text{Time A} \times \text{Utility A} = \text{Time B} \times \text{Utility B}$$

Time trade-off thus establishes that 10 years lived with utility 0.5 are equivalent to 5 years lived with a perfect utility of 1.0. We can use this framework to help our patient reveal his or her personal utilities for each possible health state.

For the equation above, Utility A (perfect health) is 1.0 and Time B is the maximum possible life expectancy (we'll use 10 years in this example). By choosing a quantity for Time A that is some fraction of Time B, the patient will define his or her personal value for Utility B. To illustrate this concept, let's return to our patient SM. You define A as relative perfect health (for SM this would be the health state "Surgical success") and B as life with an ileostomy. You can now frame the question to SM as follows:

> If you were faced with a future lifetime of 10 years (Time B = 10) with an ileostomy (Utility B), how much time (t) would you be willing to give up to spend your life in perfect health (Utility A)?

By framing the question in terms of "giving up" time, we have introduced the variable t, where

$$\text{Time B} - t = \text{Time A}$$

If SM states that he would give up or trade 1 year, then $t = 1$ year and Time A = 9 years. Returning to our original equation, the utility of the ileostomy (Utility B) can be solved easily:

$$\text{Time A (9 years)} \times \text{Utility A (1.0)} = \text{Time B (10 years)} \times \text{Utility B}$$

Solving for Utility B, we find the value to be 0.9. Thus, SM has revealed his personal utility for ileostomy to be 0.90. This method can be repeated for each of the intermediate health states.

Standard gamble. Probably the most commonly used and explicit form of utility assessment, this technique involves forcing the patient to choose between (1) accepting a certain health state and (2) taking a gamble to achieve a better outcome, while risking the possibility of the worst outcome.

An analogy for the standard gamble is the "Let's Make a Deal" game show, played for high stakes. The contestant (your patient) must choose between two doors. Door 1 is open so the contestant sees a certain outcome; this outcome is an intermediate health state whose utility needs to be defined. Door 2 is closed. Behind it may be the most desired outcome (perfect health), but this door also may hide instant death. Whether the contestant chooses door 1 or door 2 is dependent on the probability that door 2 holds perfect health versus the probability of instant death. The contestant will decide the value for the probability of finding a perfect outcome behind door 2 that makes door 1 and door 2 equally appealing. Using this situation, we can determine the patient's personal utility for the intermediate health outcome that appears in door 1.

Assume that behind door 1 is a certain outcome of permanent ileostomy; behind door 2 is either the best outcome, surgical success [utility(2a) = 1.0, probability(2a) = q], or immediate death [utility(2b) = 0, probability(2b) = 1–q]. For what probability (q) would SM be indifferent between the two doors?

Door 1:   Ileostomy [probability = 1.0] [Utility = ?]
Door 2:   Surgical success [probability (2a) = q] [Utility (2a) = 1.0]
          or
          Immediate death [probability (2b) = 1 – q] [Utility (2b) = 0]

As in the time tradeoff model, we can represent the choice with a simple equation:

$$[p(1) \times U(1)] = [p(2a) \times U(2a)] + [p(2b) \times U(2b)]$$

Since $p(1) = 1.0$, $U(2a) = 1.0$, $U(2b) = 0$, $p(2a) = q$, and $p(2b) = 1–q$, then $U(1)$ can be represented as:

$$1.0 \times U(1) = [q \times 1.0] + [(1 - q)) \times 0]$$

which reduces to:

$$U(1) = q$$

As shown, the equation simplifies to $U(1)$, the utility of the ileostomy, being equal to q, the probability of finding surgical success behind closed door 2. With help from the physician, the patient will determine the value of q, or conversely $(1 - q)$—the risk of immediate death—which makes the choice between the two doors a "toss-up." At this value, q is equal to $U(1)$, the utility of the intermediate outcome. Thus, the patient defines his or her utility for this outcome. Below, we will demonstrate how the physician can lead the patient through the standard gamble.

Each of these three methods for utility assessment has its relative merits. In addition, the methods have been shown to produce different results, although controversy surrounds the question of which result is most valid.[15] The visual-analog scale is the most intuitive for patients to understand, yet may bias toward lower values, as already mentioned. The time trade-off compares certain outcomes, which for some patients makes the time trade-off more comprehensible than the standard gamble.[16] The standard gamble, however, involves an element of risk that may be more realistic, yet can be difficult for some patients to understand. Use of both of these latter two methods would be valid in this decision analysis.

Although you could use either the standard gamble or the time trade-off for your patient, you decide to try the standard gamble method of utility assessment because it seems to reflect the element of risk involved in this clinical situation. You return to SM and outline the potential health states behind the two doors. You offer him the gamble with q = 0.75:

> Would you choose door 1, the certainty of an ileostomy, or would you choose door 2, gambling for the 75% chance of surgical success, while risking a 25% chance of instant death?

SM chooses door 1, the certain ileostomy, as he is unwilling to accept a 25% chance of immediate death. You increase the likelihood of surgical success to 85% and 90%, yet he still chooses door 1, the certain ileostomy. At a 95% chance of surgical success, SM states he would definitely choose door 2, risking a 5% chance of death to avoid the certain ileostomy. As you offer percentages between 90% and 95%, SM reveals that he is indifferent to the two doors at q = 92%. Thus, his utility for the outcome of ileostomy is 0.92. Repeating this process for the two states between ileostomy and surgical success reveals that SM values chronic ulcerative colitis (with the continued fear of cancer) at 0.98 and a state of postsurgical incontinence at 0.95.

The health-state of cancer-related death is more difficult to quantify because the outcome occurs in the distant future. Your review of the literature revealed that the incidence of colorectal cancer in patients with ulcerative colitis may be represented as a symmetric bell-curve, with a peak in mortality at age 55.[12] As a 40-year-old man with a life expectancy of approximately 30 years, SM would lose an average of half his life expectancy if he were to die of colorectal carcinoma. You return to the standard gamble and ask SM the following question:

> Assume that door 1 holds a certainty of 15 years of life followed by death resulting from cancer. Behind door 2 might be a normal life expectancy of 30 years in perfect health (probability = q, utility = 1.0) or immediate death (probability = 1 − q, utility = 0). For what probability (q) of finding a normal life expectancy behind door 2 would you be indifferent between door 1 and door 2?

You are surprised when he chooses a probability for perfect health, and thus a utility of cancer-related death, of 0.7. You expected SM to make q, and thus the utility of cancer-related death, equal to 0.5 because this outcome of a life expectancy of 15 years is the mid-point between instant death and a life expectancy of 30 years. We will continue discussing time preferences later. You have now assisted SM in calculating his personal utilities for the possible outcomes of the decision tree:

Surgical success = 1.00
Chronic ulcerative colitis = 0.98
Postsurgical incontinence = 0.95
Permanent ileostomy = 0.92
Colorectal cancer–related death = 0.70
Surgery-related death = 0.00

The standard gamble technique may seem like a strange method for generating patient utilities, but in reality our patient does take a gamble by undergoing the risk of surgery to reap its possible benefits. By responding to the forced choices of the standard gamble, SM has revealed the relative strengths of his preferences for these possible outcomes, which we can now incorporate into our decision tree. Notice how these quantitative utilities differ from a simple, ordinal ranking of 1 to 6.

Before we move on to calculating the results of our decision tree and determining the expected values of each arm of the tree, we should note a few shortcomings of utility assessment:

- An individual's preferences may vary with time. An ability that seems highly desirable at a young age (eg, the ability to run fast) may be less important later in life.
- A patient usually has a limited understanding of the potential outcomes that he or she has never experienced. Notice that SM has an emotional aversion to ileostomy, causing him to value the outcome at 0.92. A patient who actually lives with an ileostomy or incontinence may adjust to these lifestyles and rank them with a much higher utility.

- Some patients may be incapable of understanding and participating in these tradeoff and gambling techniques. In these patients, quantifying utilities can become problematic.
- Physicians may impose their own values on utility assessment, biasing the values away from the patient's true preferences.[2]

Determine the value of each competing strategy

After inserting the estimated probabilities and utilities of each possible outcome, we now analyze our completed tree to answer our original question, "Choose surgery or choose medicine?" The method of analyzing the decision tree is known as **expected value decision making.** We will review the "Choose surgery" portion of our decision tree (Figure 2–6) to demonstrate expected value calculations.

To calculate the expected value of a decision tree, we begin at the end of the tree and work backward, chance node after chance node, until we arrive at the beginning. The expected value of a chance node is the sum of each of its branch's probability multiplied by its utility; in other words, a weighted average of the node. The terminal branch of the "Choose surgery" section of the tree is characterized by a 0.82 probability of surgical success (U = 1.0) and a 0.18 probability of permanent incontinence (U = 0.95). To predict the average outcome, or the expected utility, we multiply

$$0.82 \times 1.0 + 0.18 \times 0.95 = 0.991$$

This calculation is called **averaging out** the chance node; its expected value is 0.991 (represented in Figure 2–6 within a rectangle adjacent to the final node in the surgical subtree). The next chance node we encounter, moving backward along the tree, involves a probability of 0.07 for an ileostomy (U = 0.92) and a probability of 0.93 of no ileostomy (expected value = 0.991, as calculated above). The expected value of this chance node is equivalent to

$$0.07 \times 0.92 + 0.93 \times 0.991 = 0.986$$

This process of working backward along the tree to determine the expected value for each arm of the tree is called **folding back** the decision tree. Practice calculating the expected value of different chance nodes using Figure 2–6, which shows the entire averaged out and folded back decision tree. The tree ultimately tells us to choose the surgical procedure because its expected utility is higher—0.984 versus 0.976.

Often, the difference between two strategies in a decision tree will appear to be small, as in this case. However, this result still reflects the optimal choice for the decision that SM faces. If the decision is structured as accurately as possible and the best possible values for probabilities and utilities are incorporated into the tree, the results of the analysis should be accepted. In this example, surgery is the rational choice.

Perform sensitivity analyses

Despite the confidence one may have in the completed decision tree, skepticism may remain regarding the results of the analysis. We might be concerned about the effect of a particular probability estimate that is based on inadequate data or one that represents the most dreaded outcome. Or, we may worry that a particular utility estimate has overly influenced the final results. To address our fears regarding the reproducibility of the conclusions and their dependence on any particular piece of datum, we turn to sensitivity analysis.

Sensitivity analysis tests the stability of an analysis over a range of probability estimates and value judgments. The process challenges the conclusions by systematically varying the values of particular probabilities and utilities used in the decision tree. The range selected should correspond to the reasonable area of uncertainty around each estimate. This enables us to assess the stability or "robustness" of the end result and determine whether the decision hinges on a particular variable.

In its simplest form, sensitivity analysis involves altering a single variable along a range of probabilities or utilities and recalculating the expected value of each strategy at each probability. Because only a single variable is varied, this form is called **one-way sensitivity**

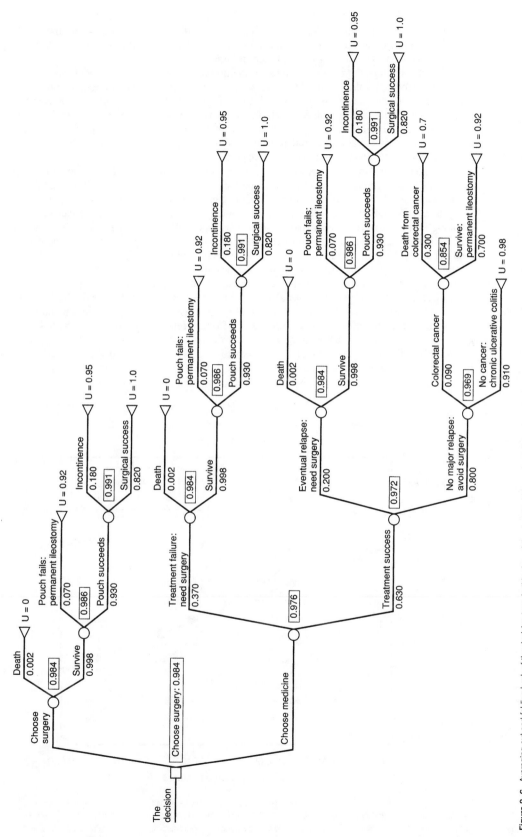

Figure 2–6. Averaging out and folding back of the decision tree. In this view of the decision tree, we see all the data needed to determine the preferred strategy. The probability for each of the branches that follows a chance node is shown beneath the branch. The utility of each terminal state is shown following its representative triangle. Knowing the probability of each branch and its utility allows us to calculate the expected value—or "average out"—each decision node from right to left (refer to description in text). The expected value of each chance node is shown in the rectangle adjacent to the node.

analysis. The expected values (in this case, expected utilities) for the surgical and medical treatment arms calculated over the wide range of possible probabilities of dying during surgery (p[surgery-related death]) are plotted in Figure 2–7.

The x-axis displays the range of values for the probability of this outcome and the y-axis shows the expected value of the "Choose surgery" and "Choose medicine" strategies at each point. Our reference estimated the risk of death to be 0.002, or 1 death per 500 cases. One-way sensitivity analysis shows that surgery is preferred over medical therapy if the risk of surgical mortality is less than 0.009, or 1 death per 111 cases. This point at which the two lines cross is called the **indifference point,** or **threshold.** Thresholds in medical decision making are discussed in detail in Chapter 3.

A second plot, Figure 2–8, represents a one-way sensitivity analysis of the probability of developing cancer (p[cancer]). We made a relatively low estimate for the likelihood of this event, 0.09, based on active surveillance with routine colonoscopy.[13] One-way sensitivity analysis reveals that surgery is the preferable strategy unless the probability of cancer developing is less than 0.04. Sensitivity analysis was repeated for the other probabilities and utilities in the decision tree, as seen in Table 2–3. Surgery had a higher expected value than medical therapy within a wide range of values for each variable.

The results of these one-way sensitivity analyses are reassuring, as they tell us that our conclusion does not hinge precariously on any one of our estimates. For example, the rate of surgical mortality in Figure 2–7 would have to be four times higher for the medical therapy to be superior. We also find that the one probability arising from expert opinion and not directly from medical literature, the probability of future relapse requiring surgery, has no impact on the overall conclusion (surgery is better than medicine for all possible values). In fact, none of the thresholds in Table 2–3 appears to be close to the "best estimate" incorporated into the decision tree. Sensitivity analysis of probabilities is more important than it is for utilities in an individual's decision tree, since the patient determined his own utilities.

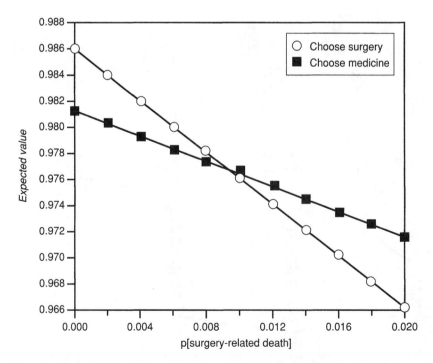

Figure 2–7. One-way sensitivity analysis of the variable p[surgery-related death], the probability of the patient dying from surgery. The effect of varying the probability of surgical mortality on the expected value of the surgery and the medical strategies is shown. Our original estimate for p[death] was 0.002. According to this figure, surgery remains preferable to medicine when p[death] is less than 0.009, the threshold value. If p[death] is greater than 0.009, medicine is preferable to surgery.

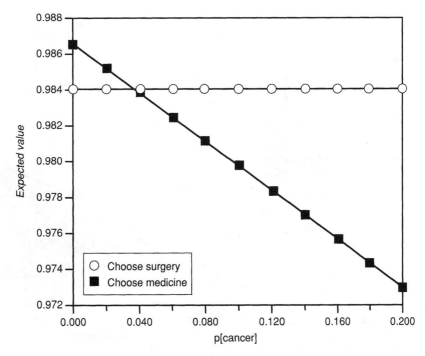

Figure 2–8. One-way sensitivity analysis of the variable p[cancer], the probability of colon cancer developing. Notice that the expected value of the surgery strategy is not affected by the probability of the development of colon cancer because proctocolectomy prevents colon cancer. We chose 0.09 as the best estimate for the likelihood of colon carcinoma developing in our patient. Above the threshold of 0.04, the surgery strategy is still preferred. For p[cancer] less than 0.04, the medicine strategy is preferred.

These utilities are inherently valid for this patient unless we misled the patient during utility assessment. When you read published decision analyses, addressed in Chapter 10, evaluating the utilities with sensitivity analysis becomes more important because you will need to determine whether your patient's personal values would change the results reported in the article.

Two-way sensitivity analysis can be used to analyze the effect of two variables simultaneously over every possible combination of values.[4] The graph of this type of plot indicates the combination of probabilities for which each strategy is preferred. In our analysis, the most crucial variables are the rates of surgical mortality and of colon cancer developing, as these probabilities are associated with the most dreaded outcomes and the lowest utilities.

TABLE 2–3. ONE-WAY SENSITIVITY ANALYSES TO TEST THE IMPACT OF EACH PROBABILITY AND UTILITY ESTIMATE ON OVERALL OUTCOME OF THE DECISION TREE.

Variable	Best Estimate	Threshold	Choose Surgery	Choose Medicine
p[ileostomy]	0.09	0.16	p < 0.16	p > 0.16
p[incontinence]	0.18	0.32	p < 0.32	p > 0.32
p[future relapse]	0.20	None	p < 1.0	N/A
U[ileostomy]	0.92	0.75	U > 0.75	U < 0.75
U[incontinence]	0.95	0.87	U > 0.87	U < 0.87
U[cancer death]	0.70	0.90	U < 0.90	U > 0.90

U[outcome] = the utility of that outcome; Best Estimate = the value for that variable incorporated into the decision tree (considered to be most representative of the true value for the probabilities and of the patient's actual preference in the case of utilities); Threshold = the value of that variable for which surgery and medicine strategies are equivalent (above and below the threshold value, one of the two strategies is preferred, as seen in the two far-right columns).

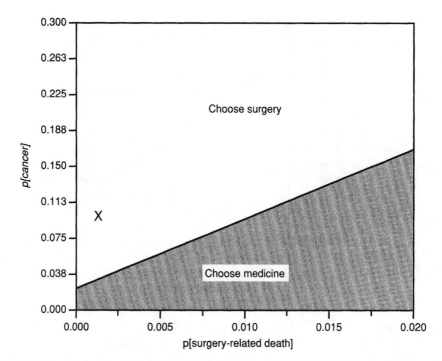

Figure 2–9. Two-way sensitivity analysis reveals the effect of altering the value of two variables simultaneously. On the x-axis is p[surgery-related death], the probability of surgical mortality. We recall from Figure 2–7 that surgery loses its advantage over medicine as p[surgery-related death] increases. On the y-axis is p[cancer], the likelihood of colon cancer developing. Figure 2–8 demonstrated that the value of the medicine strategy declines steadily as p[cancer] increases. With two-way sensitivity analysis, we may choose any two values for p[surgery-related death] and p[cancer] and determine the preferred strategy. Above the dividing line, surgery is the preferred strategy, and below it, medicine would be optimal. Our best estimate—p[surgery-related death] = 0.002 and p[cancer] = 0.09—is indicated with an X.

Two-way sensitivity analysis on these two variables is shown in Figure 2–9. Notice that as the risk of surgery-related death increases along the x-axis, medical therapy is favored; conversely, as the risk of cancer rises along the y-axis, surgery becomes preferable. Although these calculations and plots can be tedious to construct by hand, they can be created in seconds using a decision analysis software program (discussed later in this chapter).

Sensitivity analysis is a crucial step in decision analysis to test the effect of the probabilities and utilities that impact the model. The uncertainties that have the greatest impact on the decision can be investigated further to obtain more reliable estimates; thus, sensitivity analysis can help direct future research. If the results of a decision analysis are to be communicated, as in a published study, sensitivity analysis must demonstrate to the reader the stability of the conclusions. When the results of our analysis remain valid over a wide range of probabilities, we have even more confidence in the conclusions. However, in a decision analysis that we perform using our best estimates of probabilities and utilities for our individual patient, we must make a decision regardless of sensitivity analysis, and we must be prepared to accept the results of the decision tree.

ADVANCED METHODS OF DECISION ANALYSIS

Time preferences

One of the most complex aspects of decision analysis is the handling of preferences over time. We mentioned earlier that a patient's values for certain outcomes may change over time. People also value health states differently from the present to the future, usually devaluing the future relative to the present. Most would not trade a year of perfect health now for one 15 years in the future. We saw an example of this in our decision tree when our patient SM placed a utility of 0.7 on the outcome of cancer-related death, which would have decreased his life expectancy by about half. We might have expected a utility of 0.5 for this outcome, but SM showed that he was not willing to risk the near future for the promise of a lengthened life expectancy. SM, like most people, values the present greater than the future.

Placing a lower value on the future compared with the present is called **discounting.** Discounting is a systematic method for devaluing the utility of health in the future relative to the present. A standard rate of discounting used in published studies incorporating quality of life and time is 3%. Thus, a year with a given health state X is devalued by an annual rate of 3% for each year from the present in which it occurs. The formula for discounting a year in a health state, with utility = U and discount rate = D, in years (y), for example, is[17]

$$U/(1 + D)^y$$

Therefore, with a discount rate of 3%, a year spent in perfect health 10 years from now is assigned a utility:

$$1/(1 + 0.03)^{10} = 0.744$$

This year is valued at 0.744, relative to the same year in the present.

Discounting applies to money as well as to utilities, as discussed in Chapter 4. In decision analysis, the importance of discounting was recognized from observed behavior among patients who were unwilling to accept the short-term risks of a procedure (eg, surgery), although they would enjoy an overall long-term benefit in life expectancy or quality of life. A method was required to scale down these future benefits into meaningful units that we can use today. Although 3% is often used as a standard estimate, individual patients have their own intrinsic discount rates that shape their personal values of the future, relative to the present. These rates can be derived for use in an individual's decision analysis.[18,19]

As we discount utilities over time, we must also account for the amount of time that is spent with each value of utility. In clinical research, the unit of measure most used for the accounting of utilities over time is the **quality-adjusted life year,** or **QALY.** A QALY is simply calculated by multiplying the time in years by the quality as measured in utilities. For example, 5 years spent in a health state of utility 0.6 is equivalent ($5 \times 0.6 = 3.0$) to 3 years spent in perfect health, or 3 QALYs. These QALYs can then be discounted depending on how far into the future the year occurs. QALYs are used frequently in cost-effectiveness analyses and are discussed in greater detail in Chapter 4.

Markov process

Some cases in clinical medicine are too complicated to be modeled by the simple tree structure we used for our patient with ulcerative colitis. The linear structure of a standard decision tree may be incapable of representing the natural history of a complex disease. For example, to characterize the prognosis for a woman with moderate coronary artery disease, we would need to incorporate the possibility of future events at distant points of time and the gradual progression of the disease. A simple tree would have difficulty handling the complexity of time for this type of medical decision making and could not give an accurate estimate of life expectancy. The Markov model is an important method of modeling events that may occur in the future by creating a basic tree structure that cycles over fixed intervals of time.[20] For these more complex models, computer software is essential.

As in the more basic decision tree, a Markov model begins with a patient facing a difficult decision or receiving a diagnosis of a chronic disease. The model then defines a series of health states through which the patient may transition. A patient who receives a diagnosis of a hypothetical disease X may have the possible health states shown in Figure 2–10 (well, ill, and dead). The arrows in the figure demonstrate the possibilities for movement between these states. For this disease, a well person can become ill during each period or cycle, and a well or ill person could transition to death. However, once a person becomes ill with this hypothetical disease, he or she can only stay the same or die during each consecutive cycle of time.[20,21]

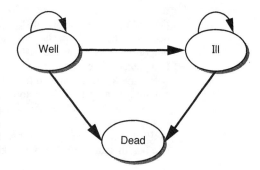

Figure 2–10. Diagram of the Markov states demonstrating the possible transitions among the health states of a chronic disease. Notice that a well person can either become ill or die. But once a person proceeds to the ill state he or she cannot return to well. Death is an absorbing state, so no person can leave this health state.

There are three types of health states in a Markov model:

1. Dynamic states: Transition is possible into one of the other states, including itself.
2. Temporary states: Outward transition is mandatory; a person cannot remain in the same state.
3. Absorbing state: No transitions can occur, ie, death.

During each cycle of the Markov model, usually 1 year, a patient has a defined probability of transitioning from his or her health state into one of the other possible states or remaining in the current state. The **Markovian assumption** is that these transition probabilities remain constant with each cycle through time. The model may continue until the patient (or cohort of patients) reaches an absorbing state, ie, death, or may continue for a fixed number of cycles.[4]

Each of these health states has a defined utility, and the computer software calculates the amount of time the patient spends in each health state. Thus, as we learned above, the software can add up the QALYs that each patient accumulates as he or she cycles through the transition states of the model, year after year, until eventual death. What's more, these QALYs can easily be discounted each cycle into the future to adjust their value to present day units. The strategy that accumulates the most QALYs (highest expected value) is the optimal choice in the decision analysis.

The Markov model is certainly more complex than the standard decision tree and may be more difficult to apply to the case of an individual patient. However, it involves the same five steps as the simple decision analysis above and the decision trees look similar. Moreover, the model is relatively easy to execute with the help of a computer and may offer important insights. The Markov model is especially useful for modeling a disease process over time and the effect of possible interventions on the progress of the disease. To answer questions regarding public health, one can simulate clinical trials with decades of follow-up that would not be feasible to conduct.[22] For a more in-depth review of the Markov process, the reader is referred to a number of excellent published reviews.[2,3,21]

Computer software in decision analysis

Decision analyses applying to individual patients, like the model we constructed in this chapter, can usually be executed with a hand-held calculator. However, several software programs have been developed to facilitate the process. These programs provide the framework for the decision tree or Markov model and can rapidly graph the results of sensitivity analysis. In addition, each is accompanied by a manual that directs the user through a sample decision analysis. As decision trees become more complex and advanced models are created, computer assistance becomes mandatory. The following software packages are frequently used by clinical researchers:

- SMLTREE (J. Hollenberg, New York, 1991)—available in PC only.
- DATA (Decision Analysis by Tree Age, Tree Age Software Inc, 1995)—available in Macintosh and in PC.

LIMITATIONS OF DECISION ANALYSIS

Most of this chapter has focused on the advantages and the strengths of decision analysis as a method for clinical decision making. But you may ask, "If decision analysis is so great and rational, why don't physicians use it more?" Let's examine five reasons why.

Clinical medicine is very complex

Often patients have multiple medical problems, making many clinical studies inapplicable to their case. It may seem very difficult to reduce "real life" into a list of outcomes that fits into a decision tree. Incorporation of new tests and therapies into an analysis may be difficult in the absence of data validating their efficacy. All these factors make clinical medicine more challenging; thus, in these situations decision analysis is more difficult, but also more necessary as an alternative to the traditional forms of clinical decision making.

The method can be laborious

Undoubtedly, decision analysis can be time-consuming, especially if a review of the literature is necessary as it was in our patient with ulcerative colitis. In an urgent and anxious situation, there may not be time or patience to complete the process. Nonetheless, the wheel need not be reinvented for each patient. Once we have structured a decision tree and gathered all the necessary clinical information, we can adapt it to similar patients in similar situations. A gastroenterologist may encounter our clinical scenario several times a year. Individual preferences need to be re-elicited and some likelihoods may bear revising, but the tree remains ready for use.

Most clinicians have limited experience with the method

This formidable obstacle is slowly being reduced. This chapter is meant to entice future experimentation and utilization of decision analysis. Excellent textbooks on the subject are included in the references at the end of this chapter.

Decision analysis cannot be performed in the absence of evidence

Clinical situations arise in which there is no evidence to direct a decision. Completing the five steps of decision analysis would be very difficult in these instances, but the techniques of formulating an explicit question and structuring the problem can still be helpful in the absence of data. In fact, sensitivity analysis may reveal that the missing data have no impact on the final decision. The skill of deconstructing a complex decision into manageable probabilities will improve "clinical judgment" to arrive at the best possible decision.

Preferences may be difficult to elicit and may change over time

As discussed previously, some patients may have difficulty revealing their preferences quantitatively. Relative preferences for certain outcomes may evolve with age. These obstacles are challenging to overcome and have varying impact on the results of the decision analysis. Sensitivity analysis can help to demonstrate the impact of the utility on the conclusion.

SUMMARY

1. Decision analysis is a rational method for medical decision making that incorporates the best available evidence and the patient's individual needs.
2. This technique is particularly suited for clinical situations that are highly complex, in which important data are uncertain, patient input is critical, or events occur at different points in time.

3. The five steps of decision analysis are
   • Formulate the question.
   • Structure the decision and build a decision tree.
   • Fill in the data (probabilities and outcomes).
   • Determine the value of each competing strategy.
   • Perform sensitivity analyses.
4. A decision tree is composed of decision nodes (clinician or patient determines the path), chance nodes (uncertain path to be determined by chance), and terminal states (outcome health states).
5. Probabilities within the decision tree can derive from:
   • Clinical studies
   • Clinical databases
   • Expert opinion/calculated guesses
6. A utility is a quantitative measure of the strength of a patient's preference for a particular health state or outcome. Methods for assessing utilities include:
   • Visual analog scale
   • Time trade-off
   • Standard gamble
7. Solving the decision tree by averaging out and folding back will reveal the optimal strategy for the clinical situation.
8. Sensitivity analysis tests the stability of the results of the decision tree by systematically varying the values of particular probabilities and outcomes incorporated within the tree.
9. Discounting is a mathematical method for devaluing the future relative to the present. Complex clinical situations that assess prognosis or that evaluate multiple health states over time should be handled with a Markov model.
10. Although decision analysis may not be practical for every clinical situation, it can be a useful, logical, and evidence-based approach to medical decision making.

REFERENCES

1. Borrowed from Browner WS: Veterans Affairs Medical Center, San Francisco, California.
2. Weinstein MC, Fineberg HV: *Clinical Decision Analysis*. Saunders, 1980.
3. Sox Jr HC et al: *Medical Decision Making*. Butterworth Heinemann, 1988.
4. Pauker SG, Kassirer JP: Decision analysis. N Engl J Med 1987;316:250.
5. Jewell DP: Ulcerative colitis. Chapter 64 in: Sleisenger MH, Fordtran JS (editors): *Gastrointestinal Diseases,* 5th ed. Saunders, 1993.
6. Pemberton JH et al: Ileal pouch-anal anastomosis for chronic ulcerative colitis: Long-term results. Ann Surg 1987;206:504.
7. Fleshman JW et al: The ileal reservoir and ileoanal anastomosis procedure: Factors affecting technical and functional outcome. Dis Colon Rectum 1988;31:10.
8. Present DH et al: 6-Mercaptopurine in the management of inflammatory bowel disease: Short- and long-term toxicity. Ann Intern Med 1989;111:641.
9. Sandborn WJ: A review of immune modifier therapy for inflammatory bowel disease: Azathioprine, 6-mercaptopurine, cyclosporine, and methotrexate. Am J Gastroenterol 1996;91:423.
10. Provenzale D et al: Prophylactic colectomy or surveillance for chronic ulcerative colitis? A decision analysis. Gastroenterology 1995;109:1188.
11. Ekbom A et al: Ulcerative colitis and colorectal cancer: A population-based study. N Engl J Med 1990;323:1228.
12. Gyde SN et al: Colorectal cancer in ulcerative colitis: A cohort study of primary referrals from three centres. Gut 1988;29:206.
13. Lennard-Jones JE et al: Precancer and cancer in extensive ulcerative colitis: Findings among 401 patients over 22 years. Gut 1990;31:800.
14. Beck JR et al: A convenient approximation of life expectancy. Parts I and II. Am J Med 1982;73:883.
15. Read JL et al: Preferences for health outcomes: Comparison of assessment methods. Med Decis Making 1984;4:315.
16. Petitti DB: *Meta-analysis, Decision Analysis, and Cost-effectiveness Analysis: Methods for Quantitative Synthesis in Medicine.* Oxford University Press, 1994.

17. Chapman GB, Elstein AS: Valuing the future: Temporal discounting of health and money. Med Decis Making 1995;15:373.
18. Redelmeier DA et al: Probability judgment in medicine: Discounting unspecified possibilities. Med Decis Making 1995;15:227.
19. Johanneson M et al: A note on QALY's, time tradeoff, and discounting. Med Decis Making 1994;14:188.
20. Beck JR, Pauker SG: The Markov process in medical prognosis. Med Decis Making 1983;3:419.
21. Sonnenberg FA, Beck JR: Markov models in medical decision making: A practical guide. Med Decis Making 1993;13:322.
22. Weinstein MC et al: Forecasting coronary heart disease incidence, mortality, and cost: The coronary heart disease policy model. Am J Publ Health 1987;77:1417.

TREATMENT & TESTING THRESHOLDS

Stephen W. Bent, MD • Daniel J. Friedland, MD

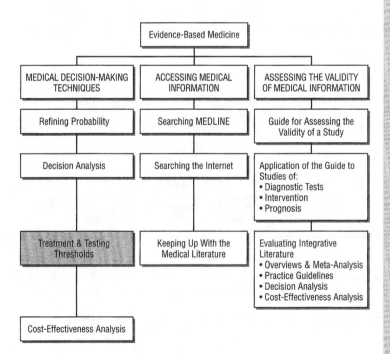

```
                    ┌─────────────────────────┐
                    │  Evidence-Based Medicine │
                    └─────────────────────────┘
```

MEDICAL DECISION-MAKING TECHNIQUES	ACCESSING MEDICAL INFORMATION	ASSESSING THE VALIDITY OF MEDICAL INFORMATION
Refining Probability	Searching MEDLINE	Guide for Assessing the Validity of a Study
Decision Analysis	Searching the Internet	Application of the Guide to Studies of: • Diagnostic Tests • Intervention • Prognosis
Treatment & Testing Thresholds	Keeping Up With the Medical Literature	Evaluating Integrative Literature • Overviews & Meta-Analysis • Practice Guidelines • Decision Analysis • Cost-Effectiveness Analysis
Cost-Effectiveness Analysis		

THE TREATMENT THRESHOLD: TO TREAT OR NOT TO TREAT

Introduction

Medical providers are constantly presented with decisions about whether to initiate treatments for specific diseases. In some cases, these decisions are quite simple. For example, if it is known for certain that the patient has a disease and that the treatment for the condition has no associated risks, treatment is the obvious choice. More often, these decisions involve a greater complexity. The reasons are twofold. First, many diagnoses cannot be established with complete certainty, and second, all treatments are associated with risks. Providers must therefore determine the likelihood that a patient actually has a given disease and whether the benefit of treating that disease outweighs the risk of the treatment's side effects.

Threshold analysis is useful in this setting primarily because it allows the physician to examine this process of making decisions when there is uncertainty. Key factors that affect these decisions are identified and analyzed. As a result, using threshold analysis, physicians may feel more confident in their decision making and understand how and why their decisions change with different patients, different diseases, and different treatments.

What is a threshold?

A **threshold** is a level, point, or value above which something will take place and below which something will not take place.

What is a treatment threshold?

A **treatment threshold** is a probability of disease above which we treat for the disease and below which we do not treat. In the figures of this chapter, the treatment threshold is represented as Rx.

How is the treatment threshold useful?

The treatment threshold helps guide the decision to treat. If a patient's probability of disease is greater than the treatment threshold, treatment is indicated. If a patient's probability of disease is lower than the treatment threshold, treatment is not indicated. Let's look at a case scenario.

> In your office, you have just examined a woman who was bitten by a tick. After obtaining a history and performing a physical examination, you estimate that her probability of Lyme disease (infection with *Borrelia burgdorferi*) is 30%. You remember reading an article in *The New England Journal of Medicine* that calculated the treatment threshold for Lyme disease to be 3.6%.[1] Because her probability of Lyme disease is greater than the treatment threshold, you determine that she should be treated.

This case information is illustrated in Figure 3–1. The bar graph shows a range of disease probability, with the patient's **probability of disease** indicated as p = 30% and denoted with an X. When X lies to the right of the treatment threshold, treatment is recommended.

> The next patient you see was also bitten by a tick. After examining him, you estimate his probability of Lyme disease to be 1% (p = 1%). Because his probability of Lyme disease is below the treatment threshold, you decide that he should not be treated.

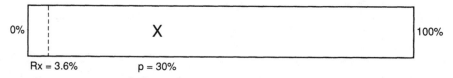

Figure 3–1. The bar represents the probability of disease from 0% to 100%. The "X" within the bar represents the patient's probability of disease, noted below the bar as "p = 30%." The treatment threshold is represented by a dashed line and labeled as "Rx."

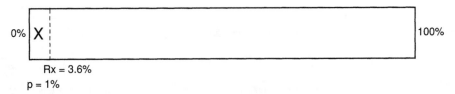

0% X 100%

Rx = 3.6%
p = 1%

Figure 3–2. The bar represents the probability of disease from 0% to 100%. The "X" within the bar is the patient's probability of disease, noted below the bar as "p = 1%." The treatment threshold is represented by a dashed line and labeled as "Rx."

This case information is also represented graphically (Figure 3–2). Note that now X is to the left, below the treatment threshold. These case examples model the process that many caregivers use every time they decide whether or not to treat patients. This process requires the ability to estimate a probability of disease (as discussed in Chapter 1) and the ability to understand a treatment threshold and how it is determined.

What determines the treatment threshold?

The treatment threshold (Rx) is determined by the costs and benefits of treatment. The treatment threshold is often confused with the patient's probability of having the disease. Note that the factors that determine a patient's probability of disease do not play a role in determining the treatment threshold, as the following case example shows.

> You are working in a pediatric clinic where you see a 7-year-old boy who is complaining of a sore throat that has lasted for 3 days. On examination, the boy has no fever but has swollen tonsils with a mild white exudate. He has no lymphadenopathy. No culture equipment is available. You are trying to decide whether to treat the patient for strep throat or just assure the family that this is a viral illness and that the boy will be well in a few days.

What is your estimate of this patient's probability of having strep throat? What is the treatment threshold for strep throat? (See Figure 3–3.)

There are two distinct probabilities that you are asked to estimate in this case example. The first probability that you must estimate is the patient's probability of disease (strep throat). This probability is determined by features of the history and physical examination that are known to be associated with strep throat (tonsillar exudate, lymphadenopathy, fever). In this case, you might estimate that the patient has a probability of disease of approximately 10% (although estimates may vary widely based on the information you were given).

The second probability that you must estimate is the treatment threshold. The treatment threshold is determined only by the costs and benefits of treatment. The treatment threshold is *not* affected by the patient's probability of disease. In this example, the costs of treatment are the side effects associated with treatment with penicillin (rash, diarrhea, anaphylaxis). The benefits of treatment are the prevention of rheumatic heart disease, the avoidance of other complications of strep infection, and the reduced duration of symptoms if the patient has a true infection.

Intuitively we know that if a treatment is associated with large benefits and small costs, we are willing to recommend the treatment to patients who have even a limited chance of actually having disease (eg, giving antibiotics for Lyme disease—the costs of treatment are small, and the benefits of preventing complications of Lyme disease are considerable).

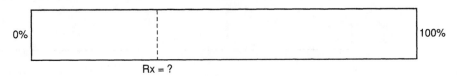

0% 100%

Rx = ?

Figure 3–3. Where on this bar graph of probability of disease would you place the treatment threshold for strep throat?

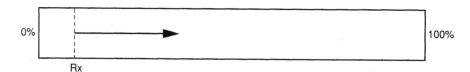

Figure 3–4. The treatment threshold, "Rx," increases (moves to the right on the probability of disease bar graph) when cost of treatment increases.

Conversely, treatments with low benefit and high cost (eg, chemotherapy for many cancers) have a much higher treatment threshold. This means that we are unwilling to treat patients unless they have a very high probability of disease. In the above case scenario, because the benefit of treating strep throat is relatively high (prevention of rheumatic heart disease and abscess formation and reduction in symptoms) and the costs are relatively low (rare severe allergic reactions), the treatment threshold is low (5%).[2]

What would happen to your treatment threshold for strep throat if you knew that the patient had an allergy to penicillin and that penicillin was the only antibiotic available? As you can see in Figure 3–4, if the cost of treatment increased (because of an increased risk for an allergic reaction), the treatment threshold would also increase. We would have to have a higher suspicion that the patient had the disease before we would be willing to subject the patient to the risks of treatment.

What would happen to your treatment threshold if you knew that in your area the incidence of rheumatic heart disease after strep throat was 25%? As you can see in Figure 3–5, if the benefit of treatment increased (increased prevention of rheumatic heart disease), the treatment threshold would decrease.

Key points to remember so far include

1. The treatment threshold (Rx) is the probability of disease above which we treat and below which we do not treat.
2. The treatment threshold is determined only by the costs and benefits of a particular treatment.
3. Around the treatment threshold, we have difficulty deciding what to do because the benefit of treating and not treating are about the same.
4. We determined the treatment threshold by intuitively thinking about costs and benefits. When costs increased, Rx increased. Conversely, if the benefits increased, Rx decreased. In the next section, we explore quantitative methods for determining the treatment threshold.

DETERMINING THE TREATMENT THRESHOLD: DECISION ANALYSIS AGAIN

So far we have not discussed the critical step of how to set the treatment threshold. You may determine Rx intuitively or use the more rigorous approach of decision analysis.

Intuitive approach

Skilled clinicians make intuitive decisions every day. When we think of treatment thresholds using an intuitive approach, we take into account the relative costs and benefits of a treatment. Consider the following case example.

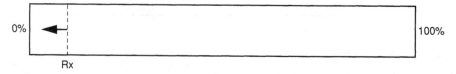

Figure 3–5. The treatment threshold, "Rx," decreases (moves to the left on the probability of disease bar graph) when the benefit of treatment increases.

You are working in a community hospital in the United States. Your computed tomography (CT) scanner is down and your ultrasound technician is ill. Your facility is hundreds of miles from another hospital. A 20-year-old man presents with abdominal pain, and you are concerned about appendicitis. Without the availability of diagnostic tests, you must decide whether to proceed to laparotomy or send the patient home.

Intuitively, you assess the costs and benefits of treatment (appendectomy). You realize that the costs of treatment are surgical morbidity and mortality and that the benefit of treatment is cure of appendicitis in those patients who have the disease (thus, preventing death and complications of a ruptured appendix).

In this situation, what is the treatment threshold for appendectomy in suspected appendicitis? For this exercise, weigh the costs and benefits and write your estimate of Rx here:
_____.

Although it is useful to think about treatment thresholds in this way, this intuitive approach is not as precise as decision analysis (discussed next) because intuitive estimates vary widely.

Decision analysis with a sensitivity analysis for probability of disease

If we return to the technique of decision analysis, we can see how the treatment threshold probability can be calculated. Although this process may appear cumbersome, it becomes relatively easy with the aid of computer-assisted programs. As you will see, simple problems can be solved easily using a hand-held calculator or graph paper.

Recall from Chapter 2 that a decision analysis involves five steps:

1. Formulate an explicit question.
2. Structure the decision.
3. Fill in the data.
4. Determine the value of alternative strategies.
5. Perform a sensitivity analysis.

Using these five basic steps, we can apply decision analysis to determine the treatment threshold as follows.

Formulating the question is simple: Should we treat or not treat?

To structure the decision, first determine all the possible outcomes of each strategy and then sequence these outcomes temporally. For both the treatment and no-treatment strategies there is the possibility that the disease is either present or absent, and this in turn influences whether the patient will live or die. For simple problems, you may find that using the format shown in Table 3–1 is helpful in constructing your decision tree.

We have simplified the process by considering only the outcomes of dying or surviving. As you become more skilled in decision analysis, you may include intermediary outcomes. For example, you might include a stroke that was experienced as a result of therapy.

Next, we can convert the table into a decision tree, as shown in Figure 3–6.

TABLE 3–1. OUTCOME OF TREATMENT AND NO TREATMENT WITH DISEASE EITHER PRESENT OR ABSENT.

Decision	Disease Status	Outcome
Treat	Present	Die as a result of treatment
		Survive after treatment
	Absent	Die as a result of treatment
		Survive after treatment
Don't treat	Present	Die without treatment
		Survive without treatment
	Absent	Survive without treatment

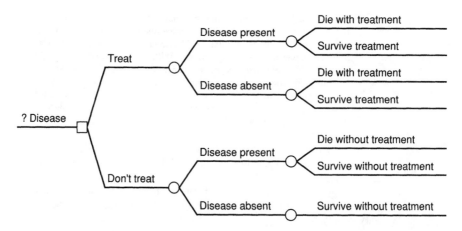

Figure 3–6. Decision tree for a patient with suspected disease. The top branch represents the possible outcomes if the patient is treated. The bottom branch represents the possible outcomes if the patient is not treated. Decision nodes are square, and chance nodes are circles. The first set of chance nodes from the left represents the probability of disease, and the second set of chance nodes represents the probability of survival after treatment or no treatment.

Now we can fill in the data. For simplicity, we will assign the utilities as follows: survival = 1 and death = 0.

When we roll back the tree to calculate the expected value of each branch (see Chapter 2, page 48), twigs that have utilities of zero do not contribute to the overall value of that branch (because the probability of that outcome multiplied by zero is zero). We can therefore simplify the tree shown in Figure 3–6 by deleting the twigs that end with death. This results in a simplified decision tree, Figure 3–7. Compare Figures 3–6 and 3–7 and see how the larger tree in Figure 3–6 was collapsed to the simplified tree in Figure 3–7.

In Figure 3–7, p is the probability of disease. Another simplification has been made in the way the data are displayed in Figure 3–7. Instead of separately filling in the utility of survival and the respective probabilities of survival, we have multiplied the two values to present the expected value of each twig as J, K, L, and M. Because the utility of survival = 1, the expected value of each twig simply equals the probability of that outcome. The expected value of each of the four twigs is thus:

J = the probability of surviving the disease after receiving the treatment.
K = the probability of surviving the treatment while not having the disease.
L = the probability of surviving the disease without treatment.
M = the probability of surviving without disease or treatment. This equals 1.0.

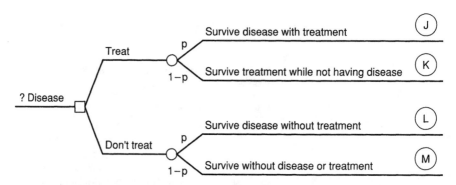

Figure 3–7. Simplified decision tree for a patient with suspected disease. The top branch represents the possible outcomes if the patient is treated. The bottom branch represents the possible outcomes if the patient is not treated. The probability of disease is denoted by "p." "J," "K," "L," and "M" are the expected values of each outcome.

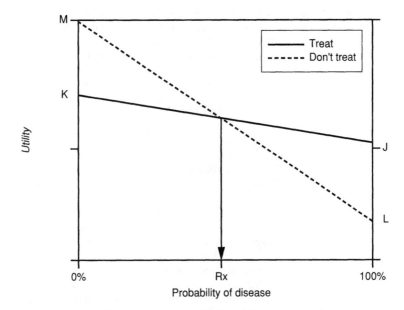

Figure 3–8. Expected utility as a function of probability of disease (also known as sensitivity analysis). Expected utility is shown on the y-axis, and probability of disease is shown on the x-axis. The expected utilities of the "Treat" and "Don't treat" options vary as the probability of disease varies to generate two straight lines. "M" and "K" are expected utilities of the "Don't treat" and "Treat" options when the chance of disease is 0%. They are equal to the probability of surviving without disease or treatment and the probability of surviving treatment while not having the disease, respectively. "L" and "J" are the expected utilities of these options when the chance of disease is 100%. These utilities are equal to the probability of surviving the disease without treatment and the probability of surviving the disease with treatment, respectively. "Rx" is the treatment threshold.

Therefore, the only pieces of information that you need obtain in a literature search to perform this *simple* threshold analysis are the above probabilities in J, K, and L. (If you choose to perform a more complex analysis involving intermediary outcomes, additional information from the literature would be required.)

Now we determine the expected value (the overall utility) of the "Treat" and "Don't treat" branches. We do this by simply rolling back the tree as explained in Chapter 2.

Utility of the "Treat" arm = pJ + (1 − p)K; rearranged, this = (J − K)p + K
Utility of the "Don't treat" arm = pL + (1 − p)M; rearranged, this = (L − M)p + M

The goal of threshold analysis is to determine the probability of disease (p) at which the utility of the "Treat" and "Don't treat" arms are equivalent (this *is* the treatment threshold). We determine this mathematically by hand or by applying sensitivity analysis for the probability of disease.

Note that the expected utility for the "Treat" arm = (J − K)p + K and the expected utility for the "Don't treat" arm = (L − M)p + M. These are each equations for straight lines in the form y = mx + b, where "y" is the expected utility of the respective arm and "x" is the probability of disease. A sensitivity analysis simply plots the utility for each arm over a range of disease probabilities. The graphical representation of the sensitivity analysis, Figure 3–8, illustrates a number of key points.

1. The preferred decision is that with the greatest utility. This preferred decision is represented by the uppermost lines on the graph. Therefore, at low probabilities, "Don't treat" is the preferred decision. At high probabilities, "Treat" is the preferred decision.
2. M − K represents the difference in utility between not treating patients without disease (ie, at 0 % probability) and treating patients without disease. This difference therefore represents the net harm of treating well patients.
3. J − L represents the difference in utility between treating patients with disease (ie, at 100% probability) and not treating patients with disease. This difference represents the net benefit of treating patients with disease.

4. At the intersection of the lines, the utility of the decisions "Treat" and "Don't treat" is equivalent. Thus, the corresponding probability, where the utility of treatment versus no treatment is equivalent, represents the treatment threshold (Rx).

At the treatment threshold, the equations for the utility of each arm are equivalent. Therefore, at the treatment threshold, $(J - K)p + K = (L - M)p + M$. This is rearranged to solve for p, which at this probability is Rx:

$$Rx = (M - K)/[(M - K) + (J - L)]$$

From key points 2 and 3 above, note that: $M - K$ represents the net cost of treating nondiseased patients and that $J - L$ represents the net benefit of treating diseased patients. Thus, substituting for $M - K$ and $J - L$ in the above equation, we demonstrate that Rx is

$$cost/(cost + benefit)$$

5. Note what happens to Rx when the magnitude of harm of treating well patients (ie, $M - K$) increases. As M and K splay apart, Rx increases. Alternatively, when the magnitude of benefit of treating diseased patients (ie, $J - L$) increases, J and L splay apart and Rx decreases. This is congruent with the formula Rx = cost/(cost + benefit). If costs increase, the treatment threshold probability increases. If benefits increase, the treatment threshold probability decreases.

Let's return to our example of appendicitis. Because no diagnostic tests are available, we have only two options: treat or do not treat. The decision is structured in the tree in Figure 3–9.

To make the treatment threshold applicable to medical practice in the United States, the relevant mortality rates were found in the literature.[3]

1. The surgical mortality for acute appendicitis is 0.24%
2. The surgical mortality for operating on a patient with a normal appendix is 0.14%
3. The mortality for patients who are discharged from the hospital and later undergo surgery because a perforated appendix is 1.66% (we are assuming that all such patients will be able to return for surgery)

With the utility of survival = 1, the expected utility for each of the outcomes is therefore:

J = the probability of surviving appendicitis after surgery = 0.9976 (1 − 0.24%).
K = the probability of surviving surgery while not having appendicitis = 0.9986 (1 − 0.14%).

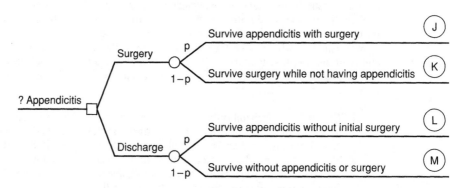

Figure 3–9. Decision tree for a patient with suspected appendicitis. The top branch shows the possible outcomes if surgery is chosen, and the bottom branch shows the possible outcomes if hospital discharge is chosen. The probability of appendicitis is denoted by "p." "J," "K," "L," and "M" are the expected utilities of each outcome.

L = the probability of surviving appendicitis without initial surgery = 0.9834
(1 − 1.66%).
M = the probability of surviving without appendicitis or surgery = 1.0.

These data may be plotted on graph paper by marking the points M and K on the vertical axis, representing 0% probability of appendicitis, and J and L on the vertical axis, representing 100% probability of the disease (Figure 3–10). Straight lines are then drawn to connect J and K as well as L and M. The intersection of these lines at the specific probability of appendicitis indicates the treatment threshold.

Alternatively, you may calculate the treatment threshold by hand using a calculator and the above cost/(cost + benefit) equation (Rx = (M − K)/[(M − K) + (J - L)]).

The cost of treatment (M − K) is the probability of surviving without appendicitis or surgery subtracted from the probability of surviving surgery while not having appendicitis; thus, = 1.0 − 0.9986 = 0.0014. The benefit of treatment (J − L) is the probability of surviving appendicitis after surgery subtracted from the probability of surviving appendicitis without initial surgery (and return with a ruptured appendix); thus, = (J − L) = 0.9976 − 0.9834 = 0.0142.

The treatment threshold = (M − K)/[(M − K) + (J − L)] = cost/(cost + benefit) = 0.0014/(0.0014 + 0.0142) = 0.09 = 9%. How does this compare with the treatment threshold that you calculated intuitively?

Your mathematically calculated result suggests that if you have no diagnostic tests available and your estimated probability of disease is less than 9%, you should discharge the patient from the hospital. On the other hand, if your estimated probability of disease is greater than 9% you should perform appendectomy. Let's consider the same treatment threshold for appendicitis, but now in the context of rural Africa.

Now, in rural Africa, you don't have any imaging equipment, and the nearest hospital is thousands of miles away. Without diagnostic tests available, you must decide whether to perform appendectomy or discharge the patient. There are no primary data available for this situation, so you extrapolate from the above data, making a couple of assumptions:

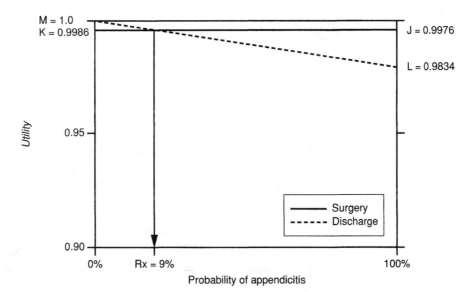

Figure 3–10. Expected utility of surgery versus hospital discharge for patients with suspected appendicitis. Expected utility is shown on the y-axis, and for each strategy is plotted against the probability of appendicitis, shown on the x-axis. The intersection of these lines is the treatment threshold, "Rx," at which the expected utility of both outcomes is equal. At probabilities of appendicitis less than 9%, discharge is the preferred option, and at greater probabilities, surgery is the preferred option.

1. The surgical mortality with limited resources would be 10 times that of the above surgical mortality. Thus the surgical mortality for acute appendicitis is 2.4% and the mortality for operating on a patient with a normal appendix is 1.4%.
2. Half the patients discharged with appendicitis die. The mortality for patients who are discharged from hospital is therefore 50%.

The expected utility for each of the outcomes is therefore calculated to be:

J = the probability of surviving appendicitis after surgery = 0.976 (1 − 2.4%).
K = the probability of surviving surgery while not having appendicitis = 0.986 (1 − 1.4%).
L = the probability of surviving appendicitis without initial surgery = 0.5 (1 − 50%).
M = the probability of surviving without appendicitis or surgery = 1.0.

As before, these data can be graphed in a sensitivity analysis, as shown in Figure 3–11. Alternatively, as before, you may calculate the treatment threshold by hand.

$$\text{The cost of treatment } (M - K) = 1 - 0.986 = 0.014$$
$$\text{The benefit of treatment } (J - L) = 0.976 - 0.5 = 0.476$$

Thus, you find that the treatment threshold = $(M - K)/([M - K] + [J - L])$ = cost/(cost + benefit) = 0.014/(0.014 + 0.476) = 0.029 = 2.9%.

Note that with the assumptions about a rural African clinic, the treatment threshold is lower than it is for the United States scenario. In the rural clinic, the costs of treatment have increased (from an expected net utility of 0.0014 to 0.014). This acts to increase the treatment threshold. However, because half the patients who are discharged from the rural clinic die compared with only 1.66% of patients in the United States, the benefits of surgery have also increased (from an expected net utility of 0.0142 to 0.476). This acts to decrease the treatment threshold. Because the benefits have increased much more than the costs, the treatment threshold has decreased.

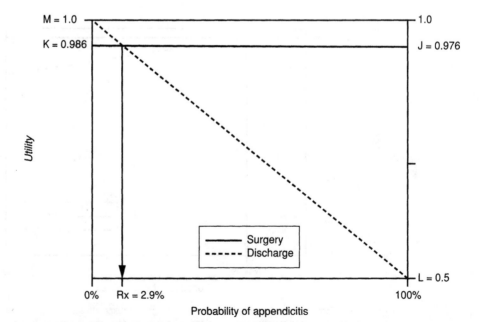

Figure 3–11. Graph of the expected utility of surgery versus discharge for patients with suspected appendicitis in rural Africa. The intersection of the lines "Surgery" and "Discharge" yields the treatment threshold (Rx) of 2.9%.

THE DECISION TO TEST & THE TESTING THRESHOLDS: WILL THIS TEST CHANGE MY TREATMENT DECISION?

Will the posttest probability cross the treatment threshold?

The concept of the treatment threshold is a tool we can use for deciding whether patients should be treated for diseases when there is uncertainty about the diagnosis. However, as all medical providers are aware, there are literally thousands of diagnostic tests that may change our estimation of a patient's probability of disease (see Chapter 1). It follows that the next issue we need to consider is whether or not we need to order diagnostic tests. When faced with the decision to order a diagnostic test, providers have three choices:

1. Do not order the test and do not treat the disease.
2. Order the test.
3. Treat for the disease without testing.

Diagnostic tests are often ordered without much thought. Some clinics order routine complete blood counts (CBCs) and measurement of electrolytes for all patients, emergency departments may order abdominal films for most or all patients with abdominal pain, and some physicians may order strep throat cultures for all patients with a sore throat. This type of test ordering is very expensive and can be misleading and even dangerous to patient care. For example, if a prostate specific antigen (PSA) test is ordered for a 40-year-old patient seen in your clinic and the test result indicates borderline elevated levels of PSA, the patient may be subjected to an array of invasive, expensive, and painful tests even though the elevated level is likely a normal variant.

Thus, the premise of this section is that *if the test result will not change the management of the patient, the test should not be ordered.* Let's return to a case scenario.

You are back with the 20-year-old patient who is seen in your US hospital because of abdominal pain. This time, however, imaging tests are available. After obtaining a history and performing a physical examination, you estimate that his pretest probability of appendicitis is 25%. You consider ordering a KUB (flat and upright abdominal x-ray) to help you determine whether the patient has appendicitis. You have three options:

1. Do not order the KUB and do not treat the patient for appendicitis.
2. Order the KUB.
3. Treat the patient for appendicitis and do not order the KUB.

How do you decide?

All tests can be evaluated using a three-step approach that applies concepts discussed earlier in this chapter.

Step 1

Find the treatment threshold. In the above example, we know that the treatment threshold for appendicitis is 9%. Techniques for determining the treatment threshold are discussed in the previous section.

Step 2

Determine the patient's pretest probability of disease. In this case, the pretest probability, estimated according to the patient's symptoms and signs, was given to you as 25%. (Techniques for determining probability are discussed in Chapter 1.) Where is this probability in relation to the treatment threshold? Because the patient's probability of disease is greater than the treatment threshold, you would treat the patient for appendicitis if no additional diagnostic testing were available.

Step 3

Using likelihood ratios for the given test, determine whether testing will change what you do for the patient. In this example, the likelihood ratios (LRs) for a KUB in the diagnosis of appendicitis are LR(+) = 4.0 and LR(−) = 0.67.[4]

Therefore, using the principles outlined in Chapter 1, first convert the pretest probability to a pretest odds (odds = probability/[1 − probability]).

Pretest probability = 25%
Pretest odds = 0.25/(1 − 0.25) = 0.33

Next, multiply the pretest odds by the largest and smallest LR for the test to generate a posttest odds. (If the test is dichotomous, this is simply the LR for the positive and negative test results.)

If the test result is negative, posttest odds = pretest odds × LR(−) = 0.33 × 0.67 = 0.22
If the test result is positive, posttest odds = pretest odds × LR(+) = 0.33 × 4.0 = 1.32

Finally, convert the posttest-odds to a posttest probability (probability = odds/[odds + 1]).

If the test result is negative, posttest probability = 0.22/(0.22 + 1) = 18%
If the test result is positive, posttest probability = 1.32/(1.32 + 1) = 57%

Now you are ready to ask yourself the key question: Has the posttest probability crossed the treatment threshold? Using the probability bar in Figure 3–12, we can see how the KUB changes the pretest probability to the posttest probabilities. Figure 3–12 shows the possible posttest probabilities based on a negative or positive result KUB in the setting of suspected appendicitis. A negative result on KUB would not move the posttest probability across the treatment threshold (Rx) and therefore would not change your decision to treat this patient for appendicitis. A positive test result would raise the patient's posttest probability, but again, it would not change your decision to treat this patient for appendicitis. The KUB is therefore not a useful test in this situation.

The key point is this: *Order a test only if the test result has the potential to cause the probability of disease to cross the treatment threshold.*

Let's return to the case at hand.

Because you have made the above calculations and have decided not to order a KUB on your patient with suspected appendicitis, you consider instead ultrasonography of the abdomen. Is this a useful test in this situation?

Let's use the same three-step method.

Steps 1 & 2

These steps are the same as above.

Step 3

Using the extremes of the test results, determine whether testing will change what you do for the patient. First, convert the pretest probability to a pretest odds (odds = probability/[1 − probability]).

As above, for a pretest probability of 25%, the pretest odds = 0.33

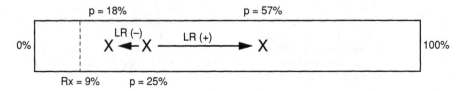

Figure 3–12. Probabilities of appendicitis before and after KUB. The center "X" shows the pretest probability of appendicitis, recorded as "p = 25%" below the bar. The arrows indicate how far the pretest probabilities move to posttest probabilities after obtaining a positive or negative result on KUB, labeled with LR(+) and LR(−), respectively. Posttest probabilities are recorded above the bar. Note that the posttest probabilities do not cross the treatment threshold (Rx).

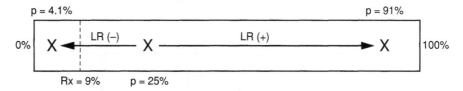

Figure 3–13. Probabilities of appendicitis before and after ultrasonography of the abdomen. Arrows indicate the movement of the pretest to the posttest probabilities based on a positive (LR(+)) or negative (LR(–)) test result. Note that the posttest probability for a negative abdominal ultrasound crosses the treatment threshold (Rx).

Next, multiply the pretest odds by the largest and smallest LR for the test to generate the posttest odds. For ultrasonography of the abdomen in suspected appendicitis, LR(+) = 29, and LR(–) = 0.13.[5,6]

If the test result is negative, posttest odds = pretest odds × LR(–) = 0.33 × 0.13 = 0.043
If the test result is positive, posttest odds = pretest odds × LR(+) = 0.33 × 29 = 9.6

Finally, convert the posttest odds to a posttest probability (probability = odds/[odds + 1]).

If the test result is negative, posttest probability = 0.043/(0.043 + 1) = 4.1%
If the test result is positive, posttest probability = 9.6/(9.6 + 1) = 91%

Now you again ask yourself the key question: Has the posttest probability crossed the treatment threshold? The probability bar in Figure 3–13 shows how the abdominal ultrasound changes the pretest probability.

In this case, you see that normal findings on ultrasonography of the abdomen would lower the posttest probability of disease below the treatment threshold. Your posttest probability would therefore be low enough for you to not perform surgery in this patient. This diagnostic test is therefore useful, because it has the potential to change your treatment decision. If the findings on ultrasonography were abnormal, posttest probability would increase, but the test would still not change the treatment decision.

This three-step method is all you need to evaluate any diagnostic test and determine whether it is useful in a specific clinical situation. This concept can also be extended and used to define a range of pretest probabilities over which testing will be useful.

Let's return to the most recent example of appendicitis. We know that a negative result on ultrasound will cause the posttest probability to cross the treatment threshold. But will the negative result cause the posttest probability to cross the treatment threshold if the pretest probability is 30% instead of 25%? How about if the pretest probability is 40%, or even 50%? What we really want to know is the *range of pretest probabilities over which testing with ultrasonography is useful*. Within this range of pretest probabilities, the test result has the potential to cause the posttest probability to cross the treatment threshold.

This range of probabilities in which testing is useful is bounded by the testing thresholds. The testing thresholds are defined in the following two sections.

Lower testing threshold

The lower testing threshold (T_L) is the probability of disease above which you test and below which you withhold testing and treatment. As shown in Figure 3–14, at all points below

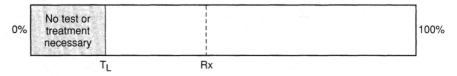

Figure 3–14. The lower testing threshold, T_L, is shown with a solid line, and the treatment threshold, Rx, is shown with a dashed line.

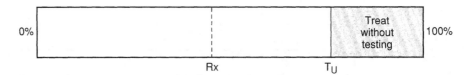

Figure 3–15. The upper testing threshold, T_U, is shown with a solid line, and the treatment threshold, Rx, is shown with a dashed line.

T_L, even a positive test result would not cause the posttest probability to cross the treatment threshold (Rx). At all points between T_L and Rx, a positive test result could cause the posttest probability of disease to cross Rx; therefore, testing in this range is useful. In our current example, there will be some patients with abdominal pain who you believe have an extremely low pretest probability of appendicitis. In some patients, this probability will be so low, that even a positive finding on ultrasound will not cause you to treat the patient for appendicitis. In that situation, the pretest probability of appendicitis is below the lower testing threshold (T_L).

The key point about T_L is this: *When the pretest probability is below this threshold, the test result will not change your decision not to treat.*

Upper testing threshold

The upper testing threshold (T_U), is the probability of disease above which you treat without testing and below which you test. As shown in Figure 3–15, at all points above T_U, even a negative test result would not cause the posttest probability to cross the treatment threshold (Rx). At all points between T_U and Rx, a negative test result could cause the posttest probability to cross Rx, therefore, testing in this range is useful. In our current example, there will be some patients with abdominal pain who you believe have an extremely high pretest probability of appendicitis. In some patients, this probability will be so high that even a negative ultrasound result will not stop you from treating the patient for appendicitis. In that situation, the pretest probability of appendicitis is above the upper testing threshold (T_U).

The key point about T_U is this: *When the pretest probability is above this threshold, the test result will not change your decision to treat.*

The implication of these upper and lower testing thresholds is this: Order or perform a test only if the test result will cause the probability of disease to cross the treatment threshold. This implication is demonstrated in Figure 3–16. As shown in this figure, everyone with a pretest probability between the two test thresholds should receive the diagnostic test (unless, as discussed later, the test is very costly or dangerous).

The next section explains how to determine these testing thresholds.

CALCULATING THE TESTING THRESHOLDS: LIKELIHOOD RATIOS REVISITED

When you use the information from above, calculating the testing thresholds is relatively simple. Testing thresholds are determined by three factors:

1. The treatment threshold
2. The test characteristics (likelihood ratios)
3. The utility (or "dysutility") of the test

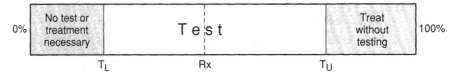

Figure 3–16. The upper and lower testing thresholds (T_U and T_L) together on the probability of disease bar.

An important point is that testing thresholds are different for every test (eg, KUB vs ultrasonography). Because the utility of the test usually contributes very little to the determination of the testing thresholds, we will set this third factor aside for now. Essentially, testing thresholds can be calculated by using only the treatment threshold and the largest and smallest likelihood ratios for a given test. We use the largest and smallest likelihood ratios because they reflect the maximal amount that a test can affect the placement of the posttest probability, thereby giving us the full range in which testing can be useful.

As seen in Figure 3–17, the testing thresholds represent two pretest probabilities. The lower testing threshold (T_L) represents the lowest pretest probability at which application of the most positive test result causes the posttest probability to equal the treatment threshold. Mathematically, T_L (in odds) $\times$ LR (for the most positive test result) = Rx (in odds). Therefore, T_L (in odds) = Rx (in odds)/LR (for the most positive test result).

The upper testing threshold (T_U) represents the highest pretest probability at which the most negative test result causes the posttest probability to equal the treatment threshold. Mathematically, T_U (in odds) $\times$ LR (for the most negative test result) = Rx (in odds). Therefore, T_U (in odds) = Rx (in odds)/LR (for the most negative test result).

There are thus three parts to determining T_L and T_U:

1. Determine the treatment threshold probability and convert it to odds.
2. Divide the treatment threshold odds by the largest and smallest LR for the test to calculate T_L and T_U (in odds), respectively.
3. Convert T_L and T_U from odds to probability.

For the above case example in which the treatment threshold for appendicitis is 9%, what are the testing thresholds for KUB and ultrasound?

KUB

First, determine the treatment threshold probability and convert it to odds.

Rx = 9%, or 0.09, converted to odds = probability/(1 − probability) = 0.09/(1 − 0.09) = 0.099

Next, divide the treatment threshold odds by the largest and smallest LR for the test to calculate T_L and T_U (in odds), respectively. Recall that KUB is a dichotomous test for the diagnosis of appendicitis, with LR(+) = 4.0 and LR(−) = 0.67. Therefore,

$$T_L = 0.099/4.0 = 0.025 \text{ (in odds)}$$
$$T_U = 0.099/0.67 = 0.15 \text{ (in odds)}$$

Finally, convert T_L and T_U from odds to probability (probability = odds/[odds + 1]).

T_L (probability) = 0.025/(1 + 0.025) = 0.024. The lower testing threshold is therefore 2.4%
T_U (probability) = 0.15/(1 + 0.15) = 0.13. The upper testing threshold is therefore 13%

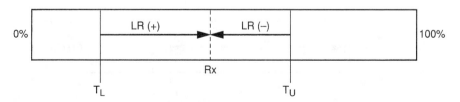

Figure 3–17. The upper and lower testing thresholds (T_U and T_L, shown as solid lines) are shown in relation to positive and negative likelihood ratios (LR(+) and LR(−)) and the treatment threshold (Rx).

Ultrasonography

First, determine the treatment threshold probability and convert it to odds.

As above, Rx converted to odds = 0.099

Next, divide the treatment threshold odds by the largest and smallest LR for the test to calculate T_L and T_U (in odds), respectively. Recall that ultrasonography is a dichotomous test for the diagnosis of appendicitis, with LR(+) = 29 and LR(−) = 0.13. Therefore,

$$T_L = 0.099/29 = 0.0034 \text{ (in odds)}$$
$$T_U = 0.099/0.13 = 0.76 \text{ (in odds)}$$

Finally, convert T_L and T_U from odds to probability (probability = odds/[(odds + 1]).

T_L (probability) = 0.0034/(1 + 0.0034) = 0.0034. The lower testing threshold is therefore 0.34%
T_U (probability) = 0.76/(1 + 0.76) = 0.43. The upper testing threshold is therefore 43%

Figure 3–18 compares the testing thresholds of ultrasonography of the abdomen with that of KUB in the diagnosis of appendicitis. The test characteristics of ultrasonography are such that it has both higher and lower testing thresholds than does KUB for the diagnosis of appendicitis. This means that ultrasonography, compared with KUB, will change the decision to treat or not to treat over a broader range of pretest probabilities of appendicitis.

Now we are ready for the third factor in testing thresholds: utility. We said earlier that there are three components to testing thresholds:

1. The treatment threshold
2. The test characteristics (likelihood ratios)
3. The utility (or "dysutility") of the test

As shown in Figure 3–19, if the utility of the test is positive (in other words, if the test itself is somehow good (positive) for the patient, eg, the test provides reassurance), the testing thresholds will widen. If the utility of the test is negative (painful, dangerous, etc), the testing thresholds will narrow.

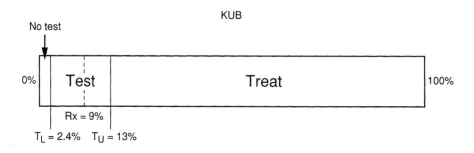

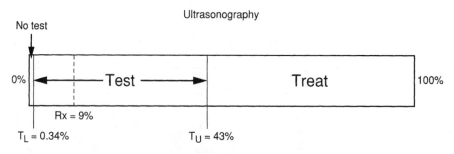

Figure 3–18. Comparison of the testing thresholds for ultrasonography of the abdomen and a KUB.

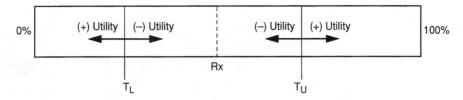

Figure 3–19. The effect of utility on the testing thresholds. The arrows show how a test with a positive utility (eg, patient reassurance) will widen the range of probabilities in which testing is useful and show how tests with a negative utility (eg, morbidity) will narrow the range of probabilities in which testing is useful.

For most tests, utilities are small and do not have much of an effect on the position of the testing thresholds. However, this is not true for a test that is very dangerous, expensive, or painful to the patient. (In situations involving these types of tests, structuring the problem using decision analysis with treatment, no treatment, and testing arms can more accurately determine treatment thresholds. Consult the text by Sox and coworkers.[4])

We have a final point about testing thresholds: This section assumes that diagnostic tests are being performed only to make a diagnosis (and change the patient's posttest probability of disease, which may affect treatment decisions). Diagnostic tests are sometimes ordered for other reasons. For example, a computed tomographic scan may be ordered before surgical resection to evaluate the exact location of a known cancer. The testing thresholds do not apply in such settings. In addition, physicians may order tests outside the testing threshold range because of medicolegal concerns. The merits of this, however, are debatable.

PUTTING IT ALL TOGETHER: A FINAL EXAMPLE USING ALL THRESHOLDS

You are taking care of a 62-year-old male veteran with stage D prostate cancer who presents to the emergency department with acute shortness of breath. His physical examination is normal except for mild tachypnea. Findings on chest x-ray are normal. Measurement of arterial blood gas shows a pO_2 of 75 and a pCO_2 of 40. You are concerned about the presence of pulmonary embolism (PE) and consider various options:

1. Should you not test and not treat?
2. Should you test with a V/Q scan?
3. Should you treat with anticoagulation without testing?

These three options define your thresholds.

Your task is to determine where the patient is relative to these thresholds so that you may decide what to do next. The thresholds are delineated with our familiar three steps.

Step 1

Determine the treatment threshold probability. This probability can be determined either intuitively or using decision analysis. First, use the intuitive method to estimate the treatment threshold probability. Think of the cost/(cost + benefit) equation. What is your treatment threshold?

Now we will use the technique of decision analysis to illustrate a more quantitative approach. How would you draw a decision tree to represent the outcomes of this patient and a decision to treat or not to treat with anticoagulation? When you have drawn your tree, compare it with the one shown in Figure 3–20.

In Figure 3–20, "p" represents the probability of pulmonary embolus, and "J," "K," "L," and "M" represent the expected utility of the four possible outcomes. Consider the three pieces of relevant information that you need to retrieve from the literature to determine the treatment threshold:

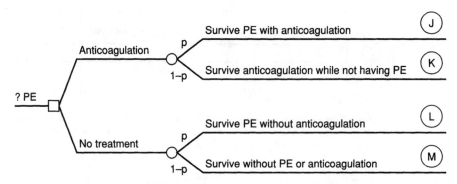

Figure 3–20. Decision tree for a patient with suspected pulmonary embolism. The top branch represents the outcomes if anticoagulation is chosen. The bottom branch represents the outcomes if no treatment is chosen. "p" is the probability of pulmonary embolism. "J," "K," "L," and "M" are the expected utilities for each branch.

1. The survival of treated PE is 91%.[7]
2. The survival without fatal hemorrhage or serious central nervous system bleeding (assumed equivalent to fatal hemorrhage) for anticoagulation alone is 99%.[7]
3. The survival of untreated PE is 70%.[7]

With the utility of survival = 1, the expected utility for each of the outcomes is therefore:

J = the probability of surviving PE after anticoagulation = 0.91.
K = the probability of surviving anticoagulation while not having PE = 0.99.
L = the probability of surviving PE without initial anticoagulation = 0.7
M = the probability of surviving without PE or anticoagulation = 1.0.

How would you plot points J, K, L, and M, and how would you determine Rx from the graph? Compare your graph to the one shown in Figure 3–21. In Figure 3–21, M and K are plotted on the vertical axis, representing 0% probability of PE, and J and L are plotted on the vertical axis, representing 100% probability of disease. Straight lines are then drawn to

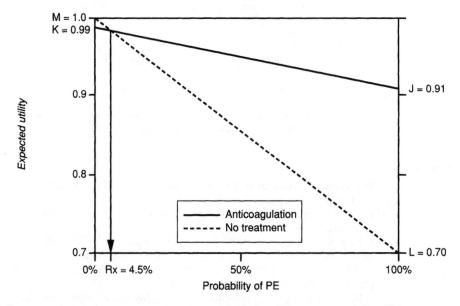

Figure 3–21. Graph plotting the expected utility of anticoagulation versus no treatment against varying probabilities of pulmonary embolism. (This graph is also known as sensitivity analysis.) The expected utilities of the points "J," "K," "L," and "M" from Figure 3–20 are shown as points on the vertical axes. The intersection of the expected utility lines is the treatment threshold, labeled "Rx."

connect J and K as well as L and M. The intersection of these lines at 4.5% indicates the treatment threshold for PE.

Alternatively, you may calculate the Rx by hand using a calculator and the cost/(cost + benefit) equation (Rx = (M − K)/[(M - K) + (J − L)]).

$$\text{The cost of treatment } (M - K) = 1 - 0.99 = 0.01$$
$$\text{The benefit of treatment } (J - L) = 0.91 - 0.7 = 0.21$$

Therefore, the treatment threshold = 0.01/(0.01 + 0.21) = 4.5%.

Step 2

Determine the patient's pretest probability of disease. On the basis of the limited case description, what is your pretest probability of disease? Is it above or below the treatment threshold? If there were no further diagnostic tests available, what would you do?

Let's say your estimation of the pretest probability of PE is 50% (this estimate may vary, but such variance often does not affect the usefulness of this technique). This probability is above the treatment threshold, so you would treat for the disease if no further diagnostic tests were available. You do, however, have a V/Q scan available, so the next consideration is whether you should use this test.

Step 3

Using likelihood ratios for a given diagnostic test, determine whether testing will change what you do for the patient. You can determine this in one of two ways. One method is to determine how the extreme LRs of the V/Q scan would change the pretest probability. Then evaluate whether the posttest probability would cross the treatment threshold. If it doesn't, the test would not change our management and would not be useful.

The other method is to determine the treatment thresholds. You can then note where the estimated pretest probability lies in relation to the no test, test, or treat zones. This relationship can then serve as the basis for your recommendation.

Using the former approach, you first convert the pretest probability to a pretest odds (odds = probability/[1 − probability]).

$$\text{Pretest probability} = 50\%$$
$$\text{Pretest odds} = 0.5/(1 - 0.5) = 1.0$$

Next, multiply the pretest odds by the largest and smallest LR for the test to generate a posttest odds. The likelihood ratios for a V/Q scan are as follows:[8]

V/Q Scan Result	Likelihood Ratio
High probability	18.3
Intermediate probability	1.2
Low probability	0.4
Normal	0.1

If the result is normal, posttest odds = pretest odds × LR (smallest) = 1.0 × 0.1 = 0.1
If the result is high probability, posttest odds = pretest odds × LR (largest) = 1.0 × 18.3 = 18.3

Finally, convert the posttest odds to a posttest probability (probability = odds/[odds + 1]).

If the test result is normal, posttest probability = 0.1/(0.1 + 1) = 0.09 = 9%
If the test result is high probability, posttest probability = 18.3/(18.3 + 1) = 0.95 = 95%

Now you are ready to ask yourself the key question: Has the posttest probability crossed the treatment threshold?

Looking at the probability bar in Figure 3–22, you can see how the V/Q scan changes the pretest probability to the posttest probabilities. From this figure, you note that a normal V/Q

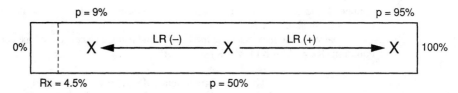

Figure 3–22. Pretest and posttest probabilities of pulmonary embolism based on normal and high probability V/Q scans. The pretest and posttest probabilities are labeled "X." Pretest probability is recorded below the bar (p = 50%), and posttest probabilities (p = 9% and p = 95%) are recorded above the bar.

scan would not cause the posttest probability of PE to cross the treatment threshold. It would therefore not affect your initial decision to recommend anticoagulation for your patient. The test is therefore not useful at this pretest probability.

Alternatively, you can use the second approach that calculates the testing thresholds. First, determine the treatment threshold probability and convert it to odds.

The Rx as determined above = 4.5%, or 0.045. Converting this to odds = probability/(1 − probability) = 0.045/(1 − 0.045) = 0.047

Next, divide the treatment threshold odds by the largest and smallest LR for the test to calculate T_L and T_U (in odds), respectively. From the table above, note that the smallest LR = 0.1 (normal scan) and the largest LR = 18.3 (high probability scan). Therefore,

$$T_L = 0.047/18.3 = 0.0025 \text{ (in odds)}$$
$$T_U = 0.047/0.1 = 0.47 \text{ (in odds)}$$

Finally, convert T_L and T_U from odds to probability (probability = odds/[odds + 1]).

$$T_L \text{ (probability)} = 0.0025/(1 + 0.0025) = 0.0025 = 0.25\%$$
$$T_U \text{ (probability)} = 0.47/(1 + 0.47) = 0.032 = 32\%$$

The thresholds are shown in Figure 3–23. As shown in this figure, your pretest probability (50%) is greater than the upper testing threshold, in the "Treat" zone. Thus, even a normal V/Q scan (which is uncommon) would not change your decision to treat this patient. The V/Q scan is therefore not a useful test in this situation. You should treat without testing or you should consider a different test (eg, pulmonary angiography). Figure 3–23 also demonstrates how other pretest probabilities of pulmonary embolism would affect the decision to treat and test. For example, for all probabilities less than 0.25%, one should not test and not treat. For all probabilities between 0.25% and 32%, the V/Q scan has the potential to cause the posttest probability to cross Rx; therefore, the test is useful in this range. For all probabilities greater than 32%, one should treat without testing or consider a different test.

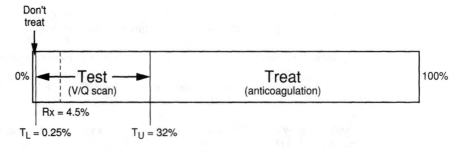

Figure 3–23. Testing thresholds for a V/Q scan in the diagnosis of pulmonary embolism. The testing thresholds (T_L and T_U) are shown as solid lines.

LIMITATIONS OF THRESHOLD ANALYSIS

The thresholds that we determine are dependent on the probabilities that we use in the decision analysis. We can assess the validity of published probabilities using the study guide in Chapter 8. However, even if we believe the published data, we need to be sure that the data are reasonable for our patient. For example, our threshold analysis for pulmonary embolism assumes that the risk of fatal hemorrhage is the same in all patients who receive anticoagulation, but patients with cancer or those who are at risk of falling may have a higher risk of fatal bleeding.

The threshold technique that we have applied only used utilities of life and death to determine the treatment threshold. Intermediary outcomes (eg, stroke), which may contribute to the overall utility of one or both treatment strategies, are not included. If we choose to consider intermediary outcomes, we need to use a more complex decision analysis.

Furthermore, our threshold technique does not take the utility of the test itself into account (eg, cost or harm of test or the reassurance it may provide) in determining the testing thresholds. If we want to include the utility of the test, we need to use a decision analysis with treatment, no treatment, and testing arms. The testing thresholds are determined using sensitivity analysis. (Decision analysis software, discussed in Chapter 2, simplifies this task.) The approach is similar to the one used to determine the treatment threshold. Recall that our goal is to optimize utility at all probabilities of disease. In Figure 3–24, the utilities for each strategy is plotted against the probability of disease. Below T_L, not treating or testing is the best strategy. Between T_L and T_U, testing provides the optimal utilities, and above T_U, one should treat without testing.

For further details on how to set up the decision analysis to determine these thresholds, refer to Chapter 2 and to the text by Sox and colleagues.[4]

Another limitation of the technique is the issue of gold standard tests. Because a gold standard test is, by definition, perfectly sensitive and perfectly specific, the test would be useful over the entire range of pretest probabilities, and all patients with any probability of disease other than 0% or 100% should receive the gold standard test. In general, if the gold standard test is economical, painless, and safe, patients should receive it. More commonly, however, the gold standard test is none of these. For example, the gold standard for the diagnosis of pulmonary embolism, pulmonary angiography, is expensive, invasive, and potentially morbid. We can determine the treatment and testing thresholds for PE that consider

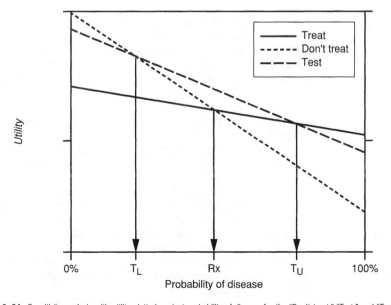

Figure 3–24. Sensitivity analysis with utility plotted against probability of disease for the "Don't treat," "Test," and "Treat" strategies. Rx = treatment threshold; T_L = lower testing threshold; T_U = upper testing threshold.

the options of a V/Q scan or pulmonary angiogram using a complex decision analysis involving four decision arms: no treatment, pulmonary angiography, V/Q scan, and anticoagulation. The approach is essentially the same as that in the preceding paragraph.

For tests with multiple levels of results, when intermediary results with likelihood ratios close to 1.0 are obtained, we still have to decide on the need for further testing. In the PE example above, an intermediate probability V/Q scan result is not helpful because the likelihood ratio of 1.2 does not change your pretest probability of disease by much. The decision to proceed to the gold standard, pulmonary angiography, depends on the overall utility of this testing strategy compared with the no treatment or anticoagulation strategies at the particular probability of PE. (Again, you may determine this probability using the more complex decision and sensitivity analysis approach previously described.)

Finally, it can be argued that if enough tests are used in sequence, almost any probability of disease can, theoretically, cross a treatment threshold if all ordered tests move the pretest probability in the same direction. Essentially, you would need to assess a summary likelihood ratio for multiple independent tests in the testing algorithm (as in Chapter 1) and use this summary value to calculate the testing thresholds. Although this may generate a broad testing threshold range, we should recognize that a series of tests often do not give concordantly positive or negative results. Furthermore, we may be reluctant to use one or more tests in the algorithm if these tests pose significant risks or costs.

Despite these limitations, the threshold technique is helpful because it highlights the important factors that determine whether we should treat, test, or simply observe the patient. This technique, even if used only qualitatively, increases our awareness of how and why we make these decisions. We can improve our ability to weigh the costs and benefits of a particular therapy to better estimate the treatment threshold. Also, our decision to order a specific test can be more rational by determining whether the test is likely to change our management of the patient.

SUMMARY

1. The treatment threshold is the probability of disease above which we treat and below which we withhold treatment. It is determined only by the costs and benefits of a given treatment.
2. The treatment threshold can be determined:
   • Intuitively
   • Using decision analysis with sensitivity analysis or a simple formula
     Note that the treatment threshold is cost/(cost + benefit), and that large benefits create low treatment thresholds and large costs create high treatment thresholds.
3. Order or perform a diagnostic test only if the test result has the potential to cause the probability of disease to cross the treatment threshold. This can be determined with a simple, three-step approach:
   • Find the treatment threshold.
   • Determine the patient's pretest probability of disease relative to the treatment threshold.
   • Using likelihood ratios for the given diagnostic test, determine whether testing will change what you do for the patient (ie, will the posttest probability cross the treatment threshold?).
4. Testing thresholds define a range of probability over which testing is useful (and can change our clinical decisions). They are determined by three factors:
   • The treatment threshold probability
   • The characteristics of the test (likelihood ratios)
   • The utility (or "dysutility") of the test
5. If a patient's pretest probability of disease lies outside the testing thresholds, testing will not change management. In this case, you should either treat, not treat, or consider a different test.

REFERENCES

1. Magid D et al: Prevention of Lyme disease after tick bites: A cost effectiveness analysis. N Engl J Med 1992;327:534.
2. Hillner BE, Centor RM: What a difference a day makes: A decision analysis of adult streptococcal pharyngitis. J Gen Intern Med 1987;2:242.
3. Velanovich V, Satava R: Balancing the normal appendectomy rate with the perforated appendicitis rate: Implications for quality assurance. Am Surg 1992;58:264.
4. Sox HC et al: *Medical Decision Making*. Butterworth-Heinemann, 1988.
5. Yacoe ME, Jeffrey RB: Sonography of appendicitis and diverticulitis. Rad Clin North Am 1994;32:899.
6. Mason JD: The evaluation of acute abdominal pain in children. Emerg Med Clin North Am 1996;14:629.
7. Quinn RJ, Butler SP: A decision analysis approach to the treatment of patients with suspected pulmonary emboli and an intermediate probability lung scan. J Nucl Med 1991;32:2050.
8. The Prospective Investigation of Pulmonary Embolism Diagnosis (PIOPED) Investigators: Value of the ventilation/perfusion scan in acute pulmonary embolism. JAMA 1990;263:2753.

SUGGESTED READING

Jernigan CA: Testing and treatment disease thresholds. Primary Care 1995;22:295.

Pauker SG, Kassirer JP: Therapeutic decision making: A cost-benefit analysis. N Engl J Med 1975; 293:229.

Pauker SG, Kassirer JP: The threshold approach to clinical decision making. N Engl J Med 1980; 302:1109.

COST-EFFECTIVENESS ANALYSIS

Leslee L. Subak, MD

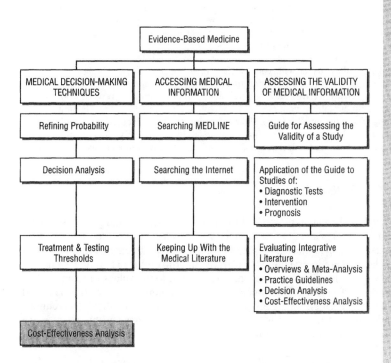

Evidence-Based Medicine

MEDICAL DECISION-MAKING TECHNIQUES

Refining Probability

Decision Analysis

Treatment & Testing Thresholds

Cost-Effectiveness Analysis

ACCESSING MEDICAL INFORMATION

Searching MEDLINE

Searching the Internet

Keeping Up With the Medical Literature

ASSESSING THE VALIDITY OF MEDICAL INFORMATION

Guide for Assessing the Validity of a Study

Application of the Guide to Studies of:
- Diagnostic Tests
- Intervention
- Prognosis

Evaluating Integrative Literature
- Overviews & Meta-Analysis
- Practice Guidelines
- Decision Analysis
- Cost-Effectiveness Analysis

You represent the Gynecology Department on a committee your health maintenance organization (HMO) has assembled to consider revision of your policy on screening mammography. Currently, you offer screening mammography to women 40–49 years of age every 1–2 years. Recently, however, new data on the effectiveness of mammography have been reported, and a national panel has recommended not screening women younger than 50.[1]

While you are contemplating these new recommendations for younger women, you have an appointment with your patient Ms Smith, a 40-year-old woman with no personal or family history of breast disease. She is asking your advice about screening mammography. She knows that death resulting from breast cancer may be preventable if the breast cancer is detected early. Like many of your patients, she has been reading about the controversy of when to begin and how often to have mammographic evaluations. The primary benefit of mammography is the possible early detection of breast cancer, leading to a reduction in mortality. If mammography is not performed, Ms Smith might have breast cancer that is found at a later stage, which carries a greater risk of death. The risks of mammography include identification of nonmalignant lesions that may lead to unnecessary biopsy and surgery. Particularly in premenopausal women, mammograms may be difficult to interpret because of the increased density of the breasts. In addition to the physical discomfort of this procedure for your patient and the emotional distress she could experience thinking that she may have cancer, there is the monetary cost that Ms Smith and her medical insurance provider must pay.

Several organizations recommend annual screening mammography in women beginning at age 40 years (American Cancer Society, American College of Radiology), others recommend screening every 1 or 2 years (National Cancer Institute), and some do not recommend screening until age 50 years (US Preventative Services Task Force, American College of Physicians, American Academy of Family Practice, Canadian Task Force). You do a literature search that shows agreement among experts that women aged 50 years and older should be offered routine screening mammography based on the results of clinical trials demonstrating a significant reduction in breast cancer mortality among screened women.[2,3] There is disagreement, however, on whether to recommend screening mammography to women aged 40–49 years.[3-5]

You are not only a conscientious physician who wants to provide the best care for your patients but also a policy maker with your HMO, which wants to provide the best care possible at a reasonable cost. Are screening mammograms for women younger than 50 effective? Are they cost-effective? How will you advise your committee on when to begin screening mammography at your HMO? How will you inform and advise Ms Smith about screening mammography? Because there is uncertainty in the medical community on the optimal clinical strategy for screening mammography in women younger than 50 years, this is a perfect setting for decision analysis and cost-effectiveness analysis.

INTRODUCTION TO COST-EFFECTIVENESS ANALYSIS

In Chapter 2 we developed an analytic method for medical decision making that used decision analysis. Decision analysis can assist clinicians in making rational decisions that reflect both the best available evidence and a patient's individual preferences. After each possible strategy for a health care intervention is determined, probabilities for future events are identified and values placed on the outcomes that are tailored to the values of an individual patient or to the values of society. This process facilitates a comparison of the risks and benefits of each alternative. Often we are also interested in the cost of medical interventions and want to include costs in the comparison of alternative strategies. In this chapter, we will use the same methods as those used in decision analysis (see Chapter 2). In addition, we will include costs as part of the outcome measure.

Cost-effectiveness analysis systematically compares decision options in terms of their monetary cost and effectiveness. The technique of cost-effectiveness analysis has been used in areas other than medicine for decades and was refined for use in business. The evaluation of costs in relation to benefits in medicine began in the 1960s for the treatment of end-stage renal disease.[6] Since then, systematic comparison using cost-effectiveness analysis has contributed to the evaluation of specific health care interventions. The results of cost-effectiveness analyses alone usually do not make health policy decisions. Rather, evaluations that include costs provide additional pieces of evidence that may contribute to the decision-making process.[7]

The primary function of cost-effectiveness analysis is to show the relative value of alternative interventions for improving health. It measures the net cost of providing a service as well as the effectiveness of the service. The result of cost-effectiveness analysis is the monetary cost per unit of effectiveness, expressed as the cost-effectiveness ratio (C/E). The numerator of the ratio, costs (C), includes both costs and savings associated with an intervention. For example, the cost of a smoking cessation program may result in future savings because of a reduction in the need for medical care for chronic lung disease and lung cancer. The denominator of the ratio, effectiveness (E), is expressed as a single unit, such as years of life saved. Although life years is a commonly used effectiveness measure for cost-effectiveness analyses, many health care interventions have minimal effect on the length of life but have substantial effect on quality of life. These interventions may be best evaluated using quality-adjusted life years (QALYs). Ideally, the measure of effectiveness in cost-effectiveness analysis is broadly defined to include the most clinically relevant outcomes. The C/E is thus commonly presented as dollars per year of life gained or dollars per QALY gained.

Cost-effectiveness analysis is particularly valuable to compare different interventions for a specific condition and, on a broader scale, may allow comparison of alternative uses of societal resources. Medical care almost always has an economic impact, paid either directly by patients, by insurance companies, or by the whole of society. Patients may pay a copayment or lose wages while out of work during the medical interventions. Insurance companies pay directly for services provided, often at a preset rate, and society may pay through the Medicare program or through increased prices for goods and services that indirectly support medical care. Because there are not enough resources to support all of the medical care possible, choices must be made between alternative uses of resources.[8]

Cost-effectiveness analysis facilitates difficult resource allocation decisions and may allow valid comparisons between alternative uses of resources. By placing quantitative values on costs and effectiveness, cost-effectiveness analysis can help to identify the less expensive of two strategies that have similar effectiveness, identify the more effective of strategies that have a similar cost, or compare the cost per unit of effectiveness. Economic analyses thus provide information that can assist policy makers to weigh alternatives and decide which option best serves their needs. For instance, if funding is available for only one preventative medicine program, a health care insurance company may use the results of cost-effectiveness analyses to choose between funding a program for smoking cessation or one for family planning education. The federal government may use cost-effectiveness analyses to decide on funding allocation to large programs, such as education, public welfare, or defense.

In this chapter, we will give a broad introduction to cost-effectiveness analysis, develop a cost-effectiveness analytic model to evaluate screening mammography in women 40–49 years of age, and use the results to formulate a plan for Ms Smith's management as well as your HMO's protocol for mammography. Our aim is to provide a general understanding of this research method rather than an exhaustive manual of how to perform analyses that incorporate costs. For more detailed understanding, directed reading is strongly encouraged.[6-16]

THE FIVE STEPS OF COST-EFFECTIVENESS ANALYSIS

A cost-effectiveness analysis uses the same five steps of decision analysis presented in Chapter 2. The fundamental difference is that in step 3 of cost-effectiveness analysis, costs are measured and added to the analysis, allowing calculation of the cost-effectiveness of the alternative health care options. Recall that the five steps of the analysis are

1. Formulate an explicit question.
2. Structure the decision.
3. Fill in the data.
4. Determine the value of alternative strategies.
5. Perform sensitivity analyses.

Formulate an explicit question

Before any analysis begins, the research question must be identified and defined. Three factors are integral to the research question: the alternative strategies being compared, the time frame of the analysis, and the perspective of the analysis.

Comparison of alternative strategies

The cost-effectiveness ratio (C/E) summarizes in one number information on costs and health outcome or effectiveness. Although the C/E for any single strategy can be calculated, the power of cost-effectiveness analysis lies in comparing one strategy with another by estimating the incremental differences between the strategies. The traditional model of cost-effectiveness analysis is to compare the existing strategy of health care with a new or different strategy. For example, we could compare yearly versus every-3-years Papanicoulou smear for the prevention of cervical cancer. The incremental C/E reflects the additional cost per unit of benefit of one strategy compared with another.

The incremental C/E is calculated by ranking individual strategies from lowest C/E to highest C/E. Incremental costs are then calculated as the additional costs of one strategy compared with the next least expensive strategy. Incremental benefits are the difference in effectiveness of one strategy compared with the next more expensive strategy. The incremental C/E is the difference in costs divided by the difference in effectiveness between two strategies.

In our case scenario of screening mammography for women 40–49 years, the important issues are (1) whether breast cancer screening beginning at age 40, rather than at age 50 years, extends life and (2) what the cost of the extended life time is. Because the current accepted strategy is screening mammography beginning at age 50 years, the relevant finding is the **incremental** cost-effectiveness of screening mammography beginning at 40 years of age. We thus express the two reasonable alternative strategies as:

Choose screening mammography ≥ 40 years or choose screening mammography ≥ 50 years

More specifically, in the "Screening mammography ≥ 40 years" strategy, women will undergo screening mammography every 18 months from 40 to 49 years of age, then biennially (every other year) beginning at age 50. In the "Screening mammography ≥ 50 years" strategy, women will not have screening mammography from 40 to 49 years of age but will begin biennial screening at age 50. The 18-month screening interval for women 40–49 years of age is based on the average screening interval of a recent meta-analysis that found a statistically significant reduction in breast cancer mortality.[3] The individual randomized controlled trials with screening intervals of 12, 18, and 24 months failed to demonstrate a significant reduction in breast cancer mortality.[3,17] The screening interval is consistent with guidelines of several organizations that recommend screening every 1–2 years. The biennial screening interval for women ≥50 years and older is chosen because the reduction in breast cancer mortality is similar to annual screening.[17]

Time frame

The time frame of a cost-effectiveness analysis is the period of time during which costs and benefits are measured. It should be long enough to capture the future health outcome and the economic impact of an intervention. This time period may be very brief or may extend throughout a patient's life.[6] The time frame for our scenario is 40 years of age until death, since the effects of mammographic screening occur during this period.

Perspective

The perspective of an analysis is the viewpoint from which the analysis is conducted. Perspective depends not only on who benefits from a health care intervention but also on who pays for it.[6,9,10] Because the patient is most directly affected by illness and medical treatment, effectiveness is usually viewed from the patient perspective.[7] Costs may be viewed from the patient, program, payor, or societal perspective.

A cost analysis from the **patient perspective** is conducted from the viewpoint of an individual. Patients bear different economic burdens for their illness. If an individual has health care insurance, her economic burden may be minimal, usually limited to copayment and charges not covered by insurance, plus costs incurred by illness or treatment, including time missed from work and transportation for medical care. From the patient perspective, the cost of a mammogram is how much she has to pay for the test, including out-of-pocket expenses, transportation, and lost wages, if any, from missed work.

The **program perspective** is that of a hospital, institution, managed care plan, or health maintenance organization. Only costs paid by the program are considered. The cost of a mammogram in the program perspective reflects the true cost of providing the service: the costs of labor, overhead, and supplies.

The **payor perspective** is often used in medical cost-effectiveness analysis. The payor may be a public or private insurer, such as Medicare or Blue Cross/Blue Shield, or an individual company that funds its own medical insurance. Costs in this perspective include contracted reimbursement for specific services and patients' sick-leave or disability time that is covered by the payor. With the payor perspective, expenditures not covered by the payor (eg, transportation and wages lost by a supportive family member) are not considered in the analysis. The cost of a mammogram from the perspective of the insurance company is the amount of money the company pays the hospital for performing mammography.

The **societal perspective** is also often used for cost analyses. Costs that affect everyone in society are included, regardless of who pays. In the societal perspective, costs include the total net cost of medical and other payments for the use of resources as well as the patient's lost productivity (time away from work). This perspective may also include reimbursement for unpaid caregivers. Although it is often difficult to quantify its varied benefits and costs, the societal perspective has the advantage of balancing one group's gain with another's loss. For example, if a state-sponsored program pays for screening mammograms, thereby reducing the cost of the test for insurers, both the increased state expenditure and the insurance company savings are included in the societal perspective. The cost of a mammogram from the societal perspective is how much society pays for the test, often estimated using national data sets or Medicare reimbursement and standardized average wage rates.[12]

Costs are most often evaluated from either the societal perspective, since the economic impact of illness is usually felt by all of society, or the payor perspective, since public or private insurers pay most of the health care bill.[9,10] A societal perspective will be used in the analysis of screening mammography.

Structure the decision

As in Chapter 2, we structure our decision by identifying the possible outcomes of each strategy and creating a decision tree. The decision tree represents the logical sequence of events over time, including additional interventions, complications resulting from interventions, and changes in state of health. Although there is no limit to the potential complexity of most clinical scenarios, the aim of creating a decision tree is to reduce a complex decision to its most important components. (See Chapter 2 for a detailed description of decision tree modeling.)

The easiest way to structure our decision is to use a simple decision tree of our statement "Choose screening mammography ≥ 40 years or choose screening mammography ≥ 50 years" (Figure 4–1).

The figure shows a simplified version of the decision tree with the analysis beginning at 40 years of age and continuing through death. Outcome health states include the terminal branches on the right side of the tree: "Well," "Alive, breast cancer," "Dead, breast cancer," or "Dead, other causes." At the end of the analysis, we will determine the number of women in each health state and the costs of breast cancer screening, diagnosis, and treatment. Although a simple decision tree can provide an estimate of the number of women in each health state at the end of the analysis, it does not permit detailed accounting (1) of intervening events between the start and end of the study, (2) of events occuring over time, (3) of time spent in each health state, or (4) of discounting.

Thus, in our case scenario of mammographic screening, a simple decision tree is insufficient. Instead we will use a **Markov process** to include events that may occur at different times in the future (as described Chapter 2, pages 53–54). A Markov process is a state-transition model that cycles over fixed intervals of time (usually yearly or monthly), allowing patients

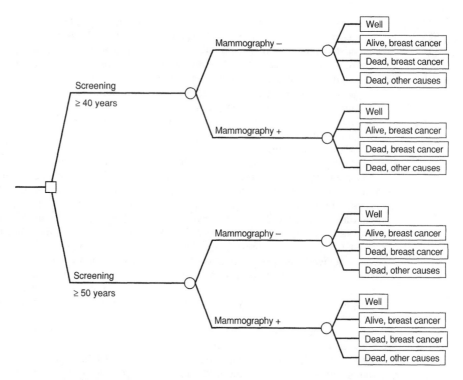

Figure 4–1. Simple decision tree of "Choose screening mammography ≥ 40 years or choose screening mammography ≥ 50 years." The tree models two breast cancer screening strategies for women: screening mammography beginning at 40 years and screening mammography beginning at 50 years. The subsequent structure indicates the mammographic results (negative [normal] or positive [abnormal]) and the terminal health states: well, alive with breast cancer, death from breast cancer, or death from other causes. Recall that a square represents a decision node, and a circle represents a chance node. The large rectangle represents an outcome.

to move back and forth from one state of health to another.[18–20] An example of a Markov process is provided in Figure 4–2, which shows the health states and possible transitions included in our screening mammography scenario. Note that the health states are the same as those used in the simple tree: "Well," "Alive, breast cancer," "Dead, breast cancer," or "Dead, other causes." All women beginning the analysis ("Baseline" time) are in the "Well" health state. The arrows in the figure demonstrate the possibilities for movement between these states. During each time period, a well woman can be diagnosed as having breast cancer, a woman with breast cancer may continue to live with or die of breast cancer or other causes, and a well woman could transition to death. Death is considered an absorbing state: Once a woman is dead, she cannot change to a different health state. Each cycle of the analysis is analogous to a snapshot of the cohort during a brief period of time. By moving through cycles of the analysis, the behavior of the cohort can be observed over time.

A **Markov analysis,** then is a decision model that contains Markov processes as elements of the larger structure.[19] Figure 4–3 shows that our Markov analysis for screening mammography beginning at age 40 years versus screening beginning at age 50 years is similar to the simplified decision tree in Figure 4–1, except that each arm of the tree includes a Markov process. This enables us to create a model in which women cycle through the decision at specified intervals during which transitions between the four outcome states may be accounted for.

After structuring the decision we next incorporate the relevant data.

Fill in the data

The relevant data that are incorporated in the Markov analysis are probabilities of events that we assign to each chance node as well as the outcome measures for cost and effectiveness. In addition, we will need to incorporate the concept of discounting. The specific

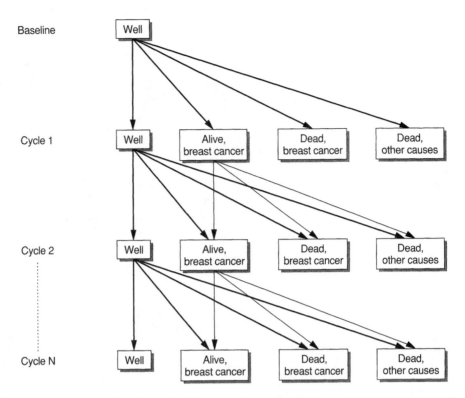

Figure 4–2. Health states and transitions in the Markov process. The arrows indicate how a woman may move between health states during each cycle.

probabilities, costs, life expectancies, patient preferences, and ultimately the cost-effectiveness finding for our case scenario are from a rigorously performed cost-effectiveness analysis of screening mammography by Salzmann and colleagues[21] that readers are encouraged to review in detail. The general issues of incorporating data in a cost-effectiveness analysis are the focus of this section.

Probabilities

After chance nodes are identified in the decision tree, probabilities are assigned to each node—these probabilities represent the probability of the event occurring. The goal of assigning probabilities is to find the most accurate estimate of the probability for each event in the decision tree.[22] This best estimate is called the **baseline estimate** and an analysis that uses baseline estimates is called the **baseline analysis.** Probabilities may be obtained, in order of desirability, from randomized controlled trials, cohort studies, case-control studies, and expert opinion. References for each probability and the baseline probability used in the analysis should be explicitly stated.

In our analysis, the key probability is the likelihood of the outcome state "Alive, breast cancer," which is influenced by whether or not screening mammography has been performed.

Outcomes

Outcomes of cost-effectiveness analyses include measures of costs and effectiveness.

Costs. Specific costs are identified and estimated for the economic component of cost-effectiveness analysis. It is important to distinguish between "cost" and "charge" as well as the different types of costs. **Cost** is defined as the consumption of a resource that otherwise could have been used for another purpose, whereas **charge** is the amount on the bill.[7] Costs include the economic resources used to provide a service, including all goods, services, and other resources consumed for a particular health care strategy, its side effects, and other

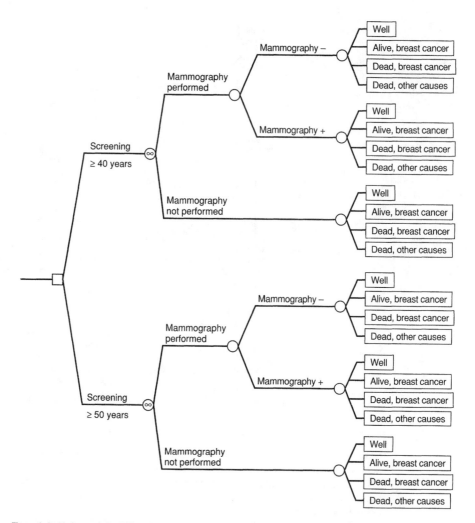

Figure 4–3. Markov analysis of "Choose screening mammography ≥ 40 years or choose screening mammography ≥ 50 years." The Markov process is represented by a Markov node (infinity symbol within a circle), which graphically depicts the point at which the cohort cycles through the tree at regular intervals. With each cycle, a woman may have mammography performed, which may be positive or negative, or not have mammography performed. At the end of each cycle, a woman will be in one of the four health states as was depicted in Figure 4–2: well, alive with breast cancer, dead from breast cancer, and dead from other causes.

current or future consequences of it. Cost, therefore, may include tests, drugs, supplies, health care personnel and medical facilities. Costs are either direct or indirect. **Direct costs** are resources consumed because of the intervention.[7] The cost of medical tests, medical and surgical therapies, hospitalizations, and physician fees, for example, are direct costs. **Indirect costs,** sometimes called productivity or opportunity costs, are losses in productivity because of illness or death.[10,12] These include time lost from work for medical examinations, procedures, or recovery for the patient and for his or her caretakers. Indirect cost may also include the value of wages lost due to death.

Cost varies by perspective. The cost of mammography to a patient, for example, is the amount the patient has to pay; cost to a hospital is the amount of resources allocated to provide the service or the true cost; cost to the insurance company is the hospital's charge for the service; and cost to society includes all direct and indirect costs. Charges, on the other hand, are set by the marketplace or regulation and may not reflect the true cost of providing a product or service.[10] They often vary by facility and geographic location. Although a charge is on average approximately double the cost, the charge for a specific medical test may be less than, the same, or more than the cost.

Cost-effectiveness analysis should attempt to identify and incorporate cost whenever possible since this number is more generalizable than charge and more accurately reflects resource use. Some health care providers have comprehensive accounting systems that allow for identification of every resource used in the treatment of an individual patient. This method, called microcosting, represents the true cost of providing medical care.[12] Although these costs may vary by geographic region, they provide an excellent measure of resource use. Unfortunately, however, it is rare to find such a system in use and most hospitals can identify only charges, not costs. An alternative approach is gross-costing, which estimates the cost of an event—for example, a hospitalization for mastectomy—by assigning a national average figure such as the Medicare-derived (diagnosis-related group [DRG]) reimbursement rate.[12] Gross-costing is usually simpler to perform and is less sensitive to geographic variation in cost than is microcosting.[12] A third commonly used method to estimate cost is the cost-to-charge ratio.[12] This ratio is an average of all costs divided by charges for services provided by the institution or group. Multiplying the charge for a specific medical procedure by the cost-to-charge ratio provides a crude estimate of cost. Use of the cost-to-charge ratio may not reveal the true cost because this ratio may vary by geographic region, institution, and the time and type of the test or intervention.

The costs used in Salzmann and colleagues' analysis are direct costs of screening mammographic evaluations, evaluating abnormal mammographic examinations, and treating breast cancer.[21] All costs are inflated to 1995 dollars. The cost of screening mammography ($106) and evaluating abnormal mammograms ($345) are based on the National Cancer Institute's national survey of mammography facilities. Costs of treatment are calculated by screening status and age, with the assumption that women in the screened group have, on average, lower stage of disease at diagnosis than women who were not screened. This assumption is based on the surveillance, epidemiology, and end results data from 1982. Treatment costs are based on data from the Group Health Cooperative, a staff model HMO with 388,000 members in Washington state. The total cost of breast cancer treatment in a subject younger than 50 years is $41,065 in the screened group and $41,563 in the unscreened group. The total cost of treatment in a subject 50 years of age or older is $33,576 in the screened group and $35,258 in the unscreened group. The analysis does not take indirect costs into account.

Effectiveness. Measures of effectiveness depend on the type and objectives of the analysis. Two common types of medical cost analyses are **cost-effectiveness analysis** and **cost-benefit analysis**. These analyses are frequently mislabeled and the terms are often misused.[8] The primary difference between cost-effectiveness analysis and cost-benefit analysis is the outcome measure. In cost-effectiveness analysis, measurements of effectiveness may be any unit of output, often life years gained, number of lives saved, or number of disease cases diagnosed. Cost is usually measured in monetary units (eg, dollars) but may be measured in nonmonetary units, such as number of hospital days, number of procedures, or hours of physician time. Because cost-effectiveness analysis does not require that measures of effectiveness be defined by economic value, it emphasizes health effects rather than economic impact of interventions or programs. In cost-benefit analysis, both costs and outcomes (benefits) are measured in the same economic or monetary unit, usually dollars.[8,10] Cost-benefit analysis converts years of life or quality outcomes into monetary values. In this approach, an individual's value to society is based on productivity or future wages. If the value of benefits is greater than costs, a program is cost-saving and therefore desirable. Inherent in this approach is the emphasis on economics that equates a human life or state of health with wage-earning potential and, at best, represents the minimum value a life is worth. However, wage estimates that differ by age, gender, and race raise troubling issues of fairness. This approach therefore has limited use in health care decision making and is rarely used.[6,7]

Clinical effectiveness should be expressed in the most appropriate and convenient units for the analysis. These can be categorized as measures of **mortality** (life years gained, number of lives saved), **morbidity** (complications or procedures avoided, days of work lost, quality of life related to various clinical conditions), **disease identification and therapy** (number of cases diagnosed, number of cases treated appropriately), and a combination of **morbidity and mortality** (quality-adjusted life years).

When the measure of effectiveness is quality of life, called **utility** (or patient preference), the method is a **cost-utility analysis** (a type of cost-effectiveness analysis). Utilities represent the subjective value people place on health states, such as disability or pain, and allow calculation of QALYs.[22] Quality-adjusted life years is the aggregate of time spent in each health state multiplied by the utility of that state. QALYs are one of the most frequently used measures of effectiveness in cost-effectiveness analyses. (See Chapter 2, pages 44–48 and 53, for a more detailed description of utilities and QALYs.)

In Salzmann and coworkers' analysis of breast cancer screening, the primary measure of effectiveness is life expectancy (years of life gained). In addition, QALYs are calculated using utility values derived from a small Australian study: 1 for "Well," 0.8 for "Alive with breast cancer," and 0 for "Death."[21]

Discounting

The value of both costs and patient preferences (utilities) may vary over time, and we tend to place a lower value on the future compared with the present in both. Discounting is a systematic method to calculate the present value of money that will be spent and the health states that will occur in the future.[8,10] Costs, for example, may occur in the present or future and their value depends on when they are incurred. In general, most people prefer to have $100 today instead of $100 in 10 years. Conversely, most of us would prefer to pay $100 in 10 years instead of today. This same time preference is true for utilities. We place a higher value on present compared with future health: Most people value a year of perfect health now more than they value a year of perfect health in 10 years. With most intervention programs, cost expenditures and health consequences occur at different times. For example, a program to combat tobacco addiction has a large immediate cost, but the health benefits may be seen 10 or 20 years after a person stops smoking. In cost-effectiveness analysis, it is possible and desirable to adjust for this differential timing of costs and health consequences by expressing all future costs and health consequences in terms of their present value.

To account for the time preference of money, for example, future costs are discounted to present value with the formula:

$$C_p = C/(1 + D)^y$$

where C_p = present cost, C = future cost, D = discount rate, and y = time period. At a discount rate of 5%, for example, the present value of $100 spent 1 year from now is

$$\$100/(1 + 0.05)^1 = \$95$$

and the present value of $100 spent 2 years from now is

$$\$100/(1 + 0.05)^2 = \$91$$

If expenditures occur at different times in the future, the present value can be calculated as:

$$C_p = C_0 + C_1/(1 + D)^1 + C_2/(1 + D)^2 + \ldots + C_n/(1 + D)^n$$

where C_p = present value, $C_0, C_1,\ldots, C_n$ = future costs, and D = discount rate. For example, at a discount rate of 5% per year, the present value of $100 spent now, another spent 1 year from now, and another spent 2 years from now is

$$\$100 + \$100/(1 + 0.05)^1 + \$100/(1 + 0.05)^2 = \$100 + \$95 + \$91 = \$286$$

In cost-effectiveness analysis, utilities are usually also discounted to present value with the same formulas (see Chapter 2, pages 52–53). Discounting utilities, however, is controversial since health is not a tradable resource that can be invested for future gain. As we've stated, however, most people would not trade a year of perfect health now for a year of perfect health 10 years from now. The reason for discounting future life years is that they are being valued relative to dollars: since a dollar in the future is discounted relative to a present dollar, so must a year of life be discounted.[8] The same discount rate used for costs should be used for utilities, usually 3–5%.[12] Discounting is easily done with computer programs for cost-effectiveness analysis, which allow discounting of each cycle of the analysis at an assigned discount rate.

Inflation, the continuous revaluation of currency, is different from discounting, which quantifies society's time-preference for money.[8] If the inflation rate for health care is the same as the general inflation rate for goods and services, inflation can be disregarded in cost-effectiveness analysis. This is because the payment for inflated future health care services will be in dollars that have increased at the general inflation rate. In practice, inflation is usually not included in cost-effectiveness analysis.

The analysis of Salzmann et al of screening mammography in women younger than 50 uses a discount rate of 3% for costs and utilities.[21]

Determine the value of alternative strategies

When all probabilities, costs, and measures of effectiveness (life expectancy and utilities) are inserted in the screening mammography decision tree, the original decision to "Choose screening mammography ≥ 40 years or choose screening mammography ≥ 50 years" can be addressed. In each yearly cycle, women without a diagnosis of breast cancer will undergo either screening mammography or not, based on the screening schedule of their group. The screening strategy influences a woman's probability of transitioning to a different health state during each yearly cycle of the Markov analysis. Each year, women may remain in the same health state, receive a diagnosis of breast cancer, or die. The model may continue for a specified number of cycles or until a woman reaches a state in which no transition can occur, ie, death. We can analyze the costs and effectiveness of each screening strategy using detailed accounting facilitated by computer software (as mentioned in Chapter 2, page 54). The computer program takes into account the *probability* of being in each health state (well, alive with breast cancer, dead due to breast cancer, or dead due to other causes), the life expectancy and utilities of each health state, the cost accrued with breast cancer detection and treatment and also discounts each annual cycle.

Since our mammography scenario is calculated using a Markov analysis that is facilitated by computer software, we will not present here a detailed example of folding-back each arm of the decision tree as was done in Chapter 2. The average cost-effectiveness and incremental cost-effectiveness of beginning screening mammography at 40 compared with 50 years of age are derived by calculating the final tally of costs measured in dollars and effectiveness measured in years of life or QALYs for each strategy.

We will now discuss the calculation of total costs and effectiveness for each arm of the tree, incremental costs and effectiveness, and the incremental cost-effectiveness ratio (C/E).

Total costs & effectiveness

We can now calculate the total costs in 1995 US dollars and the effectiveness in total years of life and quality-adjusted life years (QALYs) of our alternative strategies: Screening mammography ≥ 40 years or screening mammography ≥ 50 years. Total costs and outcomes for a woman who participates in each strategy are presented in Table 4–1.[21]

Because a woman begins the analysis at 40 years of age, she would live, on average, 24.228 additional years, discounted at 3%, if she underwent the "Screening mammography ≥ 50 years" strategy. Note that the "Screening mammography ≥ 40 years" strategy is more costly and slightly more effective. The QALYs indicate the years of life adjusted for quality.

TABLE 4–1. TOTAL COSTS, LIFE YEARS, AND QALYS FOR EACH STRATEGY.*

Strategy	Cost ($)	Effectiveness	
		Life Years	QALYs
Screening ≥ 50 years	3,407	24.228	24.021
Screening ≥ 40 years	4,083	24.234	24.027

* Reprinted with permission from Salzmann P et al: Cost-effectiveness of extending screening mammography guidelines to include women 40 to 49 years of age. Ann Intern Med 1997;127:955.

A year of life with breast cancer has a lower value than a year of life without breast cancer, which explains why total QALYs are less than total life years.

The cost-effectiveness of a health care strategy is traditionally expressed as the cost-effectiveness ratio (C/E). This ratio summarizes in one number information on costs and health outcome or effectiveness. The units of the C/E depend on the units of the numerator and denominator. The numerator of the ratio, costs, is usually expressed in dollars, and the denominator, effectiveness, may be expressed in any appropriate measure, usually in years of life or QALYs. However, simply dividing each strategy's total cost by its total effectiveness (ie, the average cost-effectiveness of each strategy) does not reveal the benefit of switching from one strategy to the other.[23] This ratio is therefore usually not helpful in describing the cost-effectiveness of a particular strategy.

Incremental cost & effectiveness

Incremental cost-effectiveness represents the additional cost incurred and effectiveness gained when one health care option is compared with another. One strategy is usually the current practice and the other strategy is usually a different existing or newly developed practice. Incremental costs and effectiveness are the differences between the two strategies in costs and effectiveness or the extra cost per unit of effectiveness. Below, incremental costs and effectiveness of one option (screening mammography $\geq$ 40 years) related to another (screening mammography $\geq$ 50 years) are calculated by subtraction.

Incremental cost (1995 dollars) = \$4,084 − \$3,407 = \$676
Incremental effectiveness (years of life) = 24.234 − 24.228 = 0.0064 years
Incremental effectiveness (QALYs) = 24.027 QALYs − 24.021 QALYs = 0.0061 QALYs

Note that the incremental difference in years of life and QALYs following the implementation for each strategy is the same as the years of life saved and QALYs saved when the "Screening mammography $\geq$ 40 years" strategy is used. The life years saved by using the "Screening mammography $\geq$ 40 years" strategy is equivalent to 2.3 days (0.0064 years × 365 d/y) at an incremental cost of \$676.

The C/E for a given strategy is often compared with the C/E of an alternative strategy. This comparison of C/Es for two or more strategies is called the incremental cost-effectiveness ratio, which is measured as the difference in costs divided by the difference in effectiveness between the two methods. This is calculated as follows:

$$\text{Incremental C/E} = \frac{\Delta \text{ Cost}}{\Delta \text{ Life Expectancy}} = \frac{\text{Cost}_1 - \text{Cost}_2}{\text{Life Expectancy}_1 - \text{Life Expectancy}_2}$$

where Cost_1 and Life expectancy$_1$ are the cost and effectiveness of the new strategy, and Cost_2 and Life expectancy$_2$ are the cost and effectiveness of the existing strategy. The same calculation is performed for incremental cost per QALY. We are now ready to calculate and compare the incremental cost-effectiveness of the "Screening mammography $\geq$ 40 years" strategy with the "Screening mammography $\geq$ 50 years" strategy.

The incremental C/E of "Screening mammography $\geq$ 40 years or screening mammography $\geq$ 50 years" is computed by the following division:

$$\text{Cost per life saved} = \frac{\$4,083 - \$3,407}{24.234 - 24.228 \text{ years}} = \frac{\$676}{0.0064 \text{ years}} = \$105,625$$

$$\text{Cost per QALY saved} = \frac{\$4,083 - \$3.407}{24.027 - 24.021 \text{ QALYs}} = \frac{\$676}{0.0061 \text{ QALYs}} = \$110,820$$

Hence, a policy that uses the "Screening mammography $\geq$ 40 years" strategy will cost approximately \$105,625 for each life year gained and \$110,820 for each quality-adjusted life year gained compared with a policy that uses the "Screening mammography $\geq$ 50 years" strategy.[21]

This method of calculating incremental costs, effectiveness, and cost-effectiveness can also be used when several alternative strategies are being compared. Both cost and effectiveness are measured as "net" changes from the next less costly strategy (Table 4–2). For example, if we also consider a strategy of no mammographic screening in *any* women called "No screening," we can calculate the incremental cost-effectiveness of adding biennial mammographic screening for women 50 years of age or older.[21] (Although women in the "No screening" strategy do not receive screening mammograms, they do undergo mammography as a diagnostic test if a breast mass is found.)

The incremental cost-effectiveness—the incremental cost divided by the incremental effectiveness—was $21,400 when biennial mammographic screening was performed for women 50 years of age and older compared with no screening. Annual mammographic screening for women 40 years of age and older was associated with $105,625 per year of life saved compared with screening only for women 50 years and older. This method of presenting data allows us to evaluate costs and benefits of strategies as they are added in a stepwise fashion.

We have used the example of one woman participating in each strategy. Commonly, analyses use a large cohort of subjects (10,000–1,000,000) participating in each strategy. Although the incremental cost-effectiveness will be the same for any size cohort, the total costs and effectiveness varies with a change in cohort size. The total costs and effectiveness thus reflects the overall burdens and benefits to society as utilization of a particular strategy increases.

Interpretation of the cost-effectiveness ratio

The term "cost-effective" should be used only when an intervention provides a benefit at an acceptable cost. If a strategy is less costly and more effective, it "dominates" the alternative option and will always be the better choice. In general, a strategy may be called cost-effective when, compared with its alternative, it is

- Less costly or cost-saving with an equal or better outcome
- More effective and more costly, with the added benefit worth the added cost
- Less effective and less costly, with the added benefit of the alternative not worth the added cost.

The determination of when added benefit is worth the added cost is made by our society and depends on societal values and availability of resources. Worth is a relative term that may change over time and with different perspectives (eg, patient, program, payor, societal). Although the explicit quantification of acceptable cost for a given benefit is very difficult to define, useful benchmarks are medical interventions society chooses to implement or not implement.[12] Many health care programs that are widely used and funded have incremental cost-effectiveness ratios in the range of $30,000 to $50,000, which therefore represents a currently acceptable incremental C/E.[12]

When we apply this range of ratios to our mammographic screening example, screening for women 50 years of age and older compared with no screening mammography provides

TABLE 4–2. INCREMENTAL COST-EFFECTIVENESS OF "SCREENING ≥ 50 YEARS" VERSUS "NO SCREENING" AND "SCREENING ≥ 40 YEARS" VERSUS "SCREENING ≥ 50 YEARS" STRATEGIES.*

Strategy	Total Cost ($)	Total Effectiveness (life years)	Incremental Cost ($)	Incremental Effectiveness (life years)	Incremental Cost-effectiveness ($ per life years)
No screening	2703	24.195	N/A	N/A	N/A
Screening ≥ 50 years	3407	24.228	704	0.0329	21,400
Screening ≥ 40 years	4083	24.234	676	0.0064	105,625

* Reprinted with permission from Salzmann P et al: Cost-effectiveness of extending screening mammography guidelines to include women 40–49 years old. Ann Intern Med 1997;127:955.

benefits at an acceptable cost to society ($21,400 per year of life saved). The addition of mammographic screening for women between 40 and 50 years of age, however, provides benefits at a very high cost compared with screening beginning at 50 years ($105,625 per year of life saved).

We have answered several of the initial questions posed in our case scenario. On the basis of the best available data at the time of the analysis, screening mammograms for women younger than 50 are minimally effective, on average adding 2.3 days of life per woman, at a cost of $676 per woman. This results in an incremental cost-effectiveness of $105,625. What our committee decides to do with these results depends on the priorities and resources of our HMO. Using the $50,000 cutoff, we would choose to begin mammographic screening at 50 years.

You can provide these same effectiveness findings to Ms Smith: Screening mammograms for women younger than 50 may add 2.3 days of life, on average, by preventing breast cancer–related death. However, it is important to note that these estimates represent the *average* benefits to a population of women and may not reflect an individual's benefit. An individual patient's preferences and ability to pay will affect her decision making. Because the benefits are so small, Ms Smith tells you that she would be willing to pay only a small amount for the test. If her cost is only a $5 copayment, she would consider having the mammogram. If, however, she has to pay more than $10, she is not interested in early mammography. Although the exact threshold of how much to pay and the magnitude of benefits will change for each patient, offering the most accurate advice is helpful.

Perform sensitivity analyses

The results of cost-effectiveness analyses are only as certain as the baseline data included. No matter how careful the analysis, the data used in cost-effectiveness analyses will include some uncertainties and potential biases. The course of illness, clinical effectiveness of testing and treatments, patient preferences for health outcomes, and costs are often very difficult to define precisely. In addition, unbiased and precise data for probabilities, utilities, and costs are usually limited, so estimations must be made. Sensitivity analysis provides a standard way to evaluate the effect of these uncertainties on cost-effectiveness analysis.

Sensitivity analysis is the process of repeatedly recalculating the incremental C/E using different values for probabilities, utilities, and costs.[24] The easiest method of sensitivity analysis is univariate, or one-way, analysis, whereby one variable at a time is varied over a plausible range. Multivariate sensitivity analysis, whereby estimates of two or more variables are varied simultaneously, should also be performed for important parameters identified in univariate analyses (see Chapter 2, pages 48–52) Variables may be evaluated over a range of the 95% confidence interval of a point estimate, over a range of values presented in the literature, or over a clinically feasible range.[25] The less confidence there is in the numeric estimate of a probability value, the wider the range should be.[24] Baseline values of the variables as well as the range over which sensitivity analyses are conducted should be explicitly stated.

Sensitivity analyses challenge the conclusions of the cost-effectiveness analysis by assessing the degree to which the findings are affected by changes in each variable (probabilities, costs, utilities). They identify variables that substantially affect the conclusions of cost-effectiveness analysis and suggest areas where better definition of values may be warranted. The difference in the C/E seen with sensitivity analyses provides an indication of how sensitive the results of the cost-effectiveness analysis may be to changes in each variable. If the cost-effectiveness analysis finding is robust or not sensitive to changes in a variable, additional precision of that parameter would be unlikely to change the results.

Figure 4–4 shows how varying several parameters in Salzmann and colleagues' mammographic screening cost-effectiveness analysis affected the results.[21] Note that varying the discount rate had the largest impact on the results. The mortality reduction expected with screening, the cost of screening mammography, and the screening interval also had a large impact on the results. Other cost and probability parameters were found to have minimal influence on the results. For the incremental C/E of screening women 40–49 years to be less than $50,000, the cost of mammography would have to be $45 or less. These one-way sensitivity analyses results reassure us that the conclusions of our cost-effectiveness analysis are fairly robust.

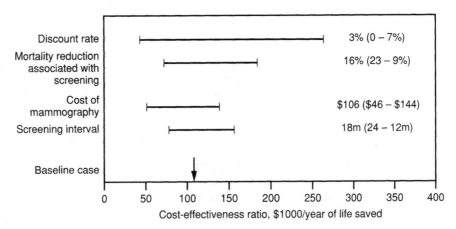

Figure 4–4. Sensitivity analyses for individual parameters in determining the incremental cost-effectiveness of screening mammography ≥ 40 years versus screening mammography ≥ 50 years. The arrow indicates the cost-effectiveness ratio in the baseline case and the bars indicate the range of the cost-effectiveness ratio when each variable is evaluated over the selected range. The baseline case estimate and range for the sensitivity analyses are presented to the right of each bar. (Adapted and reproduced, with permission, from Salzmann P et al: Cost-effectiveness of extending screening mammography guidelines to include women 40 to 49 years of age. Ann Intern Med 1997;127:955.)

LIMITATIONS OF COST-EFFECTIVENESS ANALYSIS

Although cost-effectiveness analysis can be one of many tools used to compare alternative health care strategies, it has several limitations. Cost-effectiveness analysis shares the same limitations as decision analysis, described in Chapter 2. Cost-effectiveness analysis can be laborious and complex. Reducing real-life medical problems into a structured decision tree can be very difficult, at best, and may not truly represent a patient's choices, course of illness, or health outcomes. In addition, by simplifying the course of an illness, valuable outcomes may be missed or eliminated. Nonetheless, careful structuring of the decision will include the most likely health outcomes and the process of highlighting areas of uncertainty is itself illuminating. Cost-effectiveness analysis has additional limitations that bear discussion, including the health care provider's dilemma, reliability of assumptions, comparison of strategies affecting different aspects of health, and intrinsic biases.

The health care provider's dilemma

Health care providers face an inherent conflict by serving as a primary patient advocate as well as an advocate for all patients and, therefore, society.[7] The primacy of the physician's advocacy role may be jeopardized if clinicians were charged with making decisions to achieve societal priorities that conflict with individual choices.

The final context for clinical decisions concerning the use of medical services lies in the encounter between clinician and patient. It is essential that the first commitment of the physician be to optimize care of the individual patient.[23] Yet, patient care decisions are very complex and may include some concern for cost. Almost all clinicians and all consumers of health care would agree that, at some point, extra money spent for tiny improvements in clinical outcomes is not worthwhile and represents inappropriate practice. This misspent money could have been devoted to medical care that would have achieved greater benefit or to some other meaningful societal purpose. In addition, the definition of what constitutes a "significant" benefit or cost and what benefit is "worth" what cost remains controversial and varies by perspective (eg, patient, program, payor, society). Inherent in cost-effectiveness analysis, however, is the trade-off between maximizing effectiveness and minimizing costs. Although cost-effectiveness analysis has a limited role in decision making for an individual patient, it is a valuable tool for those charged with allocating resources for groups of patients.[23]

Reliability of assumptions

Rigorous cost-effectiveness analyses are very difficult to perform, and their results are only as reliable as their assumptions. Because of insufficient data, probabilities are often difficult to determine. When clinical trial data are lacking, probabilities are often estimated by expert opinion. Costs are very difficult to determine, with few institutions having the potential to calculate actual cost. Charges, on the other hand, are relatively easy to assess but lack generalizability. Utilities vary by the method used for their quantification as well as by perspective.

These limitations may be minimized by using the best available evidence and performing sensitivity analyses over an appropriate range of values. In addition, the analysis is strengthened by choosing an appropriate perspective and logical structure of the decision.

Comparison of strategies affecting different aspects of health

An additional use of incremental cost-effectiveness analyses is to compare health care interventions for different purposes—for example, comparing the cost-effectiveness of routine varicella vaccination for all infants with annual Papanicolaou smear tests in elderly women. Each of these analyses would be incremental and compared with their accepted existing strategy, for example, no varicella vaccination and every-third-year Pap test, respectively. This comparison between interventions for different purposes is a valuable analytic tool for resource allocation. However, to make valid comparisons between various cost-effectiveness analyses, it is imperative that the methods used in the different analyses be similar.

To improve comparability between cost-effectiveness analyses, recent guidelines published by the Panel on Cost-Effectiveness in Health and Medicine[12] convened by the US Public Health Service recommend the use of a reference case—a standard set of methodological practices for cost-effectiveness studies. The reference case is from the societal perspective and "incrementally" compares the intervention of interest with existing medical practice. All costs should be evaluated in the same units (eg, 1995 US dollars) and units of effectiveness should be similar (eg, quality-adjusted life years, lives saved). In addition, discounting should be incorporated and sensitivity analyses should be performed.

Intrinsic biases

Cost-effectiveness analysis has intrinsic biases based on age and health status that should be considered.[6,7] Cost-effectiveness analyses are biased against elderly who have a higher cost per life year gained because their life years are limited compared with the life years of a younger person. Since absolute utility, rather than relative change in health status, is quantified, groups with poor baseline health status (eg, groups with lower baseline utility) will have lower QALYs and, therefore, higher cost per QALY. In addition, preventative health care does not appear as cost-effective as acute care; money is spent early for preventive care, but health benefits realized in the future are usually discounted and, therefore, lower. In acute care, both cost and benefits may be realized early and are usually minimally affected by discounting. Since discounting results in a relatively smaller number, the benefits are relatively higher and the cost-effectiveness relatively lower for acute care compared with preventive care.

SUMMARY

1. Cost-effectiveness analysis is a method of systematically evaluating outcomes in relation to costs and of identifying the relative value of alternative interventions for improving health. It may be used to determine the most efficient or productive use of limited resources, to maximize the aggregate health benefits for a population, or to minimize the cost of achieving a given health goal.

2. The five steps of cost-effectiveness analysis are
    1. Formulate an explicit question
    2. Structure the decision
    3. Fill in the data
    4. Determine the value of alternative strategies
    5. Perform sensitivity analyses
3. Important factors in formulating an explicit question are the choice of strategies to be compared, the time frame, and the perspective of the analysis. A particular strategy is usually compared with an alternative strategy, which is often the current practice or the next most expensive strategy. The time frame of a cost-effectiveness analysis is the period of time over which costs and benefits are measured. The perspective of an analysis is the viewpoint from which the analysis is conducted, including societal, payor, program, and patient perspectives.
4. The decision is structured using a decision tree composed of decision nodes (assigning the strategies being analyzed), chance nodes (characterizing an uncertain path determined by chance), and terminal nodes (defining outcome health states). A Markov analysis uses a basic decision tree structure that includes Markov processes, which cycle over fixed intervals of time, allowing patients to move back and forth from one state of health to another. Markov analysis therefore facilitates more accurate modeling of intervening events over time.
5. The key data incorporated within the analyses are probabilities of the relevant events and the outcome measures of costs and effectiveness, which may include utilities.
6. Costs are the economic resources used to provide a service (goods, services, and other resources consumed for an intervention) and are distinct from charges, which are the amounts of the bills for services. Direct costs are resources consumed because of the intervention (medical tests, therapies, physician fees), and indirect costs are losses in productivity because of illness or death (time lost from work for the patient and his or her caretakers).
7. In cost-effectiveness analyses, effectiveness may be measured by **mortality** (life years gained, number of lives saved), **morbidity** (complications or procedures avoided, days of work lost, quality of life related to various clinical conditions), **disease identification and therapy** (number of cases diagnosed, cases treated appropriately), or a combination of morbidity and mortality (QALYs, the aggregate time spent in each health state multiplied by the utility of that state). In the less commonly used cost-benefit analyses, effectiveness is measured in **monetary terms** (usually dollars).
8. Discounting is a systematic method to calculate the present value of money that will be spent and health states that occur in the future. Because people value money and optimal health more in the present than in the future, future money and utilities are discounted to their present value using a simple formula.
9. Because we are usually interested in the relative cost-effectiveness of a new strategy compared with the current accepted regimen, the most important finding is the incremental cost-effectiveness. This is the incremental cost per additional unit of effectiveness of one strategy compared with an alternative strategy, calculated as the difference in costs divided by the difference in effectiveness between the two methods.
10. A strategy may be called cost-effective when, compared with its alternative, it is (1) less costly or is cost-saving with an equal or better outcome; (2) more effective and more costly, with the added benefit worth the added cost; or (3) less effective and less costly, with the added benefit of the alternative not worth the added cost.
11. Sensitivity analysis is the process of repeatedly recalculating the cost-effectiveness result over an appropriate range of values for probabilities, costs, and utilities. Sensitivity analyses identify variables that substantially affect the results of cost-effectiveness analysis and suggest areas in which better definition of values may be warranted.
12. Although cost-effectiveness analyses may be limited in their application to decision making for individual patients, they provide additional pieces of evidence that may contribute to health policy decision making.

REFERENCES

1. National Institute of Health Consensus Development Conference: Breast cancer screening for women ages 40–49, Bethesda, Maryland, 1997. January 21–23.
2. Fletcher SW et al: Report of the International Workshop on Screening for Breast Cancer. J Natl Cancer Inst 1993;85:1644.
3. Kerlikowske K et al: Efficacy of screening mammography. A meta-analysis. JAMA 1995; 273:149.
4. Sickles EA et al: Mammographic screening for women aged 40 to 49 years: The primary care practitioner's dilemma. Ann Intern Med 1995;122:534.
5. Sox HC: Screening mammography in women younger than 50 years of age. Ann Intern Med 1995;122:550.
6. Petitti DB: *Meta-Analysis, Decision Analysis, and Cost-Effectiveness Analysis : Methods for Quantitative Synthesis in Medicine.* Oxford University Press, 1994, p. 246.
7. Weinstein MC, Fineberg HV: *Clinical Decision Analysis.* Saunders, 1980.
8. Weinstein MC, Stason WB: Foundations of cost-effectiveness analysis for health and medical practices. N Engl J Med 1977;296:716.
9. Drummond MF: Allocating resources. Int J Technol Assess Health Care 1990;6:77.
10. Eisenberg JM: Clinical economics. A guide to the economic analysis of clinical practices. JAMA 1989;262:2879.
11. Emery DD, Schneiderman LJ: Cost-effectiveness analysis in health care. Hastings Cent Rep 1989;19:8.
12. Gold MR et al: *Cost-Effectiveness in Health and Medicine.* Oxford University Press, 1996, p. 425.
13. Robinson R: Cost-effectiveness analysis. BMJ 1993;307:79.
14. Russell LB et al: The role of cost-effectiveness analysis in health and medicine. Panel on Cost-Effectiveness in Health and Medicine. JAMA 1996;276:1172.
15. Siegel JE et al: Recommendations for reporting cost-effectiveness analyses. Panel on Cost-Effectiveness in Health and Medicine. JAMA 1996;276:1339.
16. Weinstein MC et al: Recommendations of the Panel on Cost-effectiveness in Health and Medicine. JAMA 1996;276:1253.
17. Kerlikowske K: Efficacy of screening mammography among women aged 40 to 49 years and 50 to 69 years: Comparison of relative and absolute benefits. J Natl Cancer Inst, 1997;22:79.
18. Sonnenberg FA, Beck JR: Markov models in medical decision making: a practical guide. Med Decis Making 1993;13:322.
19. Naimark D et al: Primer on medical decision analysis: 5. Working with Markov processes. Med Decis Making 1997;17:152.
20. Beck JR, Pauker SG: The Markov process in medical prognosis. Med Decis Making 1983;3:419.
21. Salzmann P et al: Cost-effectiveness of extending screening mammography guidelines to include women 40 to 49 years of age. Ann Intern Med 1997;127:955.
22. Naglie G et al: Primer on medical decision analysis: 3. Estimating probabilities and utilities. Med Decis Making 1997;17:136.
23. Detsky AS, Naglie IG: A clinician's guide to cost-effectiveness analysis. Ann Intern Med 1990;113:147.
24. Krahn MD et al: Primer on medical decision analysis: 4. Analyzing the model and interpreting the results. Med Decis Making 1997;17:142.
25. Drummond MF et al: User's guides to the medical literature. XIII. How to use an article on economic analysis of clinical practice. A. Are the results of the study valid? JAMA 1997;277:1552.

2

ACCESSING MEDICAL INFORMATION

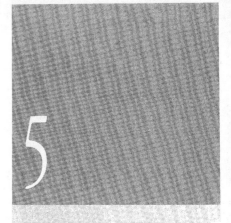

SEARCHING

MEDLINE

J. Ben Davoren, MD, PhD

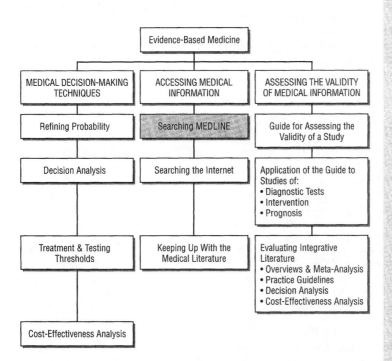

INTRODUCTION

The focus of this book is to help the individual clinician apply the most relevant published information to the care of the patient. After determining what clinical information is needed—whether it is regarding test characteristics, prognostic or risk factors, epidemiologic information, or therapeutic outcomes of varying interventions—the clinician must find and retrieve it. However, not all information is available instantaneously, and information that is available is changing constantly. Therefore, the challenge to the clinician is to not only be able to identify and scrutinize relevant existing information but also be able to do so on an ongoing basis.

The widespread availability of the personal computer has made the search and retrieval task simpler, mostly because of the speed with which information can be retrieved. But the clinician still depends on outside sources to organize the enormous amount of information that is generated worldwide. Fortunately, there are several reliable methods by which virtually the entire world's collection of peer-reviewed medical and biological scientific literature is catalogued, organized, and made available to individuals in a coherent and consistent fashion. The most well-known and comprehensive of these databases of medical literature is MEDLINE. MEDLINE is a service of the United States' National Library of Medicine (NLM) and is an acronym for their **Med**ical **L**iterature **A**nalysis and **R**etrieval **S**ystem (MEDLARS) On-Line. It is a computerized database of medical, dental, nursing, and basic life science journal articles and information accessible by searches of keywords, subjects, journal titles, authors, specific publication types, and even more specific combinations of search terms. This chapter will demonstrate how you can efficiently navigate this enormous database—nearing 10 million journal articles—to locate the highest quality, most relevant information about a particular topic of interest.

ACCESS METHODS: COMMON THREADS & SOFTWARE DIFFERENCES

MEDLINE is written in a type of code rather than in plain English, and its hierarchies—the backbone of its organizational power—are created in numbers and groupings more suitable to computer organization than to common clinical usage. This phenomenon has led to the development of a large number of specialized computer software programs that act as user-friendly interfaces for MEDLINE. These interfaces allow the user to use more familiar terms to search the database; the program invisibly converts those terms into the programming language of the MEDLARS database. Most academic medical centers have developed their own interfaces. For health care providers associated with such medical centers, these interfaces are generally easy to use, often at no or very low cost. Readers affiliated with such a center are referred to their medical librarian.

One example of such an interface that will be used in this chapter is the Melvyl system of the University of California. Most similar academic centers provide the opportunity to perform searches of the medical literature from sites either inside or outside the library, via computer networks or modem access from personal computers. We use Melvyl as our example interface specifically because it demonstrates clearly how searches are performed in a sequential, term-narrowing fashion. It shows the individual steps taken in a search by any type of searching software, even though some types of software make it look to the user as if only one step is needed. This concept will become clear with the examples to follow.

Researchers without academic affiliations have many choices for such an interface, but the most popular methods have been to use the simple and straightforward ones developed by the NLM itself, either GRATEFUL MED (a program for Macintosh or PC/Windows computers), or the new Internet versions, Internet Grateful Med and PubMed. The latter two are accessed, for free, using Web browser software, and are therefore compatible with any platform that can "surf the Web" (see page 124 and Chapter 6). GRATEFUL MED will be used for examples in this chapter, in addition to the Melvyl system. Internet Grateful Med is quite similar. All these interfaces utilize the search strategies detailed in this chapter, and each has its own set of "help" screens while the programs are actually running.

With the growth of the Internet and its popular graphical interface, the World Wide Web, a growing number of commercial services are becoming available for searching MEDLINE. See page 124 for details. Finally, there are CD-ROM versions of MEDLINE available, but they lack the advantage of on-line versions, because MEDLINE is updated weekly during most of the year.

ORGANIZATION OF THE PRIMARY DATABASE

MEDLINE is an extremely comprehensive database. Thus, the challenge for the clinician is not determining whether the information needed exists in the database—it probably does— but rather understanding how the *relevant* information is catalogued within MEDLINE. Such understanding allows the user to retrieve and perhaps even store in their own computerized database *only the relevant information.*

As noted, there are nearly 10 million distinct journal articles—clinical trials, basic science papers, reviews, editorials, individual letters—that have been catalogued by the NLM since 1966 (this is the earliest year captured in the MEDLARS database). Following the logic of older library systems (but expanding on them substantially), the primary database is set up as a hierarchy of *subjects,* with the "officially sanctioned" subject names declared "MeSH terms," a contraction of "**Me**dical **S**ubject **H**eadings." Not all "subject headings" are intuitively obvious, however. For example, "beta-blockers" are listed as "adrenergic beta antagonists." To learn how to best access individual articles, then, it is crucial to know how the NLM catalogues journal articles, not just how the article authors title or characterize them. The NLM MeSH heading hierarchy provides a standard dictionary of cataloguing terms for every article published in more than 3800 journals. Learning how particular MeSH headings are used for a specific article may feel like an overwhelming task. The search strategy discussed later in this chapter shows how this is indeed manageable by using an approach that essentially first searches for the relevant MeSH terms and subsequently searches for the relevant articles.

It is important to understand that every article is not available on MEDLINE in its entirety. Rather, each article is entered into the MEDLARS database in what is known as the "unit record." Figure 5–1 is an example of such a record for one journal article, as it appears in the Melvyl system.

You may notice that the unit record does not really resemble a journal article except for the abstract. Each individual "field" within the unit record serves as a tag by which later searches can find this particular article. Of more importance, though, as we shall see, the consistency with which these tags are applied to similar articles (by the indexers at the NLM) serves to identify essentially all other articles just like it. Each of these fields, most of which can be searched by the MEDLINE user, is identified by the two-letter abbreviation at the left. These field descriptor abbreviations are defined in Figure 5–2.

The fields that are "searchable" via most software interfaces with MEDLINE are author names; title words; journal titles and subsets; language; publication types; and, most important; MeSH headings and their optional subheadings. With use of operational commands such as "find," these headings can be used singly or in combination to locate specific journal articles and groups of articles. Combinations of fields may be searched using the Boolean operators "and," "or," and "and not." Many software programs will prompt the user to use multiple combinations of these operators to restrict searches, *because the efficient restriction of initially general search terms is the secret to obtaining relevant articles.* Some software will allow the user to input the entire search at one time, without prompts. The basic GRATEFUL MED search window is seen in Figure 5–3. This search window offers several fields that the clinician may fill in to restrict searches. Each restriction modality is discussed in detail later in this chapter.

Let's consider an example of a Boolean search statement using the Melvyl system. You could search the MEDLINE database for articles about either amiodarone *or* quinidine (both official MeSH terms as seen in our example) using the following search term:

"Find subject amiodarone or subject quinidine"

UI - 95243788
AU - Middlekauff HR
AU - Stevenson WG
AU - Gornbein JA
AD - Department of Medicine, University of California, Los Angeles, USA.
TI - Antiarrhythmic prophylaxis vs warfarin anticoagulation to prevent thromboembolic events among patients with atrial fibrillation. A decision analysis.
TA - Arch Intern Med
DP - 1995 May 8
VI - 155
IP - 9
PG - 913-20
JC - 7FS
IS - 0003-9926
LA - Eng
MH - Adolescence
MH - Adult
MH - Aged
MH - Aged, 80 and over
MH - Amiodarone/*THERAPEUTIC USE
MH - Atrial Fibrillation/*COMPLICATIONS/THERAPY
MH - Comparative Study
MH - Confounding Factors (Epidemiology)
MH - Decision Support Techniques
MH - Electric Countershock
MH - Female
MH - Human
MH - Male
MH - Middle Age
MH - Quinidine/*THERAPEUTIC USE
MH - Risk
MH - Thromboembolism/ETIOLOGY/*PREVENTION & CONTROL
MH - Treatment Outcome
MH - Warfarin/*THERAPEUTIC USE
RN - 1951-25-3 (Amiodarone)
RN - 56-54-2 (Quinidine)
RN - 81-81-2 (Warfarin)
PT - Journal Article
PT - Meta-Analysis
AB - BACKGROUND: Patients with atrial fibrillation compared with those with sinus rhythm are at increased risk for thromboembolism, often mandating therapy directed at thromboembolism prevention. However, the safest, most efficacious strategy to prevent thromboembolism associated with atrial fibrillation is unknown. We developed a decision analysis to compare the risks and benefits of two common clinical strategies to prevent thromboembolism in the patient with atrial fibrillation: (1) sinus rhythm maintenance with quinidine sulfate or with amiodarone hydrochloride after cardioversion and (2) long-term anticoagulation with warfarin sodium. METHODS: A search was conducted of the English-language MEDLINE databases of the National Library of Medicine dated 1966 through December 1992. The search was conducted by intersecting "quinidine," "warfarin," or "amiodarone" with "atrial fibrillation." Six of 249 articles concerning quinidine and five of 20 articles concerning warfarin were judged by multiple reviewers to meet predetermined inclusion and exclusion criteria. To our knowledge, no randomized, placebo-controlled trials of amiodarone therapy for atrial fibrillation have been published. Five of 112 identified articles concerning amiodarone involved nonrandomized trials that met the remaining selection criteria and were included in this analysis. RESULTS: Thromboembolic events and fatal nonthromboembolic adverse events during the course of therapy (defined as fatal proarrhythmia, fatal hemorrhage and fatal noncardiac toxic effects) were considered to have equivalent weight. The total risk during therapy, defined as thromboembolic and fatal nonthromboembolic adverse events during the course of therapy, was evaluated over a range of baseline thromboembolism risks, from 1% to 20% per patient-year. Quinidine therapy compared with no therapy was associated with increased total risk, unless baseline thromboembolism risk exceeded 11% per patient-year. Total risk during warfarin therapy was less than total risk during quinidine therapy for the entire range of baseline thromboembolism risks, from 1% to 20% per patient-year. Total risk during warfarin or amiodarone therapy was similar and less than that with no therapy for the entire range of baseline risks. CONCLUSIONS: Based on data from randomized, controlled trials of quinidine and warfarin, warfarin therapy appears to be the safest strategy for thromboembolism prevention in the patient with atrial fibrillation. The role of low-dose amiodarone therapy appears promising and warrants further study in randomized, controlled trials.
AA- Author
SB - A   SB - M   SB - X
SO - Arch Intern Med 1995 May 8;155(9):913-20

Figure 5–1. The MEDLINE unit record.

UI   Unique Identifier — The NLM identification number assigned to this one article.

AU   Author — The names of the authors of the article, currently up to 25. If you know the name of one or more authors of an article, you can quickly narrow your search, even if you are unfamiliar with the exact MeSH headings.

AD   Address — The name of the institution from whence the article was submitted.

TI   Title — The title of the article. If you know specific words in the title of one article, it may help you find related articles. Alternatively, you may find other "keywords" in the title or abstract of a given paper that may give you additional search terms/ideas.

TA   Title Abbreviation — The standard abbreviation of the journal.

DP   Date of Publication — Self-explanatory, but note that the date of entry into the MEDLINE system will be up to several months later than date of publication.

VI   Volume Issue — Self-explanatory.

IP   Issue/Part — Identifies part of journal (such as supplement).

PG   Pages — Self-explanatory.

JC   Journal Code — A unique journal code for the NLM.

IS   International Standard Serial Number — Of the journal, not the article.

LA   Language of publication — Lists the language, but also labels English vs Foreign.

MH   MeSH Headings — These are the most useful of the fields for individual searchers of the database. The NLM has a large, hierarchal "tree" system of cataloguing information, with more general MeSH headings at the top and more and more specific related terms beneath. These MeSH headings are used as index terms both in MEDLINE/MEDLARS and the *Index Medicus*. Note that the MeSH heading descriptors may be modified, as in the above example, to aid searching. The line "Atrial Fibrillation/*COMPLICATIONS/THERAPY" denotes several separate but crucially important concepts. The first part of this field, "Atrial Fibrillation," means that this article is listed under the MeSH heading Atrial Fibrillation, so that if you searched the subject of Atrial Fibrillation you would get this article. The two capitalized words that follow, separated by backslashes, are subheadings. This means that this article is not just about Atrial Fibrillation in general, but, more specifically, about the *complications of* Atrial Fibrillation, and about the *therapy of* Atrial Fibrillation. The third concept is denoted by the asterisk before the subheading COMPLICATIONS. The presence of an asterisk defines the *major emphasis of the article*, which in this case is the complications of Atrial Fibrillation; the therapeutic uses of amiodarone, quinidine, and warfarin; and the prevention and control of thromboembolism. The utility of the subheadings will become clearer in the remainder of this chapter.

RN   Registry Number — Unique numbers assigned to chemical compounds.

PT   Publication Type — This is a very helpful way to limit searches to specific types of articles, such as clinical trials, meta-analyses, multicenter studies, randomized controlled trials, and reviews.

AB   Abstract — The body of the abstract. Older abstracts may be truncated after 250–400 words, but current abstracts are printed in their entirety.

AA   Abstract Author — Relevant only if abstracted by someone other than the author(s) of the article itself.

SB   Journal Subset — Individual journals are grouped together in terms of similarities in topics/orientations or general popularity. This field is extremely useful in limiting searches to specific journal types and in eliminating other journal types. Useful subsets are cancer, dental, nursing, and "aim" (abridged index medicus, the most widely read journals). (A is aim, M is a "high priority journal," X is the cancer core.)

SO   Source — A composite of several fields above (TA, DP, VI, IP, PG), searchable by the individual searcher.

Figure 5–2. MEDLINE unit record field descriptors.

To locate articles about *both drugs together,* the term:

 "Find subject amiodarone and subject quinidine"

would give the intersection of the sets of articles about each drug. This latter search would be smaller and more specific. Note that in GRATEFUL MED, if two search terms are placed in the same field (the rectangular boxes in Figure 5–3), they are automatically linked

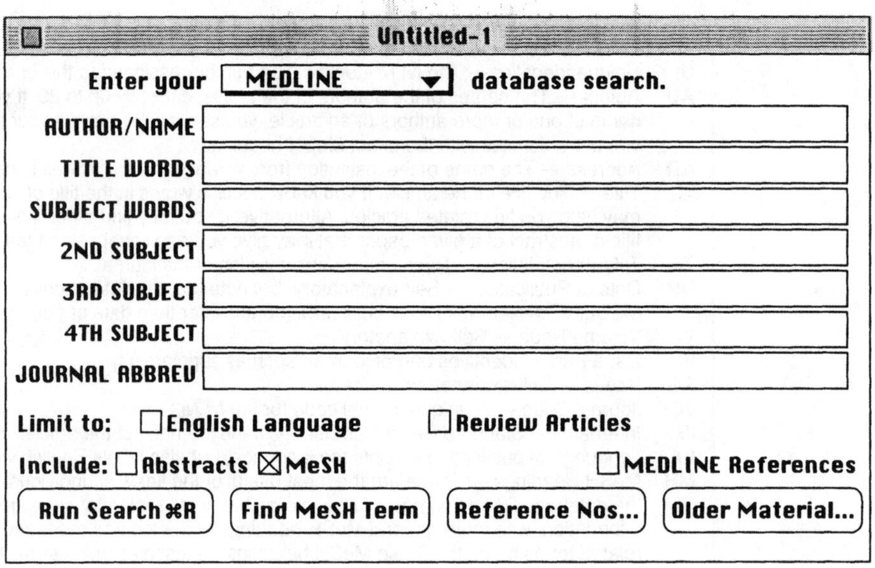

Figure 5–3. The GRATEFUL MED search window.

by "or." If they are placed in two different fields, they are linked by "and," which basically *restricts* the first term so that the retrieved articles have to include both search terms, not one or the other. Also note that in GRATEFUL MED, there is no place to state the operator command "find"; this command is assumed to exist when the fields are filled in.

SEARCH STRATEGIES

A major problem to be overcome for the MEDLINE searcher is that the terms familiar to the clinician to describe a disease, a therapy, or a particular topic of interest may not be "official" MEDLINE cataloguing terms. Searching with these non-MeSH headings will often lead to frustratingly incomplete searches. Performing a successful MEDLINE search is thus a two-stage process. The first stage is finding the right MeSH terms for the articles of interest, the second is using those MeSH terms to find *only* the articles of interest.

Regardless of how your computer screen appears, regardless of the software you use to search the primary database, the searching process always begins the same way. The steps in this process are as follows:

1. Begin with a broad set of search terms to encompass a large number of potentially relevant articles.
2. Narrow that search with modifying terms to improve its specificity.
3. Find one relevant article by reading the titles and abstracts of the articles retrieved.
4. After examining the MeSH terms under which the relevant articles are specifically catalogued, combine these MeSH terms and particular modifiers in a new re-expanded, yet highly focused search.

Begin broadly

Depending on the software you use to access MEDLINE, you may be able to begin your search with **keywords** (words in the title or abstract or suggested by the authors; or concepts that the indexers of the abstract at the NLM consider to be related or important in the published article), **title words,** or **subjects** (again, using "official" MeSH headings as the subject). Keyword or title word searches are less exacting and likely to give you more information than you need. But as you will see in the next section, there are many ways to subsequently focus a search that is too broad. In general, as mentioned before, the operational command used for any of these searches is "find," although this word is not spelled out in the GRATEFUL MED window. Either title word or keyword searches are recommended if they are options in your software package; title words are common to virtually all software options, including Melvyl and GRATEFUL MED.

To make the search as broad as possible when searching keywords and title words (but not MeSH terms), you can use "truncation" symbols. MEDLARS as well as GRATEFUL MED use a colon (:) to substitute for any number of characters or spaces. For example, the term "smok:" retrieves articles in which the terms smoke, smoking, smoker, smoked, and even Smokey the Bear appear. The colon can also be useful if you are unsure of the spelling of a term, although your results will be broader than with a more specific term. Note that individual software packages use different truncation characters; in Melvyl, you would type "find keyword smok#."

You may also initiate a search by subject. This, however, has pitfalls, because only words in "official" MeSH headings will be recognized as "subjects" in MEDLINE (but see what's on the horizon—the Metathesaurus described later in this chapter). For example, if you search the *subject* "hip fracture," you will get zero results (the official MeSH heading is "hip fractures"), but a *title word* search results in more than 1200 citations. In addition, similar subject searches end up with slightly different results, which is another reason why we will focus on finding one good article and then quickly revamping our search to find all the relevant articles that are indexed just like it. To demonstrate some of these differences, let's say we wanted to find recent articles about the therapy of chronic myelogenous leukemia (CML), with particular attention to randomized interventional trials. You might start out with a broad search, such as:

 find subject chronic myelogenous leukemia

In Melvyl, you get the response:

 Search result: 2,126 citations in the Medline database

A broader search term,

 find subject chronic leukemia

provokes this response:

 Search result: 3,798 citations in the Medline database

It seems obvious that a more generic search term would lead to a greater number of articles, but are all 2126 citations of the first search included in the 3786 of the second? How would you know? Well, as noted above, the MeSH terms are organized in a "tree structure," with more specific MeSH terms essentially "subcategories" of less specific, more comprehensive MeSH terms. These tree structures can be found in very thick MEDLINE searching handbooks but can also be found on-line in many MEDLINE searching systems and are part of the GRATEFUL MED software. Each subcategory is "collapsed" within the more senior category names, but in GRATEFUL MED each becomes visible with a mouse click on the more senior category arrow. Figure 5–4 is an example of the tree structure of leukemia, seen after a click on the "Find MeSH term" button from the main Search window of Figure 5–3. In the Melvyl system, you use the "browse" command to look at the hierarchy of available subcategories within a broader MeSH term; the result is the same. For example:

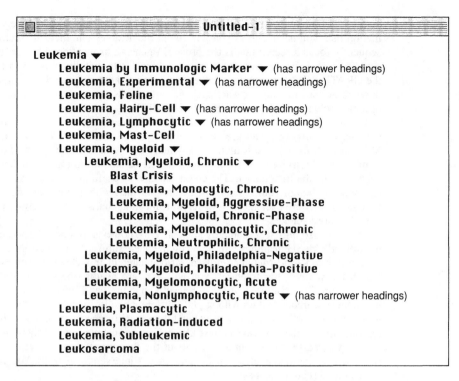

Figure 5–4. Sample tree structure. The subcategories of "Leukemia" are searched with the Explode command. Only the "Leukemia, Myeloid" category is shown in its fully exploded form.

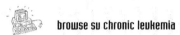

browse su chronic leukemia

gives you the following screen response:

Browse result: 9 MeSH headings in the Medline database

1. Leukemia, B-Cell, Chronic.		563 citations
2. Leukemia, Lymphocytic, Chronic. [has narrower headings]		885 citations
3. Leukemia, Monocytic, Chronic.		67 citations
4. Leukemia, Myeloid, Aggressive-Phase.		50 citations
5. Leukemia, Myeloid, Chronic. [has narrower headings]		2,000 citations
6. Leukemia, Myeloid, Chronic-Phase.		126 citations
7. Leukemia, Myelomonocytic, Chronic.		182 citations
8. Leukemia, Neutrophilic, Chronic.		26 citations
9. Leukemia, T-Cell, Chronic.		61 citations

This example reveals that the 2126 citations of items 5 and 6 are in fact all within subcategories of the "grandfather" MeSH heading in this tree structure, "chronic leukemia." "Chronic leukemia" itself looks like it should be a more specific MeSH term underlying the MeSH term "leukemia" (which is a subset of the most general related MeSH term in MEDLINE, "neoplasms"). Figure 5–4 shows, however, that "chronic leukemia" is *not* a subcategory of leukemia. This example (admittedly and purposefully a confusing one) shows how related MeSH terms are not always in perfect hierarchies. *It underscores the need to discover the best MeSH terms not by looking through a list of MeSH terms, but by finding out which MeSH terms are used to index a relevant article.* Also, note that "Leukemia, Myeloid, Chronic" is the same as "chronic myelogenous leukemia" in MEDLINE, because it is a cross-referenced term. In Melvyl, you may examine the list of cross-referenced terms by performing a "browse." Following the MeSH terms and subheading lists on the screen, a set of "used for" terms will appear. However, it is not necessary to do this step, because MED-LINE already knows to look for all those terms when you search with any one of them. In GRATEFUL MED, not only MeSH terms are cross-referenced. Some non-MeSH terms are listed in the MeSH terms window followed by an (xr), indicating that the terms are cross-referenced to a real MeSH term; for example, cancer is cross-referenced to neoplasms.

The GRATEFUL MED search window, seen in Figure 5–3, allows you to find official MeSH terms in several ways. After entering search words in any of the subject fields, you can click on the "Find MeSH Term" box, and you will be taken to a second window that shows a list of all possible MeSH terms. Fortunately, you will be taken to the MeSH terms alphabetically nearest to the search words you entered in the first screen. You can then select the most appropriate MeSH term from that list and directly replace your first search word with an official MeSH term.

Although not all MEDLINE search systems will allow further divisions of headings to be seen on the search screen, even the most specific MeSH heading can be further separated into its own components using **subheadings.** We discuss this in the next section.

Narrow your searches with specific modifiers

At the beginning of this example search, we proposed that we were going to look for articles about the therapy of CML, and, in particular, we wanted clinical trial information. So far, we have determined that there are 2126 citations (within the last 5 years, that is—the MEDLINE database is divided into components of 5 years at a time—we will revisit this concept later) about CML. But we don't want to look through all of them to find the ones relevant to our needs. We need to narrow, or focus, our search.

The reader probably already suspects that some of these 2126 articles have as their primary focus nonclinical aspects of CML (like its genetics or epidemiology) or even other diseases, that certainly not all are clinical trials, and that some may be in journals that our library does not carry. How can we further focus our search to retrieve just the relevant article citations?

The most successful approach remains trying to find one relevant article and then discovering how it is specifically indexed, rather than trying to start with "the perfect search term." To find this relevant article after searching broadly, most software packages created for MEDLINE searching allow you to narrow your search by (1) using modifiers called "check tags" (date, journal subset or title, language, or publication type) and (2) restricting title/keyword/subject search statements, using Boolean logic, with other title words, keywords, or subject statements. Most packages also allow you to use *subheading* modifiers, but these terms can modify only official MeSH headings, not keywords or title words.

Most searches are performed with a series of individual search terms, with each successive line of a search modifying the one before it in the Boolean fashion already described. To decrease the number of articles retrieved, while simultaneously increasing the specificity of your overall search, the **search modifiers** discussed next are generally used on successive lines of the search or in different fields (Figure 5–3). In GRATEFUL MED, note that not only "subjects" need go into the subject field. However, words other than "subjects" in this field may need two discrete notations: (1) a backslash (/) at the beginning of the word to tell GRATEFUL MED not to change the text to a MeSH term and (2) a parenthetical modifier to ensure recognition as something other than a MeSH term. A good example of the use of the backslash is provided in Figure 5–5, which shows that the word "explode"—a command—should not be searched as a MeSH term. Each of the important parenthetical modifiers, with examples, is discussed below.

Check tags

Check tags are MeSH terms that are applied broadly to a large number of articles. In Figure 5–1, several of the MeSH terms ("MH" in the left columns) are check tags in MEDLINE: adolescence; adult; aged; aged, 80 and over; female; human; male; and middle age. Check tags are thus a very general way to limit searches. In a Boolean modification of any search term in Melvyl, you could choose "and xs human" to make sure that no purely animal models of the disease of interest are included ("xs" stands for "exact subject," which is the way

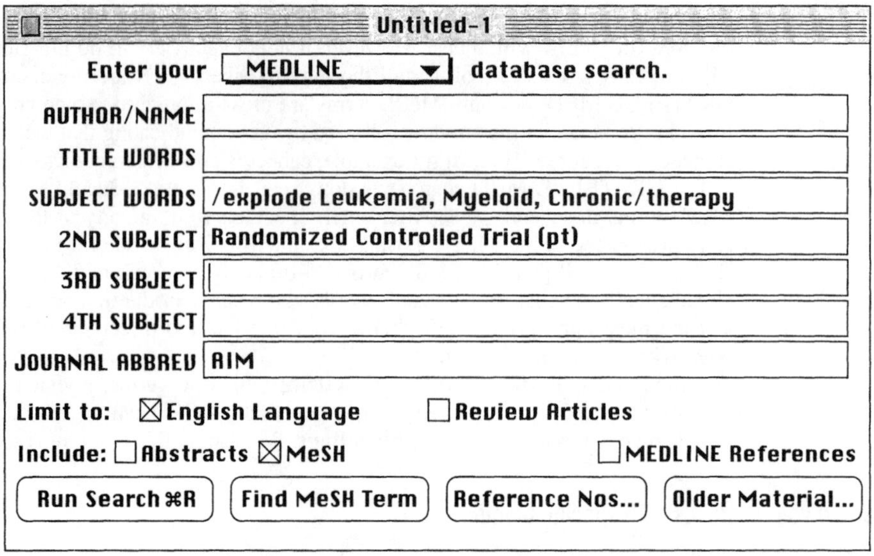

Figure 5–5. Sample exploded search in GRATEFUL MED search window.

Melvyl denotes these check tags). Articles that discuss both animal *and* human models together, however, would be found. If you wanted no animal data at all, you could limit your search with "and not xs animal." The complete list of check tags applying to species, genders, ages, article types, and monetary support categories is provided as Table 5–1. GRATEFUL MED allows you to use the check tag terms as subjects (MeSH terms) in restricting searches.

TABLE 5–1. CHECK TAG OPTIONS IN MEDLINE.

Check Tag Type	Check Tag Name	Comments
Species	Human	
	Animal	
	Mice	
	Rats	
	In vitro	
Gender	Female	
	Male	
Age	Infant, Newborn	From birth to 1 month
	Infant	Age 1–23 months
	Child, Preschool	Age 2–5 years
	Child	Age 6–12 years
	Adolescence	Age 13–18 years
	Adult	Age 19–44 years
	Middle Age	Age 45–64 years
	Aged	Age 65 and older
	Aged, 80 and over	Age 80 and older
Article type	Case Report	
	Comparative Study	
Support category	Support, Non-U.S. Gov't	
	Support, U.S. Gov't, Non-P.H.S.	
	Support, U.S. Gov't, P.H.S.	

Date

An often-overlooked modifier is the date. The MEDLARS database includes articles published beginning in 1966, although many software packages search only 3–5 years at any one time, including Melvyl and GRATEFUL MED (as their default settings). Often, you will want only very recent articles. You may choose to limit by year ("and date 1996" for 1996 publications), several years ("and date 1994–1996"), a particular month or months ("and date 3/96–5/96"), or even a single day ("and date 6/26/96") (although not all software packages allow this last option). GRATEFUL MED allows you to include any group of years in any search by clicking on the "Older Material" button in the search window (Figure 5–3). Using a parenthetical modifier technique for year of publication, you could limit your search to 1996 articles by typing the following into one of the subject lines: "/1996 (yr)."

Individual journal title

Occasionally, the searcher will want to quickly find a particular article, knowing some of the article's title words and the journal in which it was published. Some searchers may want to download the entire set of abstracts from a particular journal each time the journal is published. Individual journal titles can be searched, although to do so in the most specific manner, you must know the three-letter code of the "JC" field in the unit record (look back at Figure 5–1; *Archives of Internal Medicine* is "7FS") or know the journal's *Index Medicus* title abbreviation (in this case, Arch Intern Med). However, you can type only a portion of the journal title and retrieve a relatively small number of journals; this is the most efficient method. For example, in Melvyl, the Boolean modifier "and journal archives" would limit your search (keyword, title word, or MeSH heading) to the small number of journals with the word "archives" in their official title. GRATEFUL MED has a separate Journal Abbreviation field to limit your search if desired (see Figure 5–3), and the three-letter codes of the most-read 120 journals are included in the software (accessible from the Help menu).

Journal subsets

Most searchers will be looking not for a single journal article, however, but a series of articles about a particular topic, published in quality journals. A major point of the evidence-based medicine approach in general, and of this book in particular, is to seek only the highest quality published information, which means information published in high-quality, peer-reviewed journals. A practitioner of medicine cannot possibly read every related article published worldwide (although it usually takes a conscious effort to "lose the guilt" associated with this realization!). Furthermore, if you wish to retrieve an article after performing a search, the search will have done you no good if a retrieved article is published in a journal your local medical library does not carry. To restrict searches to journals you are more likely to retrieve, particular journal subsets can be used to modify broad initial search terms.

The journals of the MEDLINE database—about 4000 in total—are grouped into four discrete journal subsets: Abridged Index Medicus (or "aim"—the most widely read 120 journals), cancer core, dental, and nursing. Not every one of these 4000 journals, however, is in any one subset or in only one. Most medical libraries carry the aim journals, so aim is the best limiter for most searchers. The Boolean operator for this option is straightforward: "and subs aim," or "and subs dental," or "and not subs dental." In GRATEFUL MED, the particular term (eg, "aim") can be typed in the Journal Abbreviation field. To use a subject field for this, you must use a parenthetical modifier. That is, denote a subset with "(sb)." For example, if you placed the words "/nursing (sb)" into a subject field, the search would be restricted to the nursing subset.

Languages

Most readers will be interested in limiting their searches to the English language. Limiting a search with "and language English" will result in the retrieval of articles whose abstracts are in English—the remaining text of the article may or may not be in English. The list of all possible language limiters is provided in Table 5–2. In MEDLINE, all non-English

TABLE 5–2. LANGUAGE OPTIONS IN MEDLINE.

Three-letter Code	Language	Three-letter Code	Language
AFR	Afrikaans	KOR	Korean
ALB	Albanian	LIT	Lithuanian
ARA	Arabic	MAC	Macedonian
ARM	Armenian	MUL	Multilingual
AZE	Azerbaijani	NOR	Norwegian
BUL	Bulgarian	PER	Persian
CHI	Chinese	POL	Polish
CZE	Czech	POR	Portuguese
DAN	Danish	PUS	Pushto
DUT	Dutch	RUM	Rumanian
ENG	English	RUS	Russian
FIN	Finnish	SCC	Serbocroatian/Cyrillic
FRE	French	SCR	Serbocroatian/Roman
GEO	Georgian	SLO	Slovak
GER	German	SLV	Slovene
GRE	Greek	SPA	Spanish
HEB	Hebrew	SWA	Swahili
HUN	Hungarian	SWE	Swedish
ICE	Icelandic	THA	Thai
IND	Indonesian	TUR	Turkish
ITA	Italian	UKR	Ukrainian
JPN	Japanese	VIE	Vietnamese

language modifiers are also listed as "foreign," so that the database is divided not just into 44 separate language categories, but also into two main language categories, "ENG" and "FOR." GRATEFUL MED makes the selection simple; by checking the English Language box, all retrievals will be articles with English abstracts.

Publication types

The nearly 10 million articles abstracted in MEDLINE include a variety of types of articles. Many "articles" are not original publications in the usual sense, however; some are letters to the editor, editorials, or medical news summaries. Others are reviews or meta-analyses or even consensus development conferences. The publication type modifier is thus extremely powerful for limiting your search. For example, many searchers looking for general information about a topic can limit their initial search to "and pt review" to obtain review articles, which will usually have substantial bibliographies, providing the searcher with additional relevant articles. The complete list of publication type options and their corresponding codes is provided in Table 5–3.

In Melvyl, you can directly limit a search term in its Boolean search language with "and pt meta-analysis," for example. In GRATEFUL MED and other software, the syntax is different. Searches for review articles are accomplished simply by clicking in the Review box on the screen. Other publication types can be specified in the subject search fields by using the parenthetical modifier (pt). Typing "/meta-analysis (pt)," for example, results in a publication type search, not a subject search.

For the searcher interested in gathering primary published evidence regarding specific tests or therapies, limiting searches to publication types such as "clinical trial," "controlled

TABLE 5–3. TYPES OF PUBLICATIONS IN MEDLINE.*

Code	Full name	Code	Full name
ABST	Abstract	JOUR	Journal article (limit only)
BIBL	Bibliography	LEGA	Legal brief
CLAS	Classical article	LETT	Letter
CLCN	Clinical conference	MEET	Meeting report
CLTR	Clinical trial	META	Meta-analysis
CTP1	Clinical trial, phase I	MONO	Monograph
CTP2	Clinical trial, phase II	MULT	Multicenter study
CTP3	Clinical trial, phase III	NEWS	News
CTP4	Clinical trial, phase IV	NART	Newspaper article
COMM	Comment	OVER	Overall
CONG	Congress	PERI	Periodical index
CDCE	Consensus development conference	PRAC	Practice guideline
CDCN	Consensus development conference NIH	ERRA	Published erratum
CONT	Controlled clinical trial	RAND	Randomized controlled trial
CORR	Corrected and republished	RETA	Retracted publication
CURR	Current biog-obit	RETO	Retraction of publication
DICT	Dictionary	REVX	Review (limit only)
DIRY	Directory	REVA	Review academic
DUPL	Duplicate publication	REVL	Review literature
EDIT	Editorial	REVM	Review multicase
FEST	Festschrift	REVR	Review of reported cases
GUID	Guideline	REVT	Review tutorial
HISA	Historical article	SCIE	Scientific integrity review
HISB	Historical biography	TECH	Technical report
INTE	Interview	TWIN	Twin study

*Publication types marked Review plus another term are narrower types of Review. Citations indexed under these publication types are always also indexed under the more general publication type REVIEW.

clinical trial," "randomized controlled trial," or "multicenter study," can be extremely helpful. "Meta-analysis" and "practice guideline" terms may themselves lead to articles with extensive bibliographies of primary data.

Subheadings

As emphasized repeatedly in this chapter, subheading modifiers of MeSH headings provide the most powerful tools to restrict a search to only the most relevant articles about a particular topic—while simultaneously decreasing the likelihood that any relevant articles will be omitted from a search. Permitting the searcher to maximize the specificity of their searches, subheadings are used to modify MeSH terms by limiting retrieved articles to a *specific aspect* of a biomedical concept. The complete list of MEDLINE subheadings comprises Table 5–4; however, not all subheadings are applicable to each of the 16,000 MeSH headings that exist (as of December 1996). For most searches, you will discover the best subheading after finding the "one good article." But subheadings can be used in initial searches as well to help restrict the focus of the articles initially retrieved.

A few software programs, such as Melvyl, will generate, using the browse command, a display of subheadings available for each MeSH term. What follows here is the screen output list of subheadings available for "Leukemia, Myeloid, Chronic," in the format of Melvyl, by asking the computer to "display the long format" after using the browse command.

TABLE 5–4. SUBHEADINGS AVAILABLE IN MEDLINE USED TO MODIFY MeSH SEARCH TERMS.

abnormalities	epidemiology	physiopathology
administration & dosage	ethnology	poisoning
adverse effects	etiology	prevention & control
agonists	genetics	psychology
analogs & derivatives	growth & development	radiation effects
analysis	history	radiography
anatomy & histology	immunology	radionuclide imaging
antagonists & inhibitors	in adolescence	radiotherapy
biosynthesis	in adulthood	rehabilitation
blood	in infancy & childhood	secondary
blood supply	in middle age	secretion
cerebrospinal fluid	in old age	standards
chemical synthesis	in pregnancy	statistics & numerical data
chemically induced	instrumentation	supply & distribution
chemistry	isolation & purification	surgery
classification	legislation & jurisprudence	therapeutic use
complications	manpower	therapy
congenital	metabolism	toxicity
contraindications	methods	trends
cytology	microbiology	transmission
deficiency	mortality	transplantation
diagnosis	nursing	ultrasonography
diet therapy	organization & administration	ultrastructure
drug effects	parasitology	urine
drug therapy	pathogenicity	utilization
economics	pathology	veterinary
education	pharmacokinetics	virology
embryology	pharmacology	
enzymology	physiology	

Leukemia, Myeloid, Chronic.
[2,000 citations including all subheadings]

SUBHEADINGS:		citations	SUBHEADINGS:		citations
5.1	Leukemia, Myeloid, Chronic [Used alone]	160	5.16	immunology.	147
			5.17	metabolism.	123
5.2	blood.	201	5.18	microbiology.	9
5.3	cerebrospinal fluid.	3	5.19	mortality.	119
5.4	chemically induced.	9	5.20	nursing.	2
5.5	classification.	11	5.21	pathology.	596
5.6	complications.	148	5.22	physiopathology.	36
5.7	congenital.	3	5.23	psychology.	4
5.8	diagnosis.	121	5.24	radiography.	2
5.9	drug therapy.	268	5.25	radionuclide imaging.	2
5.10	economics.	1	5.26	radiotherapy.	14
5.11	enzymology.	54	5.27	surgery.	240
5.12	epidemiology.	43	5.28	therapy.	360
5.13	etiology.	36	5.29	ultrasonography.	3
5.14	genetics.	598	5.30	urine.	2
5.15	history.	2	5.31	veterinary.	2

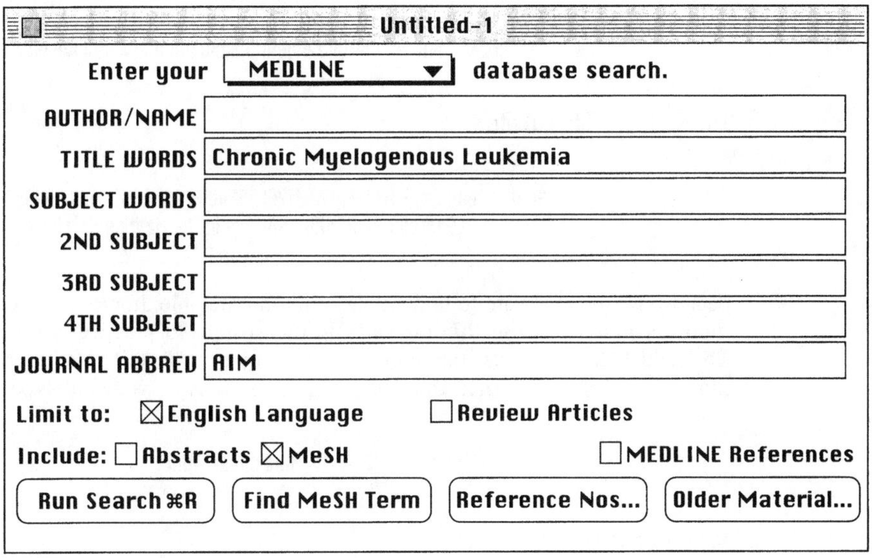

```
┌─────────────────────────────────────────────────────────────┐
│ ≣▢▦▦▦▦▦▦▦▦▦▦▦▦▦▦  Untitled-1  ▦▦▦▦▦▦▦▦▦▦▦▦▦▦▦▦ │
├─────────────────────────────────────────────────────────────┤
│                                                               │
│     Enter your  ┌ MEDLINE       ▼ ┐ database search.          │
│                                                               │
│   AUTHOR/NAME  ┌────────────────────────────────────────────┐│
│                └────────────────────────────────────────────┘│
│   TITLE WORDS  ┌ Chronic Myelogenous Leukemia ───────────────┐│
│                └────────────────────────────────────────────┘│
│  SUBJECT WORDS ┌────────────────────────────────────────────┐│
│                └────────────────────────────────────────────┘│
│   2ND SUBJECT  ┌────────────────────────────────────────────┐│
│                └────────────────────────────────────────────┘│
│   3RD SUBJECT  ┌────────────────────────────────────────────┐│
│                └────────────────────────────────────────────┘│
│   4TH SUBJECT  ┌────────────────────────────────────────────┐│
│                └────────────────────────────────────────────┘│
│ JOURNAL ABBREU ┌ AIM ───────────────────────────────────────┐│
│                └────────────────────────────────────────────┘│
│                                                               │
│  Limit to:  ☒ English Language    ☐ Review Articles           │
│  Include: ☐ Abstracts ☒ MeSH              ☐ MEDLINE References │
│  ┌ Run Search ⌘R ┐ ┌ Find MeSH Term ┐ ┌ Reference Nos... ┐ ┌ Older Material... ┐ │
│  └───────────────┘ └────────────────┘ └──────────────────┘ └───────────────────┘ │
└─────────────────────────────────────────────────────────────┘
```

Figure 5–6. Sample search in GRATEFUL MED search window.

Unfortunately, most software packages, including GRATEFUL MED, do not provide a list of subheadings available for each separate MeSH heading. However, MeSH terms that double as subheadings are denoted in the Find MeSH Term window by the suffix (sh).

The method of modifying any search with a particular subheading depends on the MEDLINE-searching software being used. In Melvyl, the user simply appends the subheading to the MeSH term—without commas or hyphens. Note, however, that some *MeSH terms* may be more than one word, separated by commas. For example, "find subject Leukemia, Myeloid, Chronic drug therapy" searches for articles on drug therapy of CML and focus on issues of therapy rather than on its diagnosis, epidemiology, genetics, or pathology. In Internet Grateful Med, the searcher is presented with a column of subheadings with "checkboxes" that can be selected with a click of the computer's mouse or equivalent. In standard GRATEFUL MED (non–CD-ROM, non-Internet), MeSH headings are modified with a backslash before and after the MeSH term, followed by the subheading—the standard format in the unit record (Figure 5–1). In our example, then, you would type "/Leukemia, Myeloid, Chronic/therapy." Alternatively, the word "therapy" could be used on a separate subject line with its parenthetical modifier (sh); eg, "/therapy (sh)" to modify a previous subject search line term, such as "Leukemia, Myeloid, Chronic." Whatever the method of modifying subheading searches available in a particular software, it is well worth using.

The student of evidence-based medicine is referred in particular to such subheadings as "adverse effects;" "complications" or "toxicity;" "diagnosis" or "prevention and control;" "radiography," "radionuclide imaging," or "ultrasonography;" and "drug therapy," "surgery," or "therapy."

After narrowing your search with modifiers, you are now in a position to find the single relevant article that will lead to others. Let's put these concepts into practice by searching for controlled trials about the therapy of CML.

Find one relevant article that leads to others: sample search

For our sample search, we'll start with a **broad approach,** using title words and limiting to the English language. Note that unless a term is specifically marked as an official MeSH heading, most software will assume the term is some form of text word (title or keyword) rather than denoting it as a subject. GRATEFUL MED gives you a single screen in which to formulate a search, and our initial search screen is shown in Figure 5–6. However, it is helpful to understand how the individual steps in this search are performed (in the background by GRATEFUL MED); therefore, we will show each Boolean limiter, using sequential narrowing terms in Melvyl:

find tw chronic myelogenous leukemia and lan eng

The Melvyl system replies:

 Search request: F TW CHRONIC MYELOGENOUS LEUKEMIA AND LANGUAGE ENGLISH
Search result: 420 citations in the Medline database

Because we usually want to find articles only in reputable, library-held journals, we should choose a **journal subset limiter** early in our search. In practice, you will usually select Abridged Index Medicus (the most widely read journals). GRATEFUL MED allows us to choose "aim" in the Journal Abbreviation field. In Melvyl, we would type:

 and subset aim

and obtain the result:

 Search request: F TW CHRONIC MYELOGENOUS LEUKEMIA AND LAN ENG AND SUBS AIM
Search result: 97 citations in the Medline database

This is still too many articles to try to read, so we must narrow the selection further. Often, only very recent articles are needed, so we can limit by **date.** In GRATEFUL MED, this option is limited to specific database years (listed by clicking the "Older Material" box); other software, such as Melvyl, allow more focused date modification, for example:

 and date 96

which leads to:

 Search request: F TW CHRONIC MYELOGENOUS LEUKEMIA AND LAN ENG AND SUBS AIM AND DATE 96
Search result: 14 citations in the Medline database

We could narrow our search even further, such as by looking just for clinical trials (a publication type). At some point, however, probably when you have retrieved between 50 and 100 citations, you will want to look at the titles and perhaps the abstracts of your citations. With some systems, you may do this while engaged on-line with MEDLINE; however, if there is a cost involved with log-on time, you will want to peruse your citations quickly. With GRATEFUL MED, you can retrieve the articles so that you may peruse them while "off-line," in the Results window. You may also print or save them to a file on your microcomputer. With Melvyl, you can scroll through the titles individually (only the first five are shown here) just by typing "display":

 display

1. Enright H; Davies SM; DeFor T; Shu X; Weisdorf D; Miller W; Ramsay NH; Arthur D; Verfaillie C; Miller J; et al. Relapse after non-T-cell-depleted allogeneic bone marrow transplantation for chronic myelogenous leukemia: early transplantation, use of an unrelated donor, and chronic graft-versus-host disease are protective. Blood, 1996 Jul 15, 88[2]:714—20.

2. Laporte JP; Gorin NC; Rubinstein P; Lesage S; Portnoi MF; Barbu V; Lopez M; Douay L; Najman A. Cord-blood transplantation from an unrelated donor in an adult with chronic myelogenous leukemia. New England Journal of Medicine, 1996 Jul 18, 335[3]167—70.

3. Wells SJ; Phillips CN; Winton EF; Farhi DC. Reverse transcriptase-polymerase chain reaction for bcr/abl fusion in chronic myelogenous leukemia. American Journal of Clinical Pathology, 1996 Jun, 105[6]:756—60.

4. Cortes J; Kantarjian H; O'Brien S; Robertson LE; Pierce S; Talpaz M. Result of interferon-alpha therapy in patients with chronic myelogenous leukemia 60 years of age and older. American Journal of Medicine, 1996 Apr, 100[4]:452—5.

5. Hochhaus A; Lin F; Reiter A; Skladny H; Mason PJ; van Rhee F; Shepherd PC; Allan NC; Hehlmann R; Goldman JM; et al. Quantification of residual disease in chronic myelogenous leukemia patients on interferon-alpha therapy by competitive polymerase chain reaction. Blood, 1996 Feb 15, 87[4]:1549—55.

For the purposes of our example (clinical articles about the therapy of CML), article No. 4 seems appropriate. We should probably look at its abstract to confirm our hunch. We can view the abstract by choosing certain display options, which are usually prominently available in most software programs. In GRATEFUL MED, for example, abstracts are seen by clicking in the Include Abstracts box before you send the search term to the MEDLINE database. Of more importance, now that we have found our "one relevant (good) article," we can determine how it—and other articles like it—are best indexed and thus retrieved in MEDLINE. To do this, we need to display this article in a format that will show the MeSH terms under which the article is indexed. In GRATEFUL MED, these terms are seen by clicking on the Include MeSH box on the search field window before the search is activated and then looking at the citations in the Results window. In Melvyl, we can display all the unit record information by typing "display long abstract" or "display MEDLINE":

display long abs 4

Author: Cortes J; Kantarjian H; O'Brien S; Robertson LE; Pierce S; Talpaz M.
Address: Department of Hematology, University of Texas, M.D. Anderson Cancer Center, Houston 77030, USA.
Title: Result of interferon-alpha therapy in patients with chronic myelogenous leukemia 60 years of age and older.
Journal: American Journal of Medicine, 1996 Apr, 100[4]:452—5.
Unique ID: 96194608.
Language: English.
Subset: Abridged Index Medicus [AIM]; Cancer Core journals.
Subject:

Age Factors.	Aged.
Antineoplastic Agents——administration & dosage.	Antineoplastic Agents——adverse effects.
*Antineoplastic Agents——therapeutic use.	Basophils——pathology.
Bone Marrow——pathology.	Chronic Disease.
Comparative Study.	Fatigue——etiology.
Follow-Up Studies.	Human.
Hydroxyurea——administration & dosage.	Hydroxyurea——adverse effects.
Hydroxyurea——therapeutic use.	Interferon Type II——administration & dosage.
Interferon Type II——adverse effects.	Interferon Type II——therapeutic use.
Interferon-alpha——administration & dosage.	Interferon-alpha——adverse effects.
*Interferon-alpha——therapeutic use.	Leukemia, Myeloid, Chronic——pathology.
*Leukemia, Myeloid, Chronic——therapy.	Leukemia, Myeloid, Philadelphia-Positive——pathology.
Leukemia, Myeloid, Philadelphia-Positive——therapy.	Middle Age.
Nervous System Diseases——etiology.	Remission Induction.
Survival Rate.	Texas.

To ensure applicability to our clinical question, let's assume we have read the abstract (it comes up with this command but is not reproduced here). We can now see the official MeSH headings, with areas of major emphasis marked by asterisks (see Figure 5–2 under "MeSH heading" for the difference between simple indexing and areas of major emphasis). The most relevant MeSH heading for our search is set in boldface type (just for our book), *now with its subheading* (therapy), separated by an em dash. We have therefore learned that the best MeSH heading is the one we saw in our "browse" command earlier. However, it is worth noting that other MeSH terms, not seen in our more general browse of chronic leukemias, may also be quite specific for CML (eg, Leukemia, Myeloid, Philadelphia-Positive) and could be used to tailor additional searches. Now, however, our task is to retrieve additional articles that are highly similar to the one we've just found.

Expand (explode) your focused subject/subheading search

The previous search's retrieved MeSH headings did not stand alone; beneath each were specific subheadings. We had the option of choosing articles specifically about the *pathology* of CML, or about its *therapy*. Use of these subheadings, identified above, increases the specificity of your search in a way that keyword or title word searching cannot. Keywords may be ideas merely "mentioned" in an abstract, trivially related to the real gist of the article. You wouldn't want your library cluttered with such "irrelevant" articles. To make the most of the high specificity lent to searches by the use of these subheadings, however, it's best to simultaneously **broaden** and **focus** the MeSH heading to which the subheading is appended. There are two ways to do this, once you have identified the MeSH term and subheading that are a major emphasis of your newly found relevant article (in the unit record format [Figure 5–1], the MeSH term denoted with an asterisk).

The first way to use this MeSH term/subheading combination is to formulate a new search, thereby limiting retrieved articles by making this combination the major focus of all the articles. In GRATEFUL MED, this is accomplished by clicking in the "Major Concepts Only" box when a specific MeSH term is used (itself obtained after clicking the "Find MeSH Term" box on the main search field window). This places an asterisk before the MeSH term during the search, ensuring that only those articles with that MeSH term asterisked in their unit records (see Figure 5–2) are retrieved. In Melvyl, the MeSH term is modified by using "major exact subject" or "MXS" as the limiter, eg, "find MXS Leukemia, Myeloid, Chronic therapy." The difference between this search and "find Leukemia, Myeloid, Chronic therapy" is that articles that are mainly about nontherapeutic aspects of CML, but that still discuss therapy, will be found in the latter but not in the former.

The second way to broaden yet focus a search is to confirm that we have the best MeSH term by making sure we have also included all MeSH headings that might be subcategories of "Leukemia, Myeloid, Chronic" in the MeSH tree structure. The command to do this is "explode." This option is available in most sophisticated MEDLINE-searching software packages. The subcategories for the MeSH term "Leukemia" is seen in Figure 5–4. Exploding "Leukemia" retrieves all articles in all of the indented subcategories shown in the figure. When you select an "explodable" MeSH term in GRATEFUL MED, the term is preferentially searched in the exploded manner, although you can "un-explode" by a mouse click in the "More Specific Terms" box in the MeSH term window (this is the window you see when you click on the "Find MeSH Term" button of Figures 5–3, 5–5, and 5–6). In Melvyl, the search term is "xxs," for "exploded exact subject." So to find all of the articles we want in our current search, we type:

 f xxs leukemia, myeloid, chronic therapy and lan eng

and obtain the result:

 Search request: F XXS LEUKEMIA, MYELOID, CHRONIC THERAPY AND LANGUAGE ENGLISH
Search result: 468 citations in the Medline database

This now represents the largest highly specific search obtainable for our example, giving you all articles about the therapy of CML in English in the last 5 years. The search was accomplished by using every MeSH term indented beneath "Leukemia, Myeloid, Chronic" in Figure 5–4, but remained highly specific by our appending the subheading "therapy" to each of those MeSH terms.

Note that in this new search we have not yet "re-limited" to journal subsets, etc. We can do this now, using the same methods described earlier. We certainly should impose these limiting factors, because in many systems, such as GRATEFUL MED, the greater the number of citations we retrieve, the more money we spend—whether or not the citations are "good."

Because our main goal has been to look at therapeutic interventions, we might want to select only randomized trials, rather than, say, review articles. Randomized trials are a publication type. In GRATEFUL MED, we can type "/randomized controlled trial (pt)" in any subject search field. In Melvyl, we continue to modify the most recent search term with another Boolean "and" term:

 and pt randomized controlled trial

and obtain:

 Search request: F XXS LEUKEMIA, MYELOID, CHRONIC THERAPY AND PT RANDOMIZED CONTROLLED TRIAL AND LANGUAGE ENGLISH
Search result: 22 citations in the Medline database

Although this is probably a very reasonable number of articles to retrieve and examine in their entirety, we could further limit the search to *particular* journal subsets. For our example, we'll use the aim (Abridged Index Medicus), although another subset, "cancer core" might also be appropriate (there is great overlap between the two subsets). In Melvyl, the next Boolean limiter in this case would be:

 and subs aim

to obtain the final result:

 Search request: F [XXS LEUKEMIA, MYELOID, CHRONIC THERAPY AND PT RANDOMIZED CONTROLLED TRIAL] AND SUBS AIM AND LANGUAGE ENGLISH
Search result: 9 citations in the Medline database

We could now review these articles to be certain, but we have probably just found the nine most important, most relevant citations published in the last 5 years about our topic, selected from more than 8 million potential citations in MEDLINE.

Figure 5–5 shows the "single-screen" version of the search we have just completed, line-by-line, in GRATEFUL MED. Note in particular the need to manually type the backslashes in the subject words field to ensure that the subheading modification of the MeSH term "Leukemia, Myeloid, Chronic" is used during the search.

BYPASSING MeSH—THE METATHESAURUS

Although the best way to refine a search remains identifying the most suitable MeSH heading modified by one or more subheadings, the NLM is currently developing (and some MEDLINE-searching software such as Internet Grateful Med uses already) an easier way to perform subject searches of the MEDLARS database: the Unified Medical Language System

(UMLS) **Metathesaurus.** This large grouping of multiple sources of knowledge preserves the main hierarchies of each system, while creating direct links of different names for the same concepts (eg, synonyms and even translations from other languages). The goal is to be able to have links between different types of databases, such as MEDLINE and an "expert diagnostic system," such as DxPLAIN (an online differential diagnosis generator developed at Harvard Medical School). For the MEDLINE searcher, this means that the more "commonplace" terms or concepts that are not themselves MeSH headings will be directly translated by the software into the proper MeSH heading during a search. Such translation already occurs, albeit on a small scale, in GRATEFUL MED, with the "cross-referenced" terms denoted by an appended "(xr)" seen in the MeSH list. But the function is not comprehensive. Regardless of the cross-referencing capabilities of future systems, finding out how a specific article is indexed will always be of great value. Still, the modified adage, "Close counts in horseshoes, hand grenades, bad breath, and MEDLINE subject searches" may soon be true!

DISPLAYING, SAVING, & PRINTING MEDLINE SEARCH INFORMATION

Once a search has been performed and appropriate articles identified, the MEDLINE searcher still needs to receive that information in a usable fashion; it must be taken "beyond the screen." This function is quite nonstandardized among MEDLINE searching software. GRATEFUL MED, which retrieves the articles during a brief search inquiry of the MEDLARS database after the searcher troubleshoots and narrows the search on their own computer, downloads the unit record information to the user's computer. The unit record can be seen in the Results window, saved to a file, or printed directly to a printer connected to the user's computer. Other software, however, including Melvyl, initially retrieves only the citations' title and author information, and it is up to the user to decide how much of the unit record information they would like to see: the title/author/journal information ("display"), complete abstracts in addition to those fields ("display abs"), or the entire "MEDLINE version," with MeSH headings, etc ("display long abs" or "display med").

There are four standard print/display options available in MEDLINE, although the interface with your computer may vary. The official "print" commands in MEDLINE—*Print* (includes authors, title, source fields), *Print Full* (adds language, MeSH headings, publication types), *Print Abstract* (adds abstract but not MeSH headings or publication type), and *Print Detailed* (every field available is printed)—are not actually commands to your printer. They are commands for MEDLINE to display this information to your screen. In practice, these commands are used rarely; your software has its own terms.

Your software also determines whether information obtained in a search is subsequently available on your hard disk or prints to an attached printer, or whether you have to take separate steps to download to your computer what is printed only to the screen. This is particularly true with most modem connections to the MEDLINE database if you do not use GRATEFUL MED. If you use the Melvyl system, for example, typing "display cont med" will cause your articles to scroll by continuously on your screen in the "MEDLINE format" (actually the print detailed command). But unless you have turned on the ability to "capture" that *screen* to *your* hard drive (using the telecommunications software you used to dial the MEDLINE database), you can't keep that information for later use. Most telecommunications software uses a "toggle on" command, usually called "file capture," "session capture," "start capture," "spool to disk," or similar wording, which you initiate just before displaying the articles you want, in the format you wish to see them, so that the screen display is brought to your computer. You do have to turn the "toggle off," however, when you're done, or everything else you type will also be added to this new file until you stop capturing.

Since all information between the "toggle on" and "toggle off" has been saved, you may have to edit your file once it is captured (you might have done several unrelated searches in one sitting). Some MEDLINE-searching systems will let you edit a "list" of references while you are connected to MEDLINE, but before you capture the file information. In Melvyl, you can type "save 1,7,19,23" if only those numbered articles are wanted of a larger retrieved set, and they become articles 1–4 of a list, which then becomes the item that should be captured.

The format in which you obtain the "list"—or any retrieved series of articles—has important implications for later use. Preferred formats should include the MeSH terms, otherwise you would have to perform another search to get them if you wanted these terms later. In fact, to ensure maximum flexibility later, it is prudent to download your search results using the longest possible format (see below). If your search software will allow it (GRATEFUL MED does not), it's advisable to send the results of your search to yourself via email (in Melvyl, simply typing "mail" brings up a series of questions regarding your email address and the format you want your list sent in). In this way, your search takes up only "virtual space." Most important, if you would like to keep the results of a search for later use, bibliographic software programs (see page 124) will decipher the MEDLINE unit record (ie, the long) format so that you can create a reference library on your hard drive. In addition, you can insert these citations, while writing a paper, for example, in word processing software, without ever having to type a single letter of them. If you choose to save your search results in GRATEFUL MED, the file on your computer will automatically contain the field information necessary for interpretation by bibliographic software programs. You should probably save every search result; you can delete these files later, but you can't go back and get what you didn't save—without spending additional time and possibly money.

TIME-LIMITED SEARCHES & FUTURE UPDATES

Although the MEDLARS database includes literature from 1966 to the present, MEDLINE is divided into separate files, each containing literature published in approximately 5-year periods. When you search "MEDLINE," the database is composed of a 5-year period, with the current year foremost (in 1997, "MEDLINE" encompasses the years 1993–1997). The back files are (as called in Melvyl and MEDLINE both) "MED90" (1990–1992), "MED85" (1985–1989), "MED80" (1980–1984), "MED75" (1975–1979), and "MED66" (1966–1974). Although many software packages search the entire database from 1966 forward, quite a few do not. The user is typically confronted with choices, however, of which database years are to be considered. In Melvyl, you would simply type "MED90" at the usual MEDLINE prompt to switch database years, and the search you have completed in the 1993–1997 database will be performed in the new database by typing "REDO." In GRATEFUL MED, all or some of the database years can be searched by clicking on the appropriate boxes viewed when the "Older Material" button on the searching window (Figure 5–3) is clicked. The GRATEFUL MED default setting is the most recent 3 years.

Searching the past literature is the typical approach, but what about the future? The clinician may be interested in having a particular search term "set" for weeks, months, or even years after the first search is performed. In individual software packages, this option varies widely. In Melvyl, for example, you can type "update" and see a menu of options. You can select the appropriate options so that the computer will weekly perform any search automatically, and the results can be electronically mailed to you; this option can be renewed every 6 months.

In GRATEFUL MED, you can save a set of search terms as a unique file on your microcomputer. When you have performed a search and quit the software, you will be asked if you wish to save the search strategy as well as the search results. The search strategy may be named in whatever fashion you wish, with limitations provided only by your computer's operating system, and the search can be rerun in the future if you desire—without having to remember exactly what combination of MeSH terms and modifiers you used before.

MEDLARS provides two other methods for redoing searches. The first is that your software may allow you to use the MEDLARS "SAVESEARCH" option, whereby you can keep search term sets you have generated, even after you log off—an option not available with Melvyl. The second is that you may have access to "SDILINE," which is the same as MEDLINE, except that it contains only the previous 1 month of articles. GRATEFUL MED has this option, too; just click on the box that says "MEDLINE" at the top of the search window (Figures 5–3, 5–5, and 5–6), and it will appear as a database choice. Thus, you can redo a search without having to wade through articles you may have seen before. You may, of course, search all of MEDLINE and simply use a date modifier to get the same result. A new database being developed at the NLM, "PREMEDLINE," will allow you to search for articles that are in press but not yet available (except for their abstracts).

SOFTWARE ACCESS TO MEDLINE

Throughout this chapter we have alluded to various computer software packages that are the tools used to search MEDLINE. Each of these tools provides slightly different methods and use different terms. There are several ways to obtain software. Readers with an academic affiliation should call their academic center's medical library. This will usually put you on the right track toward getting the institution's preferred MEDLINE-searching software, usually at low or no cost because most institutions have prepaid arrangements with NLM. You may encounter restrictions on use, however. Melvyl, for example, is restricted to persons affiliated with the University of California.

Readers who do not have such an affiliation are encouraged to pursue the new World Wide Web (WWW)-based interfaces developed by the NLM, either Internet Grateful Med or PubMed. Both of these interfaces are free (once you are connected to the Internet, anyway—see Chapter 6 for details on the WWW and how to access it) and are consistent with the tools detailed in this chapter. Either a PC/Windows or Macintosh computer, a modem or Internet connection, and a Web Browser are all that is needed.

For those who have already have an Internet connection, the NLM home page contains all the information you need about both interfaces, and is at *http://www.nlm.nih.gov/*. Internet Grateful Med, along with its user's guide, is accessible at *http://www.igm.nlm.nih.gov*. PubMed is accessible at *http://www4.ncbi.nlm.nih.gov/PubMed/*.

GRATEFUL MED is another option, although it is not free at this time. It is available for either PC/Windows or Macintosh computers. Information on obtaining an account and password can be requested by mail at MEDLARS Management Section, National Library of Medicine, 8600 Rockville Pike, Bethesda, MD 20894; by phone at 1-800-638-8480; or by electronic mail to *mms@nlm.nih.gov*.

There are many alternatives to this software, and your colleagues may have paticular preferences. Several commercial WWW sites offer free MEDLINE searching to clinicians who, in exchange for this service, are asked to provide some demographic and personal information, and who may be subjected to on-line advertising from medically related companies. Three sites in 1998 offering this free service to health care providers are "Physicians Online," "Medscape," and "Healthgate." The reader is encouraged to search for these three names with their Web browser's search engine(s), since the direct Internet protocol addresses (uniform resource locator, or URL, discussed in Chapter 6) often change. *These interfaces, however, are not nearly as robust as PubMed, Internet Grateful Med, GRATEFUL MED, or Melvyl, in separating MeSH terms, subheadings, publication types, or journal subsets.* Caveat emptor.

USE OF BIBLIOGRAPHIC SOFTWARE WITH MEDLINE

Once citations are downloaded from the MEDLINE database with whatever software package you use, you may wish to save them not only in hard copy but also in electronic form. You may want to access them later; print them out for patients, colleagues, or students; or use them as references in a manuscript. Bibliographic software, such as the popular "EndNote Plus," allows you not only to have a keyword-searchable database on a floppy or hard disk but also to effortlessly insert references into a manuscript you are typing. Once inserted in the manuscript, the citations can be formatted automatically, renumbered in order no matter when or where you add a new reference, and printed at the end of your document—without you ever having to type a single character of any reference.

The usual procedure involves downloading the full "detailed" printout style of the MEDLINE search, which has both the abstract and MeSH terms for each article. With the use of "filters" (which are, unfortunately, often separate software acquisitions—EndNote requires "EndLink"), the bibliographic software packages will read your downloaded file and import the references into its own database, creating a library of articles on your computer. You can even have separate libraries for each topic of interest to you. Thus, each citation, including the abstract, will always be available electronically and can be manipulated, printed, used in word processing software programs, etc. To keep these libraries complete, you will need to enter into them articles of which you already have a hard copy. The best way to do this is to go back into MEDLINE, find the article you already have, and download and import the MEDLINE version with MeSH headings and abstract into the bibliographic software application.

SPECIFIC SUGGESTIONS FOR ENHANCING EVIDENCE-BASED MEDICINE WITH THE USE OF MEDLINE

The student of evidence-based medicine may have noticed that some MeSH headings in our examples could prove helpful when looking for specific types of information relevant to the study of evidence-based medicine, for example, the MeSH heading "Survival Rate." We may use this heading to limit searches to *specific* aspects of therapies that can be incorporated within evidence-based medicine concepts, rather than more *general* aspects of those therapies. A list of the terms most relevant for evidence-based medicine is provided in Table 5–5. In addition, suggested readings addressing this topic appear at the end of this chapter.

TABLE 5–5. MEDLINE TERMS RELEVANT TO EVIDENCE-BASED MEDICINE.

Type of MEDLINE Term	Term	Type of MEDLINE Term	Term
MeSH Headings	Bayes Theorem	Subheadings	adverse effects
	Clinical Trials		complications
	Cost-Benefit Analysis		diagnosis
	Costs and Cost Analysis		drug therapy
	Confidence Intervals		economics
	Data Interpretation, Statistical		epidemiology
	Decision Making		etiology
	Decision Making, Computer-Assisted		methods
	Decision Support Techniques		mortality
	Decision Trees		prevention and control
	Diagnosis		radiography
	Guidelines		radionuclide imaging
	Markov Chains		surgery
	Medical Informatics Applications		therapeutic use
	Odds Ratio		therapy
	Outcome Assessment		toxicity
	Practice Guidelines		ultrasonography
	Predictive Value of Tests	Publication Types	clinical trial
	Probability		meta-analysis
	Prospective Studies		multicenter study
	Sensitivity and Specificity		practice guideline
	Survival Analysis		randomized controlled trial
	Technology Assessment, Biomedical		review
	Therapy, Computer-Assisted		
	Treatment Outcome		

COMMON PITFALLS IN SEARCHING

Searching by subject

Because the MeSH headings are hierarchically arranged in the tree structures, "subjects" are often much less complete than "exploded subjects." For example, if you search the subject "heart diseases," this will occur:

 find su [subject] heart diseases——gives 1,848 citations

whereas

 find xxs [exploded exact subject] heart diseases——gives 23,412 citations

Hence, by subject searching alone, you would miss 21,564, or *92%,* of articles about heart diseases! Another example shows why:

 "Find xxs meningitis"

will include subject headings *within* (hierarchically) the major subject of meningitis (in Melvyl, seen by "browsing" the subject Meningitis; in GRATEFUL MED, seen in the MeSH term window):

1. Arachnoiditis
2. Lymphocytic Choriomeningitis
3. Meningitis
4. Meningitis, Aseptic
5. Meningitis, Haemophilus
6. Meningitis, Listeria
7. Meningitis, Meningococcal
8. Meningitis, Pneumococcal
9. Meningitis, Viral
10. Subdural Effusion
11. Tuberculosis, Meningeal

But, if you just search "find xs (exact subject) meningitis," you will retrieve only the articles under No. 3, the minor but *specific* subject of meningitis. Articles about only listeria, for example, *will not* show up in your search. What does this mean? The official MeSH terms mean different things depending on how you enter them in a search term: **XS** is the "eXact Subject"—you want that MeSH heading and no other. **MXS** (in Melvyl) describes articles that have as their **M**ajor focus that eXact Subject (heading would have an asterisk next to it in the unit record and in a GRATEFUL MED search—see sample search, page 119). The eXploded eXact Subject (**XXS**) will give you the most comprehensive yet specific term. GRATEFUL MED's default when using MeSH terms is to explode them unless you select otherwise in the "More Specific Terms" box seen on the MeSH heading window. Finally, if you use "Meningitis" as simply a "SUbject" term (**SU**) in either Melvyl or GRATEFUL MED, you will retrieve articles under categories 3–9, since the word "meningitis" is in the subject heading of each of those MeSH terms—each of them is a "meningitis subject." The reader may note that the check tags discussed previously were also "exact subjects," that is, highly specific subject terms, and therefore cannot be exploded.

Forgetting that your current search is date-limited

Melvyl and many other MEDLINE-searching software programs search only the last 5 years of the database. But many search topics may have been better studied *before* the last 5 years. Most software will allow you to change the years of the database you search, however. See page 123 for details.

Forgetting that you may search by title word

You may get too many search results with some software in which "keyword searching" is allowed. When stuck, try to guess what the title of an article is and search using the supposed title words. This strategy can also be effective if you cannot quickly find a good MeSH term using the GRATEFUL MED MeSH terms window.

Searching for information found more easily in textbooks

Such information might include incidence, prevalence, or pathophysiology of disease, for example.

Forgetting to download the article(s) of interest with their MeSH terms and abstracts

For bibliographic software, it is crucial to download with MeSH terms and abstracts, as discussed previously. It is a main point of this chapter, in fact, to encourage the evaluation of appropriate MeSH terms as a method of refining searches effectively. Future searches using these selected MeSH terms will then proceed quickly and accurately.

SUMMARY

Let's reiterate our strategy with the following steps. Our example is based on Melvyl but uses the Boolean limitation method of many software applications. GRATEFUL MED and other applications may allow a "single-screen" search, rather than a series of steps, however (see Figures 5–5 and 5–6).

1. Start most searches with the broadest possible search terms, which will usually be a *keyword* or a *title word*. Use truncated words in your search terms to help broaden your searches. Melvyl example:

 f kw bladder cancer and kw smok#

   (for smoke, -ing, -ers, -ed)
2. From a keyword or title word search, narrow your search to fewer than 100 or so with language, publication type, date, and/or journal subset. Melvyl example:

 and lan eng and pt review and date 96 and subs aim

3. When you have narrowed your search, use the appropriate display command to scroll through the titles. If you can, save individual article titles to a list that MEDLINE will make for you with each search session. At the end of scrolling, choose the most appropriate-appearing article titles and read their abstracts by displaying (or printing) a longer format ("d long abs" or "d long abs list" in Melvyl; both the Abstract and MeSH term boxes checked in GRATEFUL MED).
4. *If the abstract looks appropriate, read the subject headings under which the article is listed.* This will refine your search and help you find out what the "true" MeSH

headings—and subheadings—are for the subject in which you are interested. You can then create a new, comprehensive, but extremely efficient search using the explode command, relevant MeSH headings (each modified by a subheading), and other modifiers that further narrow the search. Melvyl example:

 f xxs bronchitis therapy and xxs antibiotic therapeutic use and pt rand

would obtain only randomized controlled trials evaluating the therapeutic use of antibiotics in bronchitis.

5. If you have a good search statement and have used it in a time-limited database, change databases to search earlier years (1966–1992 in the 1997 version of MEDLINE). In Melvyl and some other software, you can simply "redo" the search. In GRATEFUL MED, you simply check off the desired years in the "Older Material" window. In other software, you may have to first save your search terms.

6. Once you have a list of relevant articles, you can print them in a variety of ways. If you think you may need the references or the abstracts in the future, you should display and capture your list in the longest format. This way, you'll have both the abstracts and the MeSH headings. Next, save them on your computer. This computerized, downloaded search can later import the list of references into desktop bibliographic software, such as EndNote (see page 124).

7. The first six steps are for new searches. *If you already have* a relevant article in hand, and want others like it, look the article up in MEDLINE and search its MeSH headings!

SUGGESTED READING

Lowe HJ, Barnett GO: Understanding and using the medical subject headings (MeSH) vocabulary to perform literature searches. JAMA 1994;271:1103.

McKibbon KA et al: Beyond ACP Journal Club: How to harness MEDLINE for prognosis problems [editorial]. ACP J Club 1995;123:A12.

McKibbon KA, Walker-Dilks CJ: Beyond ACP Journal Club: How to harness MEDLINE for diagnostic problems [editorial]. ACP J Club 1994;121:A10.

McKibbon KA, Walker-Dilks CJ: Beyond ACP Journal Club: How to harness MEDLINE for therapy problems [editorial] [published erratum appears in ACP J Club 1994;121:A11]. ACP J Club 1994;121:A10.

McKibbon KA, Walker-Dilks CJ: Beyond ACP Journal Club: How to harness MEDLINE to solve clinical problems [editorial]. ACP J Club 1994;120:A10.

Walker-Dilks CJ et al: Beyond ACP Journal Club: How to harness MEDLINE for etiology problems [editorial]. ACP J Club 1994;121:A10.

SEARCHING THE INTERNET

J. Ben Davoren, MD, PhD

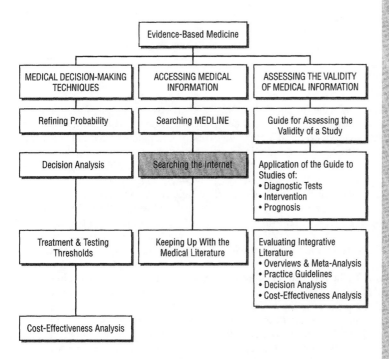

INTRODUCTION

Although the most important, best organized, and consistently updated repository of biomedical information in the world is the National Library of Medicine's MEDLINE database discussed in Chapter 5, there has been a phenomenal growth of other electronic "vaults of information" relevant to the practice of medicine. More and more, these sources, are being made available to individuals via **the Internet.** Information once available only in textbooks, journal articles, medical school course syllabi, newspaper articles, or by word of mouth now exists electronically, so that *anyone* with a personal computer and access to the Internet can obtain it. Simultaneously, anyone with the same access—physician, patient, expert, or layman—can *create* electronic "information," with or without peer review or significant censorship (at least after the highly publicized court injunction of the United States' Communications Decency Act in June of 1996).

In this chapter, we will provide a general overview of the Internet, as well as its relevance to the clinician, particularly the student of evidence-based medicine. A key point to remember is that, at the time of this writing, *the Internet is an evolving connection of computers—with changing connections, quality of information, and methods of accessibility—for which no government, organization, or group of people is responsible.*

To understand the Internet, you must understand four of its fundamental components: (1) the network of Internet connections; (2) computer hardware and software requirements; (3) connecting individual computers to the Internet; and (4) methods of transferring information via the Internet.

COMPONENTS OF THE INTERNET

The network of Internet connections

At the time of this writing, "the Internet," "the Net," and "the Web" are terms used in common conversations, newspaper headlines, and company boardrooms. These terms (the first two of which are synonymous) refer to a global network of computers linked in such a way that information can be transmitted rapidly from one computer to another—whether the recipient or sender is at a major institution of learning, a business, or a home (Figure 6–1). The information can be text, still pictures, video, or audio. Because the network is entirely electronic, information can travel at nearly the speed of light from one place to another. It is therefore possible to have minute-to-minute updates of world events, live video conferences halfway across the globe, or real-time Swan-Ganz catheter measurements sent from a patient's bedside to a consultant 6000 miles away. Although the methods used to transmit information across this system are very powerful, the Internet basically is "just wires," albeit organized very specifically.

What is now known as the Internet, really a global "network of networks," began in the late 1960s in the United States as Arpanet (Advanced Research Projects Agency), a network connecting major academic centers in the United States. Its initial purpose was to create a defense-oriented communications network that could operate after thermonuclear war. In 1986, the project was expanded and taken over by the National Science Foundation, creating NSFNet. This network can be thought of as a giant interconnected web of telephone wires (in fact, NSFNet is now defunct, with most of the wires owned by the Sprint and MCI telecommunications companies). More important than the wires is that different brands of computers, using different operating systems and software programs, can speak to each other in a common language called the **Internet Protocol** (IP). The development of IP is the key to the basic connections of the Internet. IP allows you to send electronic mail (email), pictures, text, or video to someone whose computer system may be entirely different from yours. The IP correctly translates the information so that your message arrives intact and "readable."

How does the Internet know where to send the information? Essentially, the transmission works just like a telephone call. Every computer on the network (including yours when you are "logged on") has a unique **IP address,** organized in a manner similar to the telephone number organization of country codes, area codes, and local numbers. The 14 "top-level" codes, called domain names, in the United States are listed in Table 6–1. You will note that, unlike area codes,

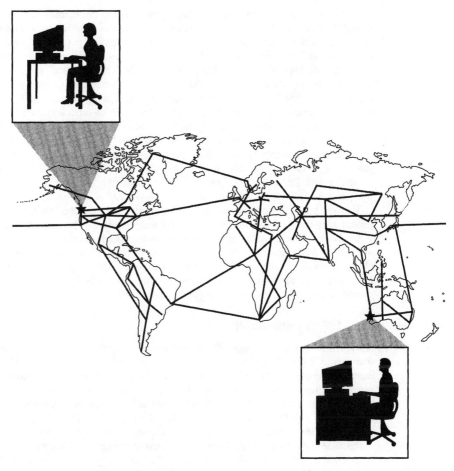

Figure 6–1. Internet connections: Worldwide and real-time. The Internet allows two or more computer users to share information simultaneously, no matter what the distance between users.

TABLE 6–1. INTERNET DOMAIN NAMES IN THE UNITED STATES.

com	Commercial sites
edu	Educational sites
int	International sites
gov	Governmental sites
mil	Military sites
net	Network sites
org	Organizational sites
firm	Businesses or firms
store	Businesses offering goods to purchase
web	Entities emphasizing world wide web activities
arts	Entities emphasizing culture, entertainment, or both
rec	Entities emphasizing recreation, entertainment, or both
info	Entities providing information services
nom	Individual or personal nomenclature

domain names are not necessarily geographic and are not usually written as numbers (although they are translated to numbers when one computer searches to contact another). A computer's IP address, such as for the main World Wide Web server (a central computer) at the University of California, San Francisco (UCSF), often stays as text, eg, *www.ucsf.edu*. Note that the top-level code appears *last*. The "ucsf" is essentially the "area code" within the greater domain of educational computers; UCSF is differentiated from other educational computers by the period between "ucsf" and "edu." All Internet-accessible computers at UCSF have addresses that end in ".ucsf.edu." Internet addresses can be even more specific, however, with individual *files*, not just individual *computers*, having their own address. This is how email works. The author's current email address, *davoren@itsa.ucsf.edu*, is merely a file on the computer "itsa" at UCSF that collects messages sent to it. Messages collect whether I am logged on the computer or not, just like a postal mailbox collects letters whether or not I am at home. Any single file on any computer with Internet access can have its own address. Because all addresses are translated into numbers, though, *blank spaces are not allowed in IP addresses.*

There is a major problem with the current organization of the Internet, however: It lacks a central repository of Internet addresses, a comprehensive "phone book" that lists who is at what address. This problem exists because the Internet lacks central control. But this may be the only way the Internet can exist, since the information available at any one address can change from day to day, making instantly obsolete any planned survey of attached computers. However, many sites serve to scour the Internet constantly for content (search engines, discussed on page 136), and several organizations describe themselves as "Internet White Pages."

Computer hardware & software requirements

All personal computers built within the last several years are capable of running programs that permit access to the Internet. Older computers (those built before 1990 or so) require extensive upgrading that is often not worth the cost. Because "built-in" hardware (central processing unit [CPU], modem, and the like) as well as software (the "programs" running the hardware) continue to be developed constantly, for specific hardware recommendations, the reader is referred to colleagues who are already connected to the Internet or to the computer magazines. However, the issues of computer speed and memory are important.

Because the speed of the Internet connection is the rate-limiting factor in information transfer, it is much more important than the "clock speed" of the computer's CPU. The faster the modem (the device that **mo**dulates and **dem**odulates computer information into "packets" that can be sent over telephone wires, the most common piece of connecting hardware for accessing the Internet), the faster you can send and receive information over phone wires. A newer wire network, called integrated services digital network (ISDN), can be obtained from many phone companies. Unlike regular phone lines, ISDN can use the fastest modems currently available.

In terms of memory, you simply cannot have too much. Specifically, invest in as much processor memory (random access memory [RAM]) or storage disk memory (hard drives and disks) as possible. Graphic and audio files, common on the Web, are huge.

Anyone who desires Internet access from a personal computer needs *at the very least* a computer with keyboard, mouse, hard disk drive, and either a modem or a direct Internet connection. Sound cards and video cards (small, specific-task computer chips that fit in your computer's housing) are highly recommended and are preinstalled in many, but not all, new computers.

Historically, software requirements to access the Internet were simple: Every modem came with a basic program that would perform the few functions required. Now, the transmission of audio, video, and spreadsheet information over the Internet has made Internet software a huge growth industry. Web browsers and email software programs (discussed later) are available for virtually any current model of computer. The reader is referred to the mass media and computer review magazines for details.

Connecting an individual computer to the Internet

The first step in being able to send and receive information via the Internet is to connect your computer to it. For this, you need a computer, a connection, and the software programs required to run your computer and make the connection. Connections can be either of two types: direct or indirect.

With a **direct connection,** your computer is "hard-wired" to a network and has an IP address assigned to it by either a company that controls the addresses or your organization, which has been allotted a set of them. In general, organizations such as hospitals and universities have their own internal network, usually called a local area network (LAN). The LAN links a number of computers together.

With an **indirect connection,** your computer needs a modem, which dials up (over a telephone line) an already hard-wired central computer called a **server.** A server "serves" stored data and files or processing power to other machines on the network. It can handle many network connections simultaneously. Direct connections are faster than indirect ones, which is most important for the transfer of large files, such as graphics or video.

If your organization is not affiliated with a "top-level" domain, like "edu," "com," or "org"—offering direct connection—you'll have to use a modem to connect to a private Internet service provider (ISP). The ISP will own and control the server you must access. The number of ISPs is increasing, some with clinician-oriented marketing strategies. Large ISPs, such as AmericaOnline, Netcom, UUNet Technologies, and PSINet, advertise regularly in PC and Macintosh magazines as well as other media. Two providers cater to clinicians: Physicians' Online and Medscape, both of which provide low-cost or no-cost access to the Internet (see page 143). Both also provide free access to MEDLINE, although the tools they use are much less powerful than most standard MEDLINE interfaces. In general, most ISPs provide the basic modem/telecommunications software, the phone numbers for your modem, identification and password codes, as well as email accounts and Web browser software (see page 134).

Methods of transferring information via the Internet

If the Internet is a network of connections, how can an individual send and receive information to and from other computers? If your computer is logged onto the Internet, it is a matter of using the right terms and addresses, then watching your computer screen. Even then, your computer doesn't do the same thing each time you're logged on. At times you may want to log on as a "dumb terminal" (whereby you use your keyboard to give commands to a remote computer, rather than your own. At other times, you may want to download a picture of the Grand Canyon so that you can print it on your printer or even email it to a friend on another computer. Even these disparate forms of interacting with the Internet presume you already know where you are going, but what if you need to navigate first?

The short answer is that once a connection is made, many different software applications and methods of transferring information can be used. However, only two are important to understand and are emphasized here: email and hypertext browsing.

Email

Email provides the simplest method of transferring information from one computer to another. In its simplest form, email is text information sent from the user at one computer to another. All email accounts, obtained from any of the domain names listed in Table 6–1, allow the user to enter the address of the recipient, type a message, and send it. In addition the user can directly reply to a message without necessarily having to re-enter the return address. Essentially all software packages that allow a user to access the Internet provide methods for obtaining an email address. Both commercial and institutional services usually assign you an email address when you register—you can customize the address, provided someone else doesn't already have the address you'd like. For example, if you're a pulmonologist signed up with AmericaOnline (the domain aol.com), you might want to have the address "lungs@aol.com."

For the practitioner of evidence-based medicine, email provides a way to directly link to experts in the field of interest and provides an electronic address to which others may submit questions or information.

A nice feature of email is that once a message is sent, you will know whether it reached its destination. In most cases, however, you will not know whether the recipient of your message read it. (Some LAN software is capable of determining this, however.) If the email did not reach its destination, it will come back to you as "undeliverable" or some equivalent, often within minutes of your sending it. Another useful feature of email is that it can act as "storage space." As discussed in Chapter 5, some MEDLINE-searching software will allow you to send the results of your search to your email account, where you can keep them for later use or subsequently copy them to your hard drive. This can be useful, for example, if you are searching MEDLINE at a library, but want the electronic version of your search result to appear on your office computer. Simply email the file(s) to yourself!

Email thus has the potential to be much more comprehensive than just including two people in a communication. In fact, multiple parties can be involved in an email communication, and the specific address of a recipient does not always have to be known. There are countless subject-specific **discussion groups**—existing entirely electronically and accessible via **mailing lists.** In these groups, a person's message is sent to a central server via mail-handling software ("**listserv**") and then back out—possibly after being screened for appropriateness by a moderator—to a list of like-minded individuals who have voluntarily subscribed to the mailing list. It is important to note that if you subscribe to a mailing list to which many others have subscribed, you will receive *a lot* of email. Two IP addresses at which you can obtain large indices of mailing lists are provided on page 144.

Hypertext: the World Wide Web is born

The rapidly expanding availability of personal computers—and their increasing capacities for hard disk storage, calculation rates, color displays with high resolution, high-quality audio and video displays, mouse-driven menus and commands instead of keyboard-based options, and high-speed modems—has entirely changed the landscape of Internet access in the 1990s. One important development was a new form of linking individual pieces of information (electronic documents) together, called **hypertext.** Hypertext allows navigation throughout much of the Internet. That portion of the Internet that can be accessed via hypertext is called the World Wide Web, WWW, or the Web.

Hypertext is best defined as a system of coding that links electronic documents together. It appears on your computer screen as highlighted (usually by color or underlining) text or graphic. This **link** is "clickable" with your mouse. For example, you may see an article on the Web about cancer therapy. In this article is a list of chemotherapeutic agents, and with each agent in the list appears the phrase, "For more information, click here." If you click with your mouse on the name of that chemotherapeutic agent, you will be directly taken to a *new* document that contains more information, just as promised. *That "jump" to a new document is the hypertext link.*

Each hypertext document may contain multiple links to other documents. A single hypertext document is usually referred to as a "Web page," and a collection of hypertext documents is a "Web site." The impressive thing about hypertext is that any given link can be connected to any other place on the Web—to the same Web site, a different part of the same Web page, or halfway across the world to an entirely unrelated Web site. The Web is thus configured as a massive connection of individual Web pages.

There are two ways to navigate the World Wide Web: with a text-only program or with a graphical interface. The text-only program, called **lynx,** is less efficient, and much less popular, than the graphical interface. Lynx uses keyboard commands only. A graphical interface is **mouse-based** and is the most common method used to navigate. Software using a graphical interface is referred to as a **Web browser.** A browser is the software required for your computer to understand that a document is written in hypertext. This just means that it translates computer code into the nice graphics and organized paragraphs of text that you see on your screen; it is not important for you to understand anything more about the code of hypertext. Browser programs simply make tasks like using email and transferring files from computer to computer user-friendly. The user can perform different tasks just by clicking a mouse on a hypertext link. The most-often cited browsers for personal computers are Netscape Navigator, Microsoft Internet Explorer, and NCSA Mosaic. All are available for different brands of personal computers, although Navigator and Explorer are by far the most common.

The best way to explain the features of hypertext and of a Browser is by example. Figure 6–2 shows one Web page, as seen using Netscape Navigator version 2.0. The components of this page are discussed next. Similarly named components exist in other browsers.

Netscape menu bar (Macintosh version)

Command bar

This Web page's title bar

Current
URL

Shortcuts

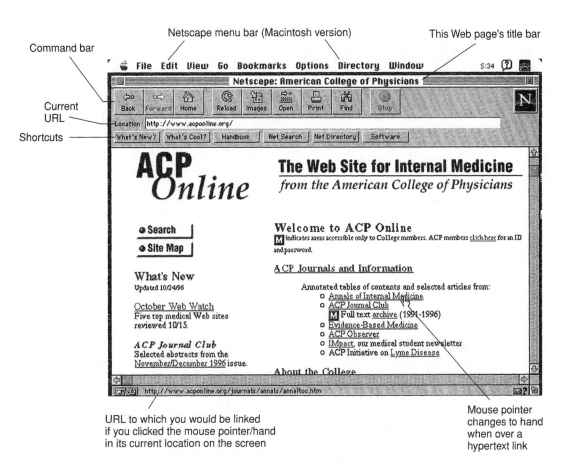

URL to which you would be linked
if you clicked the mouse pointer/hand
in its current location on the screen

Mouse pointer
changes to hand
when over a
hypertext link

Figure 6–2. Sample Web page as seen using Netscape Navigator 2.0 on a Macintosh computer.

Location & the URL. Navigating from one Web page to another is akin to a change in locale. Hence, the IP address of the Web document you are "browsing" is shown in a box labeled "location." However, location is slightly more complicated than just being an IP address. The IP address in our example document (the main page of the Web site of the American College of Physicians) is *www.acponline.org/,* but in the location box is the prefix "http://." This prefix indicates that the communications method used to access this page is the **hyper**text **t**ransfer **p**rotocol. The combination of the access method and the IP address is called the **uniform resource locator** (URL). URLs can have many characters (but again, no blank spaces). For example, I could be reached by typing *http://www.hemonc.ucsf.edu/Faculty_List/J_Ben_Davoren.html* in the "Open Location" command box (available under the File menu in Figure 6–2). This command means that you are directing the Web browser to the html document "J_Ben_Davoren," which resides within the folder "Faculty_List," which resides on the server "www.hemonc.ucsf.edu," and that you want to use the hypertext transfer protocol (http) to get there. You wish to use http because this Web page is written in **hyper**text **m**arkup **l**anguage (html). Fortunately, you rarely need to retype URLs, because you can "bookmark" them by using the "Bookmarks" pull-down menu at the very top of the window (discussed next).

Menus & title bars. The menu options and title bars of the window in Figure 6–2 apply to an Apple Macintosh but are the same in computers that run Microsoft's Windows software. Each header in the menu bar is a pull-down menu with commands that are common to almost all software, not just Internet browsers. For example, the "File" menu contains options that let you open and close new browser windows or print what you're seeing. The "Options" menu contains options that let you set the preferences of your browser (eg, which URL your "home" should be when you first launch the browser, what color the background and text should be, etc). Since these commands are common to virtually all software, we do not need to discuss them further.

One feature of browser software that is not always available in other software programs, however, is this: Browsers have additional icon options for some commands, labeled in Figure 6–2 as "Command bar" and "Shortcuts."

There are several unique commands worth mentioning. The first is a menu item labeled "Bookmarks" ("Favorites" in Explorer). Under this menu, you can quickly (one mouse click) add the URL you are currently visiting to a personalized list of others, and return to any bookmarked URL by simply clicking on it in your list. The second is the "Back" and "Forward" buttons on the command bar; these allow you to click from one already-visited Web page to another, without pages having to be linked in any pre-existing way. Third, the "Home" button takes you to whatever Web page you wish to have as the one you first see each time you launch or open the browser. When you obtain a browser, the default "home" is the home page of the company that made the browser.

Other buttons on the command bar include the "Reload" button ("Refresh" in Explorer), used to double-check that you have the most up-to-date version of a Web page. To improve access speed, your hard drive stores the last visited version of a Web page, so that when you hit the "Back" button, you will see that page quickly. However, some Web pages change literally minute-to-minute. To get the very latest version, click reload. The "Images" button will turn on or off automatic image loading. Most Web pages have a lot of slow-loading graphic images. These images can be the best part of a site, but many sites are cluttered with them, with the important information presented as text. For faster loading of these pages, turn the images load off (via the "Options" button in Explorer). Next, the "Open" button takes you to a window in which you may type in a known URL to go there directly. "Print" does just that (if you have a printer, of course). "Find" locates any desired word on the page you are currently browsing. Lastly, "Stop" is used to stop information transfer before it is completed.

Figure 6–2 also shows shortcuts to Netscape's own collection of pages ("What's New," "What's Cool," etc). "Net Search" and "Net Directory" both give you an interactive list of many search engines (see below). The "Software" button takes you to a page where you may obtain (by downloading over the network) many plug-in programs, which add functionality to your browser (see page 138).

Hypertext links. Take a look at Figure 6–2 again. Some of the information is plain text and some is underlined text. These items underlined are the hypertext links. In our example, we have placed the mouse arrow over one of them, "Annals of Internal Medicine," and the arrow has now changed to a hand, with an extended index finger. If we click our mouse here, we would be transported to the URL shown at the bottom—thus "Annals of Internal Medicine" is not only text but also a link to another Web page. Although this particular link appears as text, two other hypertext links on this page appear as graphics: the boxes on the left side labeled "Search" and "Site Map." If you placed the mouse pointer over them, you would also get the hand icon and a new URL would show up in the box at the very bottom of the page. In fact, we have done that and clicked on the "Search" graphic to get to the Web page that is seen in Figure 6–3.

Interactive web pages. Figure 6–3 demonstrates another feature of hypertext—it can be **interactive.** For example, the "Search for:" box. You can click your mouse cursor in this box and type in any keyboard characters (words for your search) and then click on the "Search" button. This initiates a search program that will check all the Web pages at this site, or even other sites if they've been indexed by the first site, for your search words. You will be instantly presented with a new page—a list of hypertext links to all those newly discovered sites.

Search engines

Once you have a Web browser installed, interacting with the Web is quite straightforward and basically involves only pointing and clicking. One setback is that the Web is not particularly organized, and as such, it can take a long time to navigate. However, it can be fun doing so, obtaining everything from the full text of a peer-reviewed journal article, to video of the current traffic conditions on the freeway you use to get home after a long day at work.

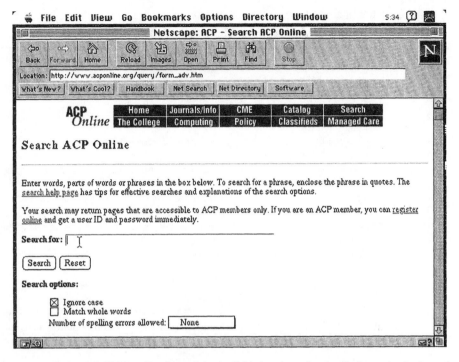

Figure 6–3. The interactive Web page. Note the search box in which text words may be entered by the user to act as keywords. Most searches like this will return keyword matches on the same Web site, not across the entire Internet.

Search engines assist in providing order to what seems like a random series of hypertext connections. Several companies, buttressed by advertising on their sites, have created methods of instantaneously searching the content of every publicly accessible Web site, using keywords that you, the searcher, offer up in their interactive keyword boxes.

The reasons why these search engines are so important are several. First, new Web pages are added every day, as are new services. Second, although most Web sites continue to have the same names (as in the title bar of Figure 6–2), their location—and thus, their URL—may change frequently. This is because some individual Web servers compete with each other in terms of what they charge the individual Web page owners to display their pages; some Web page owners may thus change Web servers to save money. This means that a site that you have "bookmarked" in your browser may not work in the future. Searching for its title, or general subject, with a search engine program, however, will probably find it (and a lot of others).

There are several premier search engines that are intuitively easy to use—once accessed. Some search engines even search for the appropriate search engine. These are listed in Table 6–2 (and are available by a click on Netscape's "Net Search" button in Figure 6–2). Several of these search engines have entire, organized sections of medicine-related information as separate, searchable subsets of the world's Web pages. For more information about how to use search engines, the reader is urged to use one of them to search the term "search engines"; many sites have detailed information about how best to use them, beyond their simple interfaces.

Beyond hypertext

It is important to note that hypertext links connect more than just hypertext documents. Clicking on a link may show you an image (like the photo of the Grand Canyon we talked about), play a song, or directly download a new software program to your computer. The browser cannot always complete each of these steps. Additional programs used to help the browser show videos, "unstuff" or "unzip" files that are transferred in compressed form,

TABLE 6–2. WORLD WIDE WEB SEARCH ENGINES.*

Search Engine Site and URL	Comments
Lycos http://www.lycos.com	Search engine provides rough order of relevance of keywords used in search term. Has "A2Z" list of medical sites
Yahoo! http://www.yahoo.com	Has specific Health & Medicine directory to speed searches
Alta Vista http://www.altavista.digital.com	Indexes full pages of more than 16 million Web sites, including newsgroups
Excite Netsearch http://www.excite.com	Indexes Web pages, including newsgroups
InfoSeek Net Search http://www2.infoseek.com	Indexes full text of Web pages, including selected newsgroups and electronic journals
Inktomi http://inktomi.berkeley.edu	Ranks searches in order of how many search terms are used on retrieved pages
WebCrawler http://webcrawler.com	America Online searcher. Indexes URL, title, and document content
WWWW—World Wide Web Worm http://www.cs.colorado.edu	Indexes hypertext, URL, and document title content
search.com http://search.com	A Meta-search engine. Uses its search engine to select the best search engine for your search
all4one http://all4one.com	Meta-search engine. Uses Alta Vista, Lycos, Yahoo, and WebCrawler simultaneously

* In general, each site searches user-provided "keywords" with an interactive form or box filled out when the search engine home page is first located.

play audio segments, etc, are usually available on line, are usually free, and are referred to as **plug-ins.** Usually, the home page of each browser—which is loaded onto your screen by default when you first launch your browser software—will direct you to specific Web sites where you can download any plug-in that you need. Figure 6–2 shows a shortcut button marked "software" that provides a link to Netscape's available plug-ins.

Nonhypertext web tools

There are a few "built-in" plug-in programs in all Web browsers that allow the use of several nonhypertext communications protocols. It's important to remember that these programs are launched automatically. You do not have to know what they do to use them, because the browser will know what protocol to use at each IP address. However, you may wish to know that the prefixes before an IP address may read "ftp://," "tel-net://," or "gopher://" in your location window when you click on a hypertext link, not just "http://." **FTP** stands for **file transfer protocol,** and is usually used to transfer either a compressed file or a software program from a Web site to your hard drive. **Telnet** is a protocol that allows you to connect with a remote computer, located anywhere in the world, with your computer keyboard. You can then use that computer's menus to locate information that is *not* hypertext-based. To download that information to your computer, however, you will have to turn on the "Session capture" command in the Telnet protocol, then display the information on your screen, remembering to turn the session capture off when completed. For more information, see the suggested reading at the end of this chapter.

Lastly, the **gopher protocol** (named after the mascot of the site of its origination, the University of Minnesota) allows you to navigate through a series of menus, in a remote computer like Telnet does, to download information. However, unlike Telnet, there are specific "gopher servers" set up across the country that have consistent menu hierarchies, making searching these sites easier than using Telnet. Telnet, ftp, and gopher protocols *can* be used to obtain information from the Internet without using a Web browser. To do this, you still need either modem access to a hard-wired computer or a direct connection to the Internet. Further explanation is beyond the scope of this chapter.

IS MEDICAL INFORMATION ON THE INTERNET VALID?

For the practitioner of evidence-based medicine, the Web provides a way to access and download text files, graphics such as blood smears and pathology slides, new computer applications, movies of real-time ultrasonography, advice and files from an expert's computer, data in MEDLINE, gopher servers, and a growing number of sites that attempt to organize all of these files in a way that is helpful to the clinician. One major difficulty is to efficiently identify valid information—because anyone with a modem and a personal computer can *post* a Web page that is not necessarily reviewed for content, style, accuracy, or ethics.

Because the Internet is an unregulated, constantly changing set of computers around the world that can communicate instantly with one another, the quality of information, particularly medical information, varies substantially from site to site. Individuals can post home pages at many educational institutions, and those individuals are solely responsible for content; advice and information given on a particular page has probably been reviewed by no one other than the person who created the page and should therefore not be taken as an educational institution's endorsement.

Nonetheless, there are "official" Web pages developed by organizations that do have a reputation at stake, including pages from high-quality, peer-reviewed journals, government institutions such as the National Institutes of Health, and many educational institutions at which individuals or groups have endeavored to create truly informative repositories of information. These sites are the real backbone of medical information on the Web, but there are also commercial medical information sites, in competition with each other, that are more aggressively and regularly updated. Identifying valid information therefore involves determining the credibility of the source. Although there are many ways to search the Web, in the end, it is up to the individual to access each site and decide whether the quality of its information is worth the trip through cyberspace.

For the student of evidence-based medicine, the Web becomes more of a starting place than a final destination. Many informative sites include references to articles that you may critically appraise using the skills discussed in Section 3 of this book (Assessing the Validity of Medical Information). Professional medical organizations may post position papers, NIH posts Consensus Statements, and academic institutions may post disease-specific tutorials. The next section presents a selection of credible resources on the Web.

THE WORLD WIDE WEB: SPECIFIC SITES & SUGGESTIONS

The following Web sites have been chosen for their relevance as Internet starting points for the student of evidence-based medicine. The Web will undoubtedly evolve, and the discussion that follows may include sites that may be out of date upon publication of this book. However, the number of services that collect and organize medically related information will only increase. And most search engines will evolve as well to improve access to these databases, which should make them easier to find. The URLs listed are correct as of April 1998. This list will be updated and expanded at our own Web site, currently at *http://www.sf.med.va.gov/Prime/Prime1.html*. If you cannot find it there, search with your browser for "Evidence-Based Medicine: A PRIME Example," or "San Francisco VA." The list will also be accessible via a link on the Appleton & Lange Web site (www.appletonlange.com).

US government sites

The National Library of Medicine (*http://www.nlm.nih.gov*): MEDLINE is not the only database available from the National Library of Medicine (NLM) that can be useful to the clinician or medical researcher. Not all of the databases can be directly searched via hypertext, but most can be searched with Grateful Med or with protocols, such as Telnet. The NLM Web site, called HyperDoc, contains detailed information about their more than 40 online databases, and several can be accessed free. The most relevant databases are listed in Table 6–3. For the practitioner of evidence-based medicine, the AIDS-related sites are notable because they include information about current clinical trials, the development of new drugs, and drug toxicities, as well as abstracts from international AIDS meetings. The

TABLE 6-3. NATIONAL LIBRARY OF MEDICINE DATABASES AVAILABLE ON-LINE.

Name	Description	Cost
NLM Home Page http://www.nlm.nih.gov	Home page of the NLM, called HyperDoc, lists multiple options for further description of available information	No
AIDSDRUGS	Currently evaluated agents in clinical trials. Includes adverse reactions, pharmacology	No
AIDSLINE	Literature database includes MEDLINE information, meeting abstracts, symposia	No
AIDSTRIALS	Information on open and closed trials, including patient eligibility and trial locations	No
CANCERLIT	Articles and abstracts about major cancer topics	No
DIRLINE	Directory of resources providing information services	No
HSTAT	Full-text clinical practice guidelines	No
INTERNET GRATEFUL MED	New MEDLINE search engine with graphical interface over the WWW	No
MEDLINE	The premier biomedical citation database	No
MeSH VOCABULARY	Thesaurus of biomedical-related terms	Yes
NIH CLINICAL ALERTS	Early release of clinical information from the NIH	No
PDQ	Advances in cancer treatments and clinical trials	No
SDILINE	Most current month of MEDLINE	Yes
TOXNET	The MEDLINE of toxicology, drugs, hazardous materials information	Yes

Health Service/Technology Assessment Text (HSTAT) database has full-text clinical practice guidelines, as well as NIH Health Clinical Alerts. The aforementioned sites are all accessible without cost, although you may need to register your name and affiliation. Hyper-Doc is well worth the trip.

The National Institutes of Health (*http://www.nih.gov*): The National Institutes of Health (NIH) is composed of a number of individual institutes (like the NLM), each with a different perspective on and orientation to clinical medicine. Nonetheless, information from all these institutes is available through this one Web site. Some health topics that can be browsed are listed in Table 6–4; other topics not listed are also available, and the site continues to grow. The practitioner of evidence-based medicine is directed particularly to the CancerNet/PDQ database. This database has frequently updated summaries of diagnostic criteria and cancer treatment options by stage and contains comprehensive bibliographies. Information is available for physicians and patients. Another important link, the NIH Consensus Development Program is a repository of NIH Consensus Statements and offers

TABLE 6-4. ON-LINE HEALTH INFORMATION AVAILABLE AT THE NIH SITE.

Name	Description
NIH Home Page http://www.nih.gov	NIH home page and master directory
CancerNet	Access to CancerLit (abstracts plus article citations relevant to cancer), the PDQ database (frequently updated, well-organized diagnosis and treatment discussions)
AIDS Related Information	Gopher server maintained by Allergy and Infectious Disease Institute of NIH
Women's Health Initiative	Description of this large prevention project, goals, and participating institutions
Bone Marrow Transplantation Unit	Information regarding current and future roles of allogeneic and autologous bone marrow transplantation
NIH Consensus Development Program	Database of NIH Consensus Statements and Technology Assessment Statements
NIH Clinical Alerts	Alerts regarding important findings from NIH-funded clinical trials
HSTAT	Database of clinical practice guidelines and reference guides for clinicians

online tests to obtain continuing medical education (CME) credit. Lastly, the HSTAT resource is available here, with its clinical practice guidelines developed by the Agency for Health Care Policy and Research (AHCPR).

Centers for Disease Control and Prevention (*http://www.cdc.gov*): The Centers for Disease Control and Prevention (CDC) constantly collects information regarding important disease entities in the United States. Their publication *Morbidity and Mortality Weekly Report* provides information for clinicians, travelers, and the general public about current trends in specific infectious diseases, common chronic illnesses, and other causes of morbidity or death. This and other information can be accessed by hypertext at *http://www.cdc.gov*. The hypertext version requires a specific free software-decoding program called Adobe Acrobat (a plug-in). This plug-in can be obtained by entering the search term "Adobe Acrobat" in your search engine page.

Academic centers & affiliations

The number of medically related sites developed by medical schools and major academic centers is growing quickly. Many are officially organized sites with tremendous resources—even online textbooks. Others contain a variety of individual pages maintained by individual physicians or other health-care providers, researchers, administrative staff, or students—therefore, the quality varies substantially. Several premiere sites in North America are described here to illustrate the types of information available. But with the use of a search engine, you can rapidly search the name of your favorite medical school or medical center, in or outside of the United States. In general, the main menu at each of these sites is comprehensive, maintained by a "webmaster" who keeps all the individual sites linked. Therefore, you usually should first search for the medical center's home page to look at its main index. Usually, the home page has the simplest URL, eg, *http://www.ucsf.edu* for the University of California, San Francisco.

There is no way to list *all* medically related Web sites in a text; only a short list of recommended sites is discussed here. The reader is strongly encouraged to tour these sites for links to other sources of information, creating personal bookmarks in your browser along the way. These 10 sites serve mainly as examples of the types of information that exist in cyberspace.

Cliniweb at Oregon Health Sciences University (*http://www.ohsu.edu/cliniweb.htm*): This site has an index of all Web pages containing clinical information that the center is aware of, using the MeSH headings of the NLM. This allows searching or browsing of Web sites in a manner similar to searching MEDLINE. There are also lists of clinical resources at US medical schools, grouped by state. Many of these contain clinically relevant disease approach summaries, including diagnostic strategies, therapies, and outcomes. Other lists include histology or pathology images. In addition, there are "homegrown" features, such as "Dr. Deloughery's Famous Handouts," which are handouts on a variety of internal medicine topics written for medical students and house staff.

Evidence-based medicine site at McMaster University (*http://hiru.mcmaster.ca/ebm*): This site includes a series of published articles, users' guides to assessing the validity of medical information, and even interactive pages. These are especially interesting because they allow you to calculate likelihood ratios, use Bayes' theorem, and analyze numbers needed to treat (a concept explained in Chapter 8), using whatever scenarios you like. The published articles are downloadable via the file transfer protocol (FTP).

Harvard Medical School (*http://www.med.harvard.edu*): This site links to all of the school's associated hospitals and departments, with "interactive patient" testing files available for study or CME credit. The "Whole Brain Atlas" contains multiple downloadable images and movies. This site also includes an extensive list of Web sites of other medical schools.

Medical College of Wisconsin International Travelers Clinic (*http://www.intmed.mcw.edu/travel.html*): With a comprehensive list of specific health and immunization recommendations for travelers by geographical destination or disease, this site links to the CDC. It provides frequently updated information about endemic diseases worldwide and also has a directory of travel clinics and physicians.

MedWeb at Emory University's Health Sciences Library (*http://www.cc.emory.edu/WHSCL/medweb.html*): MedWeb offers an index of a huge number of Internet resource sites, by biomedical specialty.

Oncolink at the University of Pennsylvania (*http://cancer.med.upenn.edu*): This site is a constantly updated source of cancer information, compiled from a variety of sources. It has disease-oriented menus, medical specialty–oriented menus, information on clinical trials, and links both to the National Cancer Institute and CancerNet. In addition, there is a large body of patient-oriented information from a variety of sources, including newsletters and first-person accounts, along with updates from news organizations and cancer conferences.

University of California San Francisco Division of General Internal Medicine (*http://dgim-www.ucsf.edu*): This site contains primary care teaching modules and interactive quizzes and links to other sites. Other UCSF sites include the Cancer Center—with lists of open clinical trials, including the full texts of protocols, consent forms, and information on contacting participating clinicians—and the Computer Graphics Laboratory, with three-dimensional molecular structures of DNA and other important biological compounds.

University of Washington Health Links (*http://www.hslib.washington.edu*): Here the viewer will find an exhaustive list of links to online journals, from *ACP Journal Club* to the *World Wide Web Journal of Biology.* Abstracts and even the full text of current issues can be read on screen or printed. There are also links to subscribable mailing lists and links to "Health MetaGuides." These sites catalogue biomedical information on the Web. The educational sites contain tutorials, such as how to interpret blood smears, with the ability to have unmarked slides presented for analysis as a self-test.

The Virtual Hospital at the University of Iowa (*http://indy.radiology.uiowa.edu/VirtualHospital.html*): This site contains multimedia teaching files and case studies including x-rays. There are also several online textbooks, mostly written in a practical handbook style. One is the *Mosby Family Practice Handbook,* which covers the essentials of "bread and butter" medicine—the causes of hypokalemia and the workup of chest pain. In addition, there are evolving areas of the site, such as physiologic imaging in three dimensions, with downloadable movies and still images.

WebPath at the University of Utah (*http://www-medlib.med.utah.edu/WebPath/webpath.html*): WebPath contains very high-quality pathology images, along with laboratory exercises, quizzes that can be scored online, tutorials correlating clinical histories with pathology, and a comprehensive list of other pathology instructional resources and multimedia educational sites in medicine.

Medical societies & published journals

A growing number of medical societies have created Web pages that both members and nonmembers may visit. In addition, peer-reviewed journals are accessible on the Web, some as full-text, others with just abstracts and editorials. What follows is a list of popular sites that demonstrate the potential for the direct dissemination of high-quality medical information. A quick search of your favorite journal title(s) or medical organization using a search engine should lead you to additional information.

American College of Physicians (*http://www.acponline.org*): This is the premiere site of its type (see Figures 6–2 and 6–3 for its home page). It offers sneak previews of the tables of contents of upcoming editions of *Annals of Internal Medicine* and the full text of featured *Annals* articles, including figures and tables. In addition, the full text of the *ACP Journal Club* is online (for members), as is their publication *Evidence-Based Medicine.* A frequently updated "WebWatch" section lists and evaluates other medically related sites. There are even discussions on the state of computers in medicine.

American Cancer Society (*http://www.cancer.org*): Mostly for patients, this site contains many valuable resources for clinicians, including professional education statements with references and scholarly discussion, general statements on the treatment of cancer, and cancer statistics. The cancer statistics—on incidence, prevalence, trends, and mortality—are the most widely quoted national statistics about cancer and are presented in great detail.

American College of Cardiology (*http://www.acc.org*): Here you will find the abstracts (and some full text) of the *Journal of the American College of Cardiology* (*JACC*) but also online CME courses online and press releases from the organization's annual meeting.

American Heart Association (*http://www.amhrt.org/*): Containing general information about heart disease and risk factors for both physicians and the general public, this site also has the abstracts of the journals *Circulation, Circulation Research, Stroke, Hypertension,* and *Arteriosclerosis, Thrombosis & Vascular Biology* at a subsite (*http://www.at-home.com/get_doc/250221/2112*).

American Medical Association (*http://www.ama-assn.org*): This site provides general information about the AMA, as well as the Web versions of the *Journal of the American Medical Association* (*JAMA*), the *American Medical News,* and each of the subspecialty Archives journal series (internal medicine, dermatology, family medicine, etc). JAMA contains one full-text article each week, including figures and tables, and the complete abstracts of the other articles. Job opportunities and other medical information are also listed.

Journal of the National Cancer Institute (*http://cancernet.nci.nih.gov/jnci/jncihome.html*): Here the viewer will find the abstract of each article published in the main journal, along with the full text of articles containing news on cancer.

The Lancet (*http://www.thelancet.com*): The viewer will find the full text of selected articles from each issue and abstracts of selected editorials and original articles.

The New England Journal of Medicine (*http://www.nejm.org*): This site contains the abstract of each week's articles and the full text of its editorials, including their usually useful references.

The public domain

The overwhelming majority of Web sites are neither official organizations nor educational sites but still contain a lot of information. Many medically related sites exist, some put together by individuals at educational institutions without official endorsement, some by groups of persons interested in alternative medical therapies, some by pharmaceutical companies, and others by physician-run enterprises. Some of these public domain sites are quite comprehensive. Because they may have funding based on advertising revenue and have bigger staffs than many educational site Web servers, public domain sites may be updated more often than official sites. It is likely that the number of medically relevant sites will increase and that the sites will probably present more advertising to the viewer. What follows is a list of frequently updated medically related sites that may be of interest to both clinicians and patients.

Medical World Search (*http://www.mwsearch.com*): This site is useful for three reasons. The first is that the authors have pre-screened thousands of web sites for relevant medical information. The second is that they have created a search engine that searches the full text of all the pages on those thousands of web sites. The third is that they have used the UMLS Meta-thesaurus to try to "map" common terms directly to MeSH terms, improving the power of your keyword searches. MEDLINE searches can also be directly done from here using the PubMed interface of the NLM.

Doctor's Guide to the Internet (*http://www.docguide.com*): This contains medical news, drug information updates, lists of medical meetings and conferences, as well as organized links to other sites. There are many well-organized sites for both patients and physicians.

Lycos Health and Medicine (*http://a2z.lycos.com/Health_and_Medicine*): The viewer will find here easy-to-search areas of medicine, all of which are links to other medically related sites. The index is searchable and very powerful.

Martindale's Health Science Guide (*http://www-sci.lib.uci.edu/HSG/HSGuide.html*): This contains an enormous list of medically oriented sites and an excellent example of one person's efforts to organize relevant information on the Web. The organization separates clinical information from basic science information extremely well. The viewer can locate everything from interactive anatomy videos to medical dictionaries in several languages.

Medical Matrix (*http://www.medmatrix.org*): This site, maintained by the Internet Working Group of the American Medical Informatics Association, is a reviewed index of medically related sites on the Web and contains numerous organized links. There are clinical practice issues, medical education sites, and specialty information sites—all well-described.

Medscape (*http://www.medscape.com*): This site is also a service that contains medical links and also provides free access to MEDLINE. Registration is required but free. There are selected online journals, with their peer-reviewed articles available as full text. The site offers a well-developed searchable index of medical headlines and health policies.

Physicians' Online (*http://www.po.com*): Meant as a physician's communication center, this proprietary online service requires free registration to use. Access cannot occur directly through a Web browser, but rather requires a separate access method. Once online, the user can obtain a free email account, search MEDLINE and other NLM databases, obtain drug and drug interaction information, see medical news, participate in discussion groups with other physicians, and obtain online CME credit. The site is paid for with advertising, so the presence of ads (mostly pharmaceutical) is noticeable.

Yahoo! Health Index (*http://www.yahoo.com/Health/*): This site also maintains organized sections of Web pages, which you can search using keyword combinations. Comprehensive and fast, with frequently updated links to other sites.

Your Health Daily (*http://yourhealthdaily.com*): A service of *The New York Times* syndicate, this site provides daily, well-written articles on current health news. "Backissues" are searchable online by categories or by keywords.

Pharmaceutical company sites

Several pharmaceutical companies have created sites that provide physician education, patient education, and more general medical information. However, these sites are strongly oriented toward the treatment of diseases for which these companies offer specific name-brand medications. The sites have obvious names (eg, *www.bayer.com, www.merck.com, www.Pfizer.com,* etc). In competition with one another, they may provide interesting information not available at other sources. For example, Roxane company has an entire series of slides about pain management that the viewer can download, along with the text descriptions of each, for further use.

Listservs

The following two sites contain the biggest indices of listservs and both describe how to subscribe to these mailing lists of like-minded individuals. Briefly, you send an email message that says "Subscribe" to the email address of a central server; all the email that is sent there is then sent to you. You can also "unsubscribe."

Health Links at the University of Washington (*http://healthlinks.washington.edu/news/newsgroups.html*): This site has health and biomedical mailing lists and discussion groups.

Tile Listservs (*http://www.tile.net/tile/listserv/medicine.html*): This site has more than 100 mailing lists noted, from attention deficit disorder to Wilson's disease.

SUGGESTED READING

Hahn H, Stout R: *The Complete Internet Reference Book.* Osborne McGraw-Hill, 1994.

KEEPING UP WITH THE MEDICAL LITERATURE

Terrie Mendelson, MD

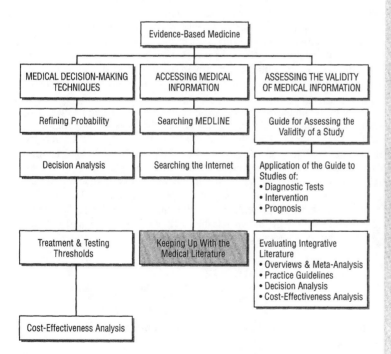

INTRODUCTION: THE MEDICAL LITERATURE AS OFFICE FURNITURE

An essential component of the practice of evidence-based medicine is the clinician's familiarity with major developments within the scope of his or her practice. The most highly esteemed clinicians and teachers maintain a solid foundation of up-to-date knowledge spanning broad areas of medicine, within which can be found the answers to particular clinical questions. Despite this laudable goal, however, it is doubtful that a single physician can be found who does not admit to being woefully behind in his or her reading—most of us, in fact, feel as though we fall further behind with every mail delivery. This sentiment is, unfortunately, rooted in fact: The volume of medical literature is expanding at a rate of greater than 7% per year,[1] doubling approximately every 10–15 years.

This evolving information may be found in a myriad of places: in the minds of expert consultants, in textbooks, in nonpeer-reviewed "throw away" magazines, in pharmaceutical company literature and advertisements, in peer-reviewed medical journals as original research articles, and in the form of published clinical practice guidelines or overviews. Physicians' attitudes about the reliability of these sources of information are intriguing. In 1994, Tunis and colleagues published the results of a survey of 2600 randomly selected members of the American College of Physicians, who were asked to rate the effect of the information source on their clinical practice.[2] Greater than 80% of respondents listed published review articles as the information source most likely to have a major effect on their practice. This category, however, did not distinguish systematic reviews from nonsystematic, narrative overviews. In descending order of importance, the physicians also cited the advice of colleagues, continuing medical education courses, published clinical practice guidelines, original research, and textbooks as having a major effect on their practice.

It is notable that among these potential sources of clinical information, only systematically researched practice guidelines, methodologically sound original research articles, and systematic reviews can be considered truly evidence-based, yet these do not comprise the major source of data that clinicians draw upon when making medical decisions.

Skilled physicians place an emphasis on using evidence-based literature found in medical journals. However, given the considerable time constraints inherent in today's health care marketplace, it is virtually impossible to read more than a tiny fraction of the 20,000 medical journals in publication. Even within the relatively narrow field of internal medicine, there are more than 10 major monthly publications containing more than 200 articles and 70 editorials.[3]

How, then, do those few individuals who are renowned for their knowledge of the literature manage to identify, read, and critically evaluate most of the relevant and important studies that are published each month? These individuals have mastered three techniques. (1) They have developed a surveillance strategy with which they identify reliable literature sources to update themselves on new developments in their areas of interest. (2) They are skilled in both searching and critically evaluating the literature to answer specific clinical questions. (3) They are disciplined enough to designate a specific time for selective reading. If you begin to develop a strategy for selective reading now, you will rapidly expand your fund of clinically useful knowledge and shrink the stacks of plastic-wrapped journals that may currently serve as your office (or bedroom) furniture.

A STRATEGIC APPROACH

A successful strategy for keeping abreast of the relevant medical literature includes the following steps:

1. Develop a surveillance strategy to keep abreast of new developments across a broad range of subjects within clinical medicine.
2. Develop expertise in finding specific information to answer focused clinical questions.
3. Establish protected time for regular reading.

Develop a surveillance strategy

Because it is extremely time-inefficient to perform a comprehensive medical literature search every time a clinical question arises, it is highly desirable to prospectively identify and critically review newly published studies that are likely to affect our clinical practice. The well-informed, evidence-based clinician should endeavor to keep abreast of major developments in several relevant areas of clinical medicine, frequently supplementing this broadly based fund of knowledge with the techniques learned in Chapters 5 and 6 for answering focused clinical questions. A successful surveillance strategy for maintaining broad familiarity with the most reliable medical literature is a cornerstone of the practice of evidence-based medicine. The following guidelines will be useful in accomplishing this goal.

Choose a small number of core journals for regular browsing

Select two or three peer-reviewed journals that publish studies within your particular field of interest and one or two general medical journals, and plan to browse these on a regular basis. Journals have widely differing standards and reputations for methodologic rigor, peer review, and statistical review. An adept reviewer of the literature will be aware of these factors as they apply to the major journals in his or her field. In developing your list of core journals, consider seeking the advice of expert clinicians, department chairs or division chiefs, expert lecturers at well-presented continuing medical education meetings, valued consultants, or a reference librarian in your medical library. When prominent faculty at our institution were informally asked to list 3–5 of the most clinically useful journals they would recommend for regular reading by others in their field, we obtained the following responses:

> Internal medicine: *The New England Journal of Medicine, Annals of Internal Medicine, Journal of the American Medical Association, British Medical Journal, The Lancet*
> Neurology: *Neurology, Archives of Neurology, Journal of Neurology, Neurosurgery and Psychiatry*
> Obstetrics/gynecology: *American Journal of Obstetrics and Gynecology, Obstetrics and Gynecology, British Journal of Obstetrics and Gynecology, Adolescent and Pediatric Gynecology, Contraception*
> Pediatrics: *Pediatrics, American Journal of Public Health, American Journal of Diseases of Children, Journal of Pediatrics, Journal of Adolescent Health*
> Surgery: *Surgery, Journal of Vascular Surgery, British Journal of Surgery, Journal of Surgical Oncology, Journal of Thoracic and Cardiovascular Surgery*

Note that the above list is incomplete and serves only as an example of a few quality journals in a number of fields of medicine. It may serve as a starting point to help you generate your own list, which likely will include journals that usually publish studies that are interesting, important, and relevant to your clinical practice.

Browse before you read

It is much more efficient to browse several journals for articles worth reading than it is to read every study in a few journals. Once you have identified 2–5 peer-reviewed journals that publish high-quality studies in areas in which you are interested, develop the habit of browsing the table of contents when each arrives. Reject immediately any articles on topics that are either uninteresting or unimportant to your areas of interest or clinical practice. Then ask yourself whether the studies that have met your first criterion will provide novel information, rather than simply support a clinical practice you already embrace. Next, read the abstract of the articles you have selected to determine whether the conclusions (if later judged valid) would be relevant to your practice. Reading the abstracts will not allow you to determine whether the conclusions are in fact valid, but it will tell you whether they are potentially useful. If not, move on to the next article. Finally, consider the authors and the study site. Are the results likely to be generalizable to your patient population? Once you have winnowed the articles that you will read, examine this small collection of studies critically, following the guidelines described in Chapter 8 for assessing the validity of a study.

Expand your literature surveillance by reading prereviewed summaries

A number of journals and organizations publish structured abstracts of articles culled from many major journals: *Journal Watch, ACP Journal Club,* and the recently published *Evidence-Based Medicine,* for example, provide brief summaries of important papers published in more than 50 American and British medical journals. The reviewers of the original articles provide commentary about the background, applicability, and limitations of the studies. Also included is the article's reference citation, which will enable you to find the original paper at the library or on-line for critical reading. Publications of this type can be invaluable in increasing your familiarity with important advances in fields outside your area of expertise, helping you increase your fund of knowledge across all fields of medicine.

Use continuing medical education courses and conferences to expand your familiarity with the medical literature

All physicians licensed in the United States are required to document attendance at accredited continuing medical education (CME) courses or conferences. As is true for medical journals, these courses provide variable degrees of evidence-based education. The best of them, however, can provide you with an opportunity to learn about the most important advances in your field from expert discussants prepared to answer questions. Several national organizations include "Updates" series at their annual meetings. The American College of Physicians presents "Updates" in all of the subspecialties of internal medicine and also provides on disk to all members a synopsis of the key studies discussed.

Expand your knowledge by reading evidence-based syntheses

Integrative literature (eg, systematic reviews, meta-analyses, and comprehensive clinical practice guidelines) can function as a very efficient tool for increasing both the breadth and depth of your knowledge about a particular aspect of clinical care.

Suppose, for example, that you wish to update yourself about the optimal therapy for congestive heart failure—a broad topic (ie, the broad question, "What is the current optimal therapy for congestive heart failure?"). You are unlikely to have browsed all the relevant articles in your small set of core journals to which you have been subscribing during the last few years. Evidence to this fact are the hundreds of articles that have been published on this subject during the last few years. Time simply does not allow you to retrieve all these articles. Furthermore, many of these articles are methodologically flawed. And even with a thorough search using MEDLINE, you are certain you will not identify *all* of the papers that are relevant to your clinical question. On the other hand, identifying and reading a well-researched publication that has integrated all the relevant research *will* efficiently update you in this area of interest. A MEDLINE search, including the terms "congestive heart failure" and "practice guideline" identifies a number of published guidelines, including one published by the Agency for Health Care Policy and Research (AHCPR). You download the 126-page "AHCPR Clinical Practice Guideline for the Management of Congestive Heart Failure"[4] from the Internet. Using the approach to evaluating the validity of integrative literature in Chapter 10, you determine that this source of information is comprehensive and evidence-based, so you spend the next 2 hours reading and learning, rather than frantically searching for missing journals in the library. You might instead have searched for a systematic review published in a respected journal or by The Cochrane Collaboration,[5] a network of worldwide teams that use quantitative techniques to produce comprehensive summaries on a wide variety of important clinical topics. The Cochrane reports, which in the earliest publications focused primarily on topics in obstetrics and perinatology, are disseminated primarily via electronic means and can be easily accessed using the skills you learned in Chapter 6.

Your update of the clinical area of interest is obviously only as current as the most recent year that studies were included in the synthesis. Nonetheless, you have been very efficient and have covered many years of voluminous material. The relatively small number of relevant articles published subsequent to the synthesis may be searched by using MEDLINE, as discussed below.

Develop expertise in finding specific information to answer focused clinical questions

Even if you have been successful in maintaining a broad fund of knowledge regarding new developments in your field using the above suggestions, you will frequently need answers to very *specific* questions.

In addition to keeping abreast and up to date with a relatively broad clinical question, **systematic reviews, meta-analyses,** and **clinical practice guidelines,** which provide the most comprehensive, rigorous review of data, are often a good starting point to answer a question about a very specific aspect of patient care. Even if the review or guideline does not answer your specific question, you might discover a specific article in the bibliography that does.

Alternatively, you may elect to find the answer by performing a MEDLINE search of **original research articles** that address the specific clinical question. The reader is cautioned to search for all relevant articles rather than stopping at the first one identified in a cursory search. If you do not find a particular study that answers your question, you may discover illuminating information by searching for a relevant **decision or cost-effectiveness analysis.** A comprehensive guideline for MEDLINE searching is presented in Chapter 5.

A number of other sources supplement the breadth and depth of your fund of knowledge.

Textbooks are the traditional source for researching medical facts or identifying treatment algorithms. The rapid pace of scientific advancement has rendered most textbooks outdated or obsolete by the time of publication, however. Although a comprehensive textbook may prove to be the best source of information about pathophysiology, disease classification, or staging, it infrequently provides up-to-date treatment information. CD-ROM versions allow for more frequent updating of text material, but the reader will still be unable to ascertain whether all relevant data were incorporated into the text's recommendations. Textbooks thus serve as a useful source for background reading, but usually do not supply truly evidence-based treatment recommendations to guide clinical practice.

Pharmaceutical company literature and **noncomprehensive overviews** published in "throw-away" journals, although readily accessible and highly readable, vary widely with regard to peer review and quality and are particularly susceptible to bias. These sources of information may provide up-to-date background reading on a subject but should not be relied upon to provide the rigorous analysis and synthesis of available data on which one guides evidence-based practice.

Establish protected time for critical reading

To reach your goal of keeping up with the medical literature, you need to start reading today. The task is daunting, because your scheduled reading time will compete for your valuable "free" time with those popular activities of sleep, social intercourse, and eating. The key to establishing a lifelong discipline of reading is to recognize that you will never have enough free time to accommodate the reading you need to do. Instead, you must identify and protect a few hours each week that you will devote to medical reading. Starting now, resolve to establish a lifelong discipline of reading regularly, selectively, and critically.

SUMMARY

1. Increase the breadth of your knowledge by developing a surveillance strategy by which you select core journals that you browse and critically evaluate those articles you find interesting, novel, and relevant. In addition, read prereviewed summaries and evidence-based syntheses and attend continuing medical education courses and conferences.

2. Increase the depth of your knowledge by answering focused clinical questions using MEDLINE and the Internet to search for individual studies, systematic reviews, meta-analyses, and rigorously assembled clinical practice guidelines.
3. Finally, to meet this challenge, establish protected time for reading.

REFERENCES

1. Price DS: The development and structure of the biomedical literature. In: Warren KS (editor): *Coping with the Biomedical Literature: A Primer for the Scientist and the Clinician.* Praeger, 1981.
2. Tunis SR et al: Internists' attitudes about clinical practice guidelines. Ann Intern Med 1994;120:956.
3. Warren KS: Qualitative aspects of the biomedical literature. In: Warren KS (editor): *Coping with the Biomedical Literature: A Primer for the Scientist and the Clinician.* Praeger, 1981.
4. Agency for Health Care Policy and Research: *Clinical Practice Guideline: Congestive Heart Failure.* US Department of Health and Human Services, Public Health Service, 1995.
5. Bero L, Rennie D: The Cochrane Collaboration. Preparing, maintaining, and disseminating systematic reviews of the effects of health care. JAMA 1995;274:1935.

3

ASSESSING THE VALIDITY OF MEDICAL INFORMATION

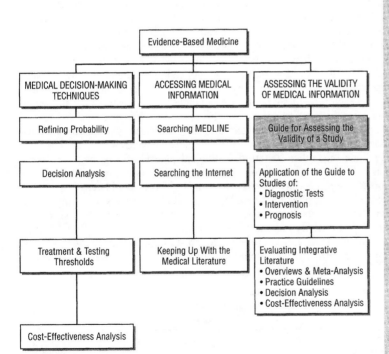

GUIDE FOR ASSESSING THE VALIDITY OF A STUDY

Daniel J. Friedland, MD

Evidence-Based Medicine

MEDICAL DECISION-MAKING TECHNIQUES	ACCESSING MEDICAL INFORMATION	ASSESSING THE VALIDITY OF MEDICAL INFORMATION
Refining Probability	Searching MEDLINE	Guide for Assessing the Validity of a Study
Decision Analysis	Searching the Internet	Application of the Guide to Studies of: • Diagnostic Tests • Intervention • Prognosis
Treatment & Testing Thresholds	Keeping Up With the Medical Literature	Evaluating Integrative Literature • Overviews & Meta-Analysis • Practice Guidelines • Decision Analysis • Cost-Effectiveness Analysis
Cost-Effectiveness Analysis		

INTRODUCTION

Scientific studies pursue truth. In evaluating a study, the initial consideration is whether the study arrived at this truth successfully. The next consideration is whether knowledge of this truth will benefit the patient.

The evaluation of truth in a study is analogous to the evaluation of the true nature of the human body. During the first session of anatomy in medical school, we faced the daunting task of discovery. The human body would reveal itself to us after a thorough, systematic dissection. The dissection process allowed us to view body structures juxtaposed, and this relationship ultimately revealed truth in the body. In the same manner, dissection of a study reveals its truth. For a successful, thorough, systematic dissection of a study or the human body, a dissection guide can be invaluable.

Creation of a single guide to evaluate the diversity of medical information is indeed a challenge. To extend the above analogy, this is akin to the design of a single dissection guide that applies not only to humans but to chimpanzees, dogs, horses, and mice as well. To simplify matters, the diversity of published medical information may be classified as shown in Figure 8–1.

Published medical research may be broadly classified as either **studies** or **integrative literature.** Studies are considered **descriptive** if they "describe" individual variables (eg, the prevalence or characteristics of a particular disease) or **analytic** if they "analyze" the association between two or more variables (eg, an intervention and mortality). The majority of studies that we evaluate are of the analytic type. **Integrative literature** is distinct in that it "integrates" information derived from individual studies within a particular framework to provide a summary finding or recommendation. Examples of integrative literature are overviews, meta-analyses, practice guidelines, decision analyses, and cost-effectiveness analyses.

Recently, the Evidence-Based Medicine Working Group (EBMWG) has undertaken the challenge to systematically evaluate this diversity of published medical research. Its approach has been published as a series of journal articles, the "Users' Guide to the Medical Literature."[1-15] Their guide contains a series of questions that are individually tailored to multiple types of studies (therapy, diagnosis, harm, and prognosis) and integrative literature (overview, decision analysis, practice guidelines, and cost-effectiveness analysis).

The guide presented in this chapter incorporates the EBMWG guide's general framework, which considers a study's validity, results, and application to patient care. Our guide, however, is fundamentally different in two main respects. First, instead of posing a different set of questions for each type of study, it poses a single set of questions for studies of risk, diagnostic tests, intervention, and prognosis. This *unified approach* is rooted in an explanation of a number of key concepts in epidemiology, medical decision making, and designing clinical research. Second, our guide attempts to place the study within a context of other relevant knowledge (eg, other literature, biological plausibility) to help us assess whether the result is believable. In other words, our guide attempts to provide a Bayesian perspective of the poststudy probability. (We'll discuss this in more detail later.)

The guide presented below applies to the evaluation of studies. It does not apply to the evaluation of integrative literature. (An approach to integrative literature is presented in Chapter 10). The guide is primarily tailored to analytic studies and is slightly modified to evaluate descriptive studies. Thus, if you are evaluating a study that *examines the association between two or more variables* you should use the analytic study guide. If, however,

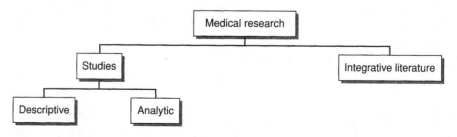

Figure 8–1. Classification of published medical research.

you are evaluating a descriptive study, which simply *describes one or more variables,* you should use the modified guide.

The outline of the analytic study guide is presented first, followed by a detailed explanation of each step. Near the end of the chapter, you will find a one-page summary that may serve as a memory aid when using this guide to evaluate analytic studies. At the end of the chapter, you will find a description and summary of the guide's modified approach to descriptive studies. In addition, you will also find these study guide summaries on the handy bookmark provided with this book.

The guide is designed to systematically evaluate a study in five steps. Infrequently, a particular question will not apply to a specific type of study. For example, in studies of diagnostic tests, you do not need to consider the issue of confounding. When a question is not applicable, simply proceed to the next question.

To facilitate understanding and proficiency with the guide, this chapter should be read in conjunction with Chapter 9, in which the guide is applied to study examples.

ANALYTIC STUDY GUIDE OUTLINE

Step 1. Do I want to evaluate the study?
Step 2. Outline the study.
Step 3. Is the study finding believable?
    A. Do the study subjects and variables accurately represent the research question?
    B. Is the finding attributable to other factors?
      • Chance
      • Bias
      • Confounders
    C. Is the finding believable within the context of other knowledge?
      • Consistency with other literature
      • Biological plausibility
      • Analogy
Step 4. What is the clinically relevant finding?
Step 5. Will the study help me in caring for my patient?
    A. Are the subjects adequately described and similar to my patient?
    B. Is the predictor variable adequately described and applicable to my patient?
    C. Will the finding result in an overall net benefit for my patient?

ANALYTIC STUDY GUIDE EXPLANATION

Step 1. Do I want to evaluate the study? (Three questions [INR])[16]

Is the research question:

Interesting? The most compelling reason for reading an article is whether it stimulates our interest. Interest provides the motivation for us to take the necessary time to evaluate the study.

Novel? A study is novel if it provides new findings or extends previous findings.

Relevant? There are three factors to consider to help you determine whether a study is relevant. First, is it an important clinical question, in terms of either prevalence of disease or resources used? Second, will the study topic apply to a patient that we might see in our clinical practice? Finally, is the research question framed in a clinically meaningful way? This often entails a consideration of the significance of the outcome. For example, a study that determines the impact of antihypertensive treatment on morbidity or mortality would be more relevant to the care of our patient than would a study that considered the impact of antihypertensive treatment on blood pressure control alone.

Step 2. Outline the study

This step constitutes the dissection. The premise of the dissection is that there is a given truth or reality in the universe that is expressed as a particular research question. This *truth* is sought by a *study,* which yields a *finding.* The outline therefore is composed of three components: the truth in the universe, the study method, and the study finding (see Figure 8–2).

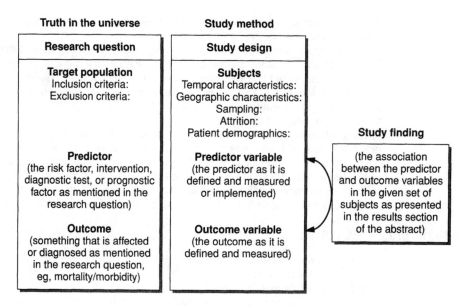

Figure 8–2. Outline for an analytic study.

The concept of **truth in the universe** is broad and expansive. A **research question** represents a particular truth in the universe that considers the association between a given predictor and the outcome in a defined target population. In an analytic study, we may identify the key components of a specific research question (predictor, outcome and target population) by considering the association of "what" with "what," in "whom." Because this format easily delineates these key components of the research question, if a particular study does not present the research question in this manner, it is helpful to reformat it as such. An example of an optimally formatted research question is, "What is the effect of the use of a steroid inhaler on mortality in adults with asthma who are older than 18 years?" Let's look at the individual components of the research question, described in detail below.

The **target population** is the complete set of persons throughout the world as defined by the main inclusion and exclusion criteria of the study. In the above research question, the target population is all adults with asthma who are older than 18 years.

The **predictor** and **outcome** are simply occurrences or events in the universe. A **predictor** is something that precedes, affects, or tests for the outcome. Predictors are thus either the risk factor, prognostic factor, intervention, or diagnostic test. It follows that an **outcome** is something that is being affected or diagnosed. Mortality and morbidity, for example, are outcomes. To identify the predictor and outcome, we simply consider the research question. For example, in the research question, "Does the use of a steroid inhaler reduce mortality in adults with asthma who are older than 18 years," the predictor is the intervention (ie, the use of the steroid inhaler), and the outcome is mortality. The specific predictor and outcome are dependent on the type of study, as shown in Table 8–1.

To evaluate a research question, the researcher chooses a particular study design, selects a group of subjects to represent the target population, and defines measurable variables to represent the predictor and outcome. This enables the researcher to evaluate the association

TABLE 8–1. PREDICTOR AND OUTCOME ACCORDING TO STUDY TYPE.

Study Type	Predictor	Outcome
Risk	Risk factor	Mortality, morbidity
Intervention	Intervention	Mortality, morbidity, cost, quality of life
Diagnostic test	Diagnostic test	Morbidity
Prognosis	Prognostic factor	Mortality, morbidity

between the predictor variable and outcome variable in a given set of subjects. The study design and manner in which the subjects and variables are selected are critical to a study's validity. These factors largely determine the study's ability to answer the "truth in the universe" research question—which considers the association between the predictor and outcome in the given target population.

In the **study method,** the type of study design, the subjects, and the variables are outlined. Each of these components is described as follows.

As mentioned in the introduction, studies are broadly classified as **descriptive** or **analytic.** Analytic studies analyze the association between a predictor and outcome variable and are classified according to one of four basic **study designs:** experimental, cohort, case-control, and cross-sectional. The prototype **experimental study** is the double-blind, randomized, controlled trial. Subjects are randomly divided into two or more groups. The researcher provides one group with a placebo and the other with an intervention and in each group measures the occurrence of an outcome variable. The "double-blinding" refers to both researcher and subject not having knowledge as to whether the placebo or intervention has been provided (eg, by using identical coded capsules, the identity of which is revealed only after completion of the trial). In the **cohort study,** subjects are observed over time and associations are made between predictor and outcome variables. In **case-control studies,** these associations are made by selecting groups according to whether an outcome is present or absent, and then within each group determining whether a given predictor variable has occurred. In **cross-sectional studies,** a group of study subjects are evaluated at a single slice in time, and associations are made between predictors and outcome variables. Detailed descriptions of these designs and their relative strengths and weaknesses have been published.[16,17] Three simple questions that serve to distinguish these basic analytic study designs are outlined in Figure 8–3.

It is usually not feasible to study all the patients in the target population. Therefore, a representative group of study **subjects** are chosen through a selection process. Upon selection, the usual process of attrition accounts for the final group of subjects analyzed. A number of key factors are included in the outline to describe the subjects used in the analysis. "Temporal characteristics" refer to the dates encompassing the recruitment period as well as the duration of follow up. "Geographic characteristics" refer to the country or city as well as type of center in which the study took place. "Sampling" is the most important aspect of study selection and describes the manner in which subjects are sampled. We first consider the number of patients screened and then the sampling method used to enroll subjects into the study (eg, subjects sampled and assigned randomly or consecutively). "Attrition" notes the subjects who drop out or who are lost to follow up. The final subjects used in the analysis are characterized by "patient demographics" that are usually presented in the first table of the study.

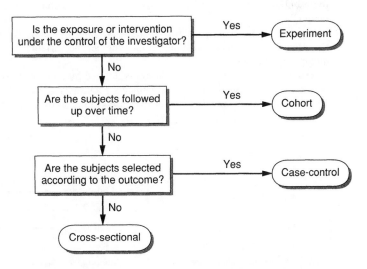

Figure 8–3. Flow diagram to help determine the basic analytic study design.

A **variable** represents the manner in which the predictor and outcome are defined and measured (or, in the case of some predictors, implemented). For example consider the research question, "Does intravenous drug use lead to an increased risk of human immunodeficiency virus (HIV) infection in the general population?" If you were evaluating such a study, in the outline you would note how the variables define and measure the predictor and outcome. The predictor variable in such a study would be the way it defined and measured the predictor, intravenous drug use. For example, the predictor variable in the study might define intravenous drug use as "the use of any intravenously administered recreational drug after 1975" and measure it in a blinded fashion using a structured interview. Similarly, as an outcome variable, HIV infection may be defined as a positive HIV antibody test, which is measured by enzyme-linked immunosorbent assay (ELISA), and confirmed by Western blot analysis.

The **study finding** is the final component of the outline. It is the association between the predictor and outcome variables in the given set of subjects as presented in the "results" section of the abstract. The magnitude of the finding is commonly presented together with its level of statistical significance (usually a p value or 95% confidence interval). In addition, in this part of the outline, you may choose to note the key statistical methods used to analyze the association.

Before you proceed to the next step, you may find it helpful to look at examples of the outlines for the three studies evaluated in Chapter 9. Once you have outlined the study, the dissection is complete! Each reader will decide whether it is more efficient to actually write the outline or to simply use it as a cognitive process for organizing the key elements of the dissection. The next step of the guide evaluates the relationships between the various components of the study outline to help us determine whether we *believe* the study finding.

Step 3. Is the study finding believable?

A. Do the study subjects and variables accurately represent the research question?

Recall that the research question considers the association between "what" and "what," in "whom" (ie, the association between the predictor and outcome in a target population). To determine whether the research question is represented by appropriate study subjects and variables, we therefore assess whether study subjects and variables accurately represent the target population, the predictor, and the outcome.

The premise of step 3A is that the subjects and variables must be accurate representations of the target population, predictor, and outcome in order for the **association** between the predictor and outcome in the given target population to be meaningful. In other words, the variables and subjects describing the "what," "what," and "whom" must be accurate representations before you can consider "the association between the what and what, in whom."

Figure 8–4 shows how we first evaluate whether the study subjects accurately represent the target population and then determine whether the variables accurately represent the predictor and outcome.

Remember that the target population is defined by a given set of inclusion and exclusion criteria. To determine whether the subjects accurately represent the target population, we therefore need to ensure that the subjects used in the analysis actually met the inclusion and

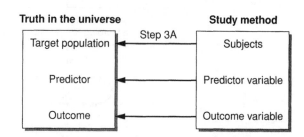

Figure 8–4. Schematic representation of step 3A.

exclusion criteria. For example, in a study that evaluated whether carotid endarterectomy decreased stroke and mortality in asymptomatic patients with carotid artery stenosis of greater than 60%, fewer than 5% of patients had stenosis of less than 60%.[18] Because only a few subjects did not meet the criteria, the subjects are therefore well representative of the target population. If, however, half the subjects had been found to have stenosis of less than 60%, they would not have been representative of the target population. The study would not have answered the given research question, but rather would have evaluated the association of "what" with "what" in a *different* "whom."

To determine whether the variables are accurate representations of the predictor and outcome, we consider how each variable was defined and measured. If the variables are inaccurate representations of the predictor and outcome, the association made between the variables will not be meaningful—no matter how rigorously the study limits the effect of chance, bias, or confounding. Suppose a study evaluates the association between Q-wave myocardial infarction (predictor) and congestive heart failure (outcome). If the researcher uses an inaccurate variable to represent the predictor, such as self-reported Q-wave myocardial infarction, rather than an electrocardiographic-based diagnosis, the association would not be meaningful. Similarly, consider a study of a diagnostic test that evaluates the use of a ventilation-perfusion (V/Q) scan (predictor) to diagnose pulmonary embolism (outcome). If the study uses as the outcome variable the "paper standard" of pleuritic chest pain, rather than the "gold standard" angiography to measure a pulmonary embolism, the reported sensitivity and specificity would not be valid.

Some people confuse step 3A, "Do the study subjects and variables accurately represent the research question?," with whether the subjects and variables can be applied to their patient population. It is important to recognize that this question is intended to determine whether the study subjects and variables appropriately represent the target population and predictor and outcome in the research question (in truth, in the universe). If the subjects and variables are accurate representations, we proceed to the next two questions (steps 3B and 3C), which evaluate whether the *association* between the predictor and outcome is valid and believable in the context of other knowledge. If we believe the finding, we then determine the clinically relevant result (step 4). In the final step (step 5), we determine whether the study can be applied to our patient (ie, whether the subjects and variables can be applied to our patient population) and whether the clinically relevant result would lead to net patient benefit.

B. Is the finding attributable to other factors?

(See Figure 8–5.)

If the subjects, predictor variable, and outcome variable accurately represent the research question, we next consider whether the association between the predictor and outcome variable is believable. To determine the validity of the association, we assess whether the predictor itself was responsible for the finding or whether the finding is attributable to other factors. If there are no other factors to explain the finding, the finding is valid.

Two issues will help you anticipate the likelihood that the finding will be explained by other factors. These are the **study design** and the study **source.**

When considering the study design, you should first determine whether a comparison or control group has been included. If not, the study design is descriptive, rather than analytic. The study can therefore only describe an outcome in a population and not analyze

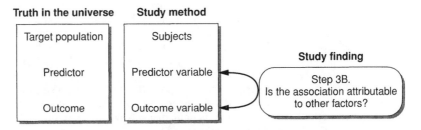

Figure 8–5. Schematic representation of step 3B.

associations. Consider an example of a study of aspirin and stroke. If the study does not include a comparison group, it only describes the number of strokes in a population a subjects taking aspirin—and we cannot draw any conclusions as to the nature of the association between aspirin and stroke. On the other hand, if the study does include a comparison group, the study is analytic and can determine whether aspirin reduces the incidence of stroke. With a comparison group, we are able to determine whether the outcome is explained by the predictor, rather than being attributable to the natural history of disease in that population.

Other factors that may provide an alternative explanation for the finding are **chance, bias, confounding,** and **effect-cause.**[16] The strength of the analytic study design is determined by its susceptibility to a number of these factors and therefore helps us anticipate the degree to which these factors might explain the finding. The strength of design is as follows:

Experimental studies > cohort studies > case-control and cross-sectional studies

The experimental and cohort study designs are usually less susceptible to bias than are cross-sectional and case-control studies. An experimental study in the form of a randomized-controlled trial is the design that is least susceptible to the effect of confounding.

Another noteworthy aspect of the study design is whether it is prospective (eg, prospective cohort) or retrospective (eg, retrospective cohort or case-control). **Prospective studies** are considered stronger because they identify a predictor variable, follow the subjects forward in time, and then determine an outcome. **Retrospective studies,** on the other hand, look back in time at the relationship between the predictor and outcome. In prospective studies, we are thus more confident that the predictor variable preceded the outcome variable (ie, that the horse came before the cart). It is important that a predictor precedes the outcome; otherwise, the finding cannot be attributed to the predictor. In fact, rather than the predictor causing the outcome, an alternative explanation is that the outcome caused the predictor (ie, rather than *cause-effect,* the finding is attributed to *effect-cause*). Consider a study that evaluates whether low serum levels of vitamin D predispose toward hip fracture. If this were a retrospective study, we might be unsure whether the predictor preceded the outcome. It is possible that rather than diminished levels of vitamin D leading to hip fracture, hip fractures result in less exposure to sunlight because patients more often stay indoors, and *this* leads to decreased levels of the vitamin. Retrospective studies, therefore, need to take additional steps to ensure the predictor precedes the outcome. In this example, we would need to ensure that the serum was collected before the subjects experienced their fractures or otherwise show that hip fractures alone do not decrease the serum level of the vitamin.

The source of the study is the other issue that helps us anticipate how hard we may have to work to assess whether a particular study finding is believable. The "source" includes the study's sponsorship, the merit of the journal in which it was published, and the authors' reputation. For example, studies that are sponsored by pharmaceutical companies and published in the "Journal of Medical Obscura" may require particularly close scrutiny to ensure that the finding is not significantly biased or confounded.

Step 3B focuses on the three major factors that provide alternative explanations that would decrease our belief in a finding: chance, bias, and confounding.

Chance (statistical significance). The role of chance in the reported association is evaluated by the following statistics.

The **p value** represents the probability that the association found between the predictor and outcome variables could have occurred by chance when in fact there is no association between the predictor and outcome. Arbitrarily, if the p value for the association was found to be less than 0.05 (ie, there was less than a 5% probability of finding an association when no association exists), it is generally considered statistically significant[16] and unlikely to be attributable to chance.

The **power** of a study records the probability of finding a specific magnitude of association between the predictor and outcome variables, if such an association exists. This value is calculated *before* the study is implemented and is determined by the number of subjects, the estimated magnitude of effect, and the precision of the measures. Arbitrarily, a power of 0.8 (ie, an 80% probability) is usually thought to be sufficient to detect a specified effect size determined before the study.[16] It has been argued that power is a statistic that is relevant only in the design phase of the study. After the study is completed, the width of the confidence interval (discussed below) is the more relevant statistic,[19] facilitating contemplation as to whether more precise variables or a greater number subjects might have enabled the researcher to find a particular association.

The **confidence interval** (CI) represents the range of values that are statistically compatible with the estimate of the study result. By convention, the 95% CI is the range of values that would not differ from the estimate provided by the study at a statistical significance of 0.05.[19] A study that reports a mortality reduction of 10% (95% CI of 5–15%) implies that the data are statistically compatible with an effect as small as 5% or as large as 15% at a significance level of 0.05. If an interval spans a relative risk or odds ratio (see step 4A for an explanation of these terms) of 1.0 or effect size of 0, the results are statistically indistinguishable from no effect and are therefore not statistically significant. The width of the CI is determined by the number of study subjects and the precision of the measurements. The narrower the CI, the more precise the result and the less likely it is attributable to chance. The CI is thus a very useful statistic. As shown in Table 8–2, the CI provides information about both the statistical significance and the precision of the finding.

Studies with an imprecise finding that is not significant lead us to question whether the finding might be significant with more precise measurements or a larger number of subjects.

A subtle point to note about defining the CI: A 95% CI does not represent a 95% probability of finding the test result in the given range of values. This would require a consideration of previous information (ie, prior probability) to help us ascertain the true probability of the effect. The CI is determined entirely by the study data. The prior probability is not at all considered in the calculation.[20]

?Bias. Bias has been defined as "any process at any stage of inference which tends to produce results or conclusions that differ systematically from the truth."[21] In other words, bias is a process during the design, implementation, or analysis of the study by which researchers, subjects, or instruments effect a spurious increase or decrease in the magnitude of the finding.

Because there is no statistical method to evaluate the effect of bias, the determination of its impact is a matter of judgment. A major bias may invalidate a study even before the analysis is performed, as there is no effective way to adjust for it statistically. However, when a major bias is identified, caution is required before dismissing the study as invalid. The direction of the bias should always be assessed because it may strengthen rather than weaken the finding (see Chapter 9, page 205).

An extensive list of biases has been catalogued.[22] Although the following approach to the evaluation of bias is not necessarily exhaustive, its systematic evaluation of the individual components of the study method and analysis should identify most significant biases (Figure 8–6). By referring to the study outline (and focusing on the "study method" and "study finding" components of Figure 8–2 in particular), you may identify biases that take place in:

1. Selecting the study subjects
2. Following up on the study subjects
3. Executing or measuring the predictor variable
4. Measuring the outcome variable
5. Analyzing the data

TABLE 8–2. EXAMPLES OF CONFIDENCE INTERVALS.

Relative Risk	Confidence Interval	Comment
1.2	0.1–9	Not significant, imprecise result
1.2	0.9–1.4	Not significant, precise result
1.2	1.1–1.3	Significant, precise result
4	1.1–8	Significant, imprecise result

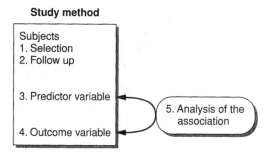

Figure 8–6. Schematic representation of the components of the study outline in which biases may occur.

BIASES IN SELECTING THE STUDY SUBJECTS. For studies of risk, intervention, and prognosis, it is important that, but for the effect of the predictor, both the study and comparison groups are equally likely to have the outcome. For example, in studies of intervention, if patients in the comparison group are in worse health than patients in the study group, comparison group patients may be more likely to have the outcome than the study group patients. This would result in the intervention appearing to be more effective than it really is. Consider a study that evaluates the ability of a new congestive heart failure medication to reduce mortality. If the intervention group recruited patients with less severe heart failure, a reduction in mortality in this group could be explained by having relatively healthier patients than the comparison group, rather than a real efficacy of the medication. In studies of intervention, one way to ensure that study and control group members have similar baseline characteristics is to first assess whether the patients have been allocated randomly (ie, in a randomized-controlled trial). Next we note the similarity of each group's baseline characteristics (usually displayed in the first table of an article) to evaluate whether the random allocation was successful.

Alternatively, for studies of risk, intervention, and prognosis, if the study and comparison group are recruited according to outcome (ie, case-control studies), the occurrence of the predictor should not be influenced by the process of group selection. Suppose, for example, a hospital population is being studied. If the study outcome makes it more likely that subjects with a given predictor are admitted, the measure of association will be distorted. Consider a study in which the prevalence of hypertension in a hospital population with acute myocardial infarction is compared with the prevalence of hypertension in a hospital group without acute infarction. If patients with a history of hypertension were more likely than those without this history to be admitted to rule out acute infarction (because emergency department physicians, believing that hypertension is a risk factor for acute infarction, had a lower threshold for admitting these subjects), there would be a spurious increase in the strength of association between a history of hypertension and acute infarction.

In studies of diagnostic tests, the most important factor in subject selection is that an appropriate spectrum of subjects are represented. **Spectrum bias** occurs if selection of the subjects results in diseased patients all having relatively advanced illness and nondiseased patients being very healthy. Since subjects with advanced disease are less likely to have false-negative test results and very healthy nondiseased subjects are less likely to have false-positive test results, such a spectrum of patients would overestimate the sensitivity and specificity of the test in a population with a broader spectrum of disease severity.[23] (An explanation of the terms sensitivity and specificity is provided in Chapter 1.)

BIASES IN FOLLOWING UP ON THE STUDY SUBJECTS. In studies of intervention, successful random allocation of subjects does not ensure that the study and control groups will have similar baseline characteristics when the data are finally analyzed. For example, if the most ill patients in the study group dropped out or were lost to follow up, at the time of analysis the study group would be healthier than the comparison group. This may result in the intervention appearing to be more efficacious then it really is.

Similarly, spurious associations can result in studies of risk and prognosis if subjects from either the study or comparison group drop out or are lost to follow up.

In studies of diagnostic tests, it is important that subjects who have negative test results still be evaluated with the gold standard. If these patients drop out of the study, the proportion of patients with both false-negative and true-negative results would be reduced. As a result, the sensitivity of the test would be overestimated and the specificity of the test would be underestimated. This is known as **verification bias.**[23]

BIASES IN EXECUTING OR MEASURING THE PREDICTOR VARIABLE. When you are determining bias in execution of the predictor variable, it is important to assess whether the study and comparison groups received the assigned therapy. If some members of the study group did not receive the intervention, while some in the comparison group did, for a truly efficacious therapy, the magnitude of the study finding may be systematically reduced. Furthermore, it is also important to determine whether the study and comparison groups experienced other interventions ("co-interventions"). For example, in a study evaluating the efficacy of a cholesterol-lowering medication on cardiac mortality, it would be important to ensure that the study group did not receive more intensive counseling on tobacco cessation or other lifestyle changes. Any study finding ascribed to the therapy might otherwise be attributable to the co-intervention.

In case-control studies in which study and comparison groups are defined by the outcome, it is important to assess bias that might occur in measuring the predictor variable. We make this assessment by ensuring that the appraisal of the predictor variable by both subject and researcher was equal between the study and comparison groups. Both the subjects' memory of an exposure and the vigor with which the researcher ascertains the exposure may lead to spurious findings. For example, in a study that evaluates the association of estrogen therapy and breast cancer, women with breast cancer may ruminate as to the disease's cause and therefore may be more likely to remember their exposure to estrogen than women without breast cancer. This is known as **recall bias** and can be assessed by verifying the subjects' report with medical or pharmacy records or determining whether the women with breast cancer reported a greater frequency of "dummy" exposures (exposures unlikely to be associated with breast cancer) than did the comparison group. Alternatively, if the research hypothesis is that estrogen *does* lead to breast cancer, the researcher might be more vigorous in eliciting a history of estrogen use in women with beast cancer. This is known as **investigator bias** and can be assessed by determining whether the interviewer was unaware of ("blinded to") the outcome variable.

Studies of diagnostic tests are also subject to investigator bias (also known as **gold standard review bias**).[23] If researchers have knowledge of the outcome variable (the gold standard test result), their interpretation of the predictor variable (the diagnostic test) may be affected. For example, in a study that evaluates the test characteristics of a V/Q scan for the diagnosis of pulmonary embolism, knowledge of the gold standard angiogram result would likely result in a concordant V/Q scan interpretation. For the angiogram that showed an embolus, the V/Q scan is more likely to be read as high probability. Similarly, knowledge of a negative angiogram makes it more likely that the V/Q scan would be read as normal. This therefore overestimates both the sensitivity and specificity of the test.

BIASES IN MEASURING THE OUTCOME VARIABLE. In the same way that a subject's memory and researcher's vigor can bias a finding in the measurement of the predictor variable, both parties may play a role in affecting the measurement of the outcome variable. If subjects are aware that they have received a particular intervention or are being observed, they may change their behavior, which then may change the frequency in which the outcome variable is noted. Consider a study in which the hypothesis that aspirin reduces cerebrovascular events is tested. A patient who was aware that he or she was taking the potentially beneficial medication might be less inclined to report subtle transient neurologic changes. Alternatively, if the researchers had knowledge of which patients received the medication, they might be less inclined to record subtle neurologic symptoms as cerebrovascular events in this group. As a result, aspirin's real efficacy would be systematically overestimated. Much of the strength of the double-blind, randomized, controlled trial comes from the "double-blinding," whereby both the subjects and researchers have no knowledge of the treatment assignment.

In studies of diagnostic tests, blinding the predictor variable is similarly important in determining the outcome variable (ie, interpreting the gold standard test result). In the example of the study evaluating the test characteristics of a V/Q scan for pulmonary embolism, knowledge of a normal V/Q scan would more likely result in the gold standard angiogram being read as negative. Conversely, knowledge of a high-probability V/Q scan would make it more likely that an angiogram would be read as positive. This is known as **index test review bias,** which overestimates both the sensitivity and specificity of the test.[23]

BIASES IN ANALYZING THE DATA. The association between the predictor and outcome variables is evaluated using statistical tests. Most clinicians, however, have a rudimentary view of statistics. Clinicians are thus often challenged to assess whether an inappropriate statistical approach or inappropriate use of a test biased the study to show a statistically significant result. A review on how to detect common statistical errors has been published[24]; detailed discussion is beyond the scope of this chapter. Reputable journals use a peer review process that often includes statisticians who may limit this type of bias.

A specific issue that arises in a randomized-controlled trial is how the groups are analyzed when members of the control group receive the intervention and members of the study group do not. Should the researcher analyze the groups according to their original assignments (ie, "intent-to-treat analysis") or according to the actual intervention that was received? Although it is unfortunate that both options probably provide spurious findings, the intent-to-treat analysis is usually preferred. The intent to treat analysis places a premium on preserving the random allocation. Consider what would happen in a study that evaluated the efficacy of a surgical intervention if a patient was too sick to receive the surgery. If this patient's outcome was analyzed on the control arm, this population of patients would now be even more ill overall and perhaps more likely to have the outcome event than the surgical group. This crossover could thus bias the result in favor of the surgery.

?Confounders. Whereas bias occurs through an *intrinsic* systematic process within the design, implementation, or analysis of a study, a confounded result is due to an *extrinsic* factor. This factor is associated with the predictor variable and is a cause of the outcome variable (see Figure 8–7).

The implication of confounding is that although the magnitude of the association between the predictor and outcome variables is real (as long as chance and bias do not play a role), it is not meaningful, because this magnitude can be explained by the extrinsic factor (the confounder). For example, how would you interpret the finding of a study that reported an association between carrying matches and lung cancer? Clearly this relationship is confounded by smoking tobacco, which is associated with carrying matches and causes lung cancer. In this case, the association between carrying matches and lung cancer is entirely explained by smoking tobacco (see Figure 8–8).

It is possible to limit the effect of confounding in either the design or the analytic phase of the study.[16] Two methods that limit its effect in the design phase are **specification** (exclusion of subjects with the particular confounder) and **matching subjects and controls** based on the particular confounder(s). Two methods that assess and adjust for confounding in the analytic phase of a study involve either **stratification** of the groups according to the confounder or **multivariate analysis.**

How do we then determine whether a study has accounted for all known confounders? A simple approach is to generate a list of all known factors that could cause the outcome. We then select from this list those factors that could also be associated with the predictor. This subset should represent a complete list of known confounders.

After generating the list of possible confounders, we consider whether the confounders were eliminated or adjusted for in the study using any of the four methods described above.

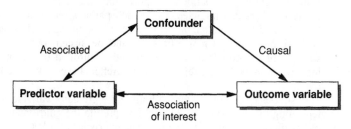

Figure 8–7. Schematic representation of confounding.

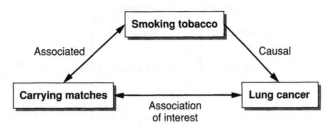

Figure 8–8. Schematic example of confounding.

Be very cautious to notice whether these methods were applied to confounders and *not* to factors in the causal pathway. For example, if a study evaluates the association between a high-fat diet and coronary artery disease, cholesterol level is *not* a confounder. A high-fat diet is not simply associated with but is rather *causal* of the cholesterol level that then causes coronary artery disease. Causal pathway is shown schematically in Figure 8–9.

If the researcher were to adjust for the cholesterol level, the ability to observe the actual association between a high-fat diet and coronary artery disease would be inappropriately eliminated.

A study obviously cannot adjust for a confounder unless it is included in the stratification or multivariate analysis. Therefore, even if a study finding has been successfully adjusted for all *known* confounders, the effect of *unknown* confounders is often questioned. This is when the randomized-controlled trial has an advantage over all other study designs. In the process of effective randomization, both known and unknown confounders should be distributed evenly between the study and control groups, thus eliminating the effect of both known and unknown confounding.

A major factor that will help you determine the degree to which a confounder is able to explain the reported association between the predictor and outcome variables is the **magnitude of the association.** The stronger the association, the less likely confounding plays a role in explaining the association.[7]

C. Is the finding believable within the context of other knowledge?
(Bayesian poststudy probability)

(See Figure 8–10.)

The first two questions asked in step 3 help you determine whether you believe the study finding based only on the study's validity. Our ultimate belief in the study finding, however, not only rests on the validity of a particular study but also includes a consideration of how the finding relates to other knowledge.

Consider that you have just read two different double-blind, randomized-controlled trials on the secondary prevention of acute myocardial infarction. The intervention in the first study is *325 mg of aspirin a day,* whereas in the second study it is a *daily glass of cranberry juice.* Both studies show a 50% reduction in acute infarction without a significant difference in side effects. Asking the first two questions in step 3, you note:

Do the study subjects and variables accurately represent the research question?

- Both studies recruit similar subjects that meet the inclusion and exclusion criteria of the same target population and both use the same definition and measure that appropriately represents acute infarction.

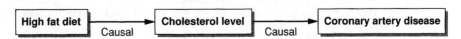

Figure 8–9. Schematic example of a causal pathway.

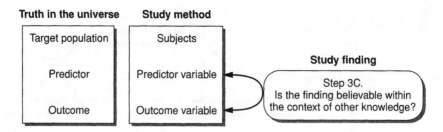

Figure 8–10. Schematic representation of step 3C.

Is the finding attributable to other factors?

- Estimations of the effect of chance are equivalent, with both studies showing a similar 95% CI for the reduction in acute infarction. The CI is narrow, suggesting that both study findings are precise and unlikely to be attributable to chance.
- The design and implementation of each study are such that there are no significant biases in either one.
- The clinical characteristics of the study and control arm, provided in the first table of each article, are evenly distributed. Thus, because the randomization was effective, you are satisfied that there will be no effect of either known or unknown confounders.

Now suppose your patient has recently experienced an acute infarction, and for the sake of this example, you can offer only one of the above therapies. Would you offer your patient an aspirin or a glass of cranberry juice a day?

Even though both studies show the same efficacy for their intervention and have equal validity, most of us would offer our patient aspirin (of the doctors I have polled so far, none has chosen cranberry juice). In determining our belief in a finding, we not only use information from the given study, but we also place the study within a context of other relevant information. This is more explicitly outlined using the principles of Bayesian theory.

Bayes' theorem is named for Thomas Bayes (1702–1761), an English clergyman and mathematician who presented his probability theory in *Essay Towards Solving a Problem in the Doctrine of Chances* (published posthumously in 1763). As defined in Chapter 1, Bayes' theorem may be simply stated: The probability of an event depends on new information about the event that is applied to previous information about the event, or alternatively,

Prestudy probability + study findings = poststudy probability
(What we thought before) + (new information) = (what we now believe)[25]

We qualitatively weigh the following factors to help us determine the prestudy probability of the finding:[26]

?Consistency with other literature. A knowledge of other research may lead to an increased or decreased prestudy probability of the finding. Although there is other literature to support the efficacy of aspirin in the secondary prevention of acute infarction, there is no such support for cranberry juice. Thus the prestudy probability for the finding is higher for aspirin than it is for cranberry juice.

?Biological plausibility. A knowledge of pathophysiology may lead to an increased or decreased prestudy probability of the finding. In the above example, although there is convincing knowledge of a physiological effect of aspirin at the biochemical level to support its secondary prevention of acute infarction, there is no such support for cranberry juice. Thus the prestudy probability for the finding is higher for aspirin than it is for cranberry juice.

We should, however, be cautious about placing too much emphasis on biological plausibility. For example, the Cardiac Arrhythmia Suppression Trial (CAST)[27] evaluated whether encainide and flecainide decreased morbidity and mortality in postmyocardial infarction patients. These drugs, which were known to decrease ventricular ectopy, surprised everyone by *increasing* mortality.

In general, previous literature with hard outcomes (eg, mortality rather than a surrogate end point of ventricular ectopy suppression) should contribute more to the prestudy probability than should biological plausibility.

?Analogy. A knowledge of analogous findings may lead to an increased or decreased prior probability of the finding. Although aspirin has been shown to be effective in the treatment and prevention of many vascular events (eg, treatment and prevention of cerebrovascular disease, treatment of acute infarction), there is no similar analogy for cranberry juice. Thus the prestudy probability for the finding is higher for aspirin than it is for cranberry juice.

Of all the factors that contribute to the prestudy probability, analogy is the weakest and contributes the least.

After estimating the prestudy probability, the application of the study finding helps us determine the poststudy probability, ie, the overall believability of the finding. Because the prestudy probability for aspirin is higher than it is for cranberry juice, the application of the equivalent findings results in an increased poststudy probability for the favorable effect of aspirin therapy. In our example, this serves as the basis for our recommendation of aspirin over cranberry juice therapy.

Although the determination of the poststudy probability, as portrayed above, is largely a qualitative process, you may also make this determination quantitatively. Take, for example, a recently published article on the reevaluation of the Global Utilization of Streptokinase and Tissue Plasminogen Activator for Occluded Coronary Arteries (GUSTO) trial using a Bayesian analysis.[28] By incorporating the prestudy information about the relative efficacy of tissue plasminogen activator (t-PA) compared with streptokinase in the setting of acute myocardial infarction, the investigators showed that the clinical superiority of t-PA demonstrated in the GUSTO trial remains uncertain.

By the end of step 3, we have determined whether we believe the association. For studies in which risk factors or interventions are evaluated, even if we believe the association, we more specifically want to know whether the risk factor or intervention actually *caused* the outcome. The factors that establish causal inference are essentially all those described above.[26] *Causation* is supported by: experimental designs; appropriate temporal relationships in which one can be certain that the predictor variable preceded the outcome variable; ensuring the absence of chance, bias, and confounders; consistency with other literature; biological plausibility, and analogy. In addition, one other factor that supports causal inference is the finding of a biological gradient or dose response, by which a graded change in the magnitude of the predictor results in a predictable change in the outcome variable. The classic example of this is the observation that the death rate associated with lung cancer steadily increases with an increasing number of cigarettes smoked.[29] This observation strongly supports the assertion that cigarettes cause lung cancer.

If we believe that the predictor is truly associated with or causes the outcome, we proceed to the next step to determine the clinically relevant finding. Then, in the final step, we ultimately consider whether the study helps us in caring for our patient.

Step 4. What is the clinically relevant finding?

(See Figure 8–11.)

Study findings are often presented in a manner that does not give you either an intuitive sense of or an ability to evaluate quantitatively the clinically relevant effect of the finding on your patient. A few key concepts and simple calculations for each study type are presented below to help you more clearly identify the clinically relevant finding for your patient. These calculations and concepts are by no means intended to be all-inclusive, but rather are intended only to serve as an initial guide to stimulate you to consider what the clinically relevant result might be. You may find some of the concepts complex at first (particularly the concepts dealing with prognosis). If you are reading this guide for the first time, you may elect to skim this section and return to peruse it in greater detail later.

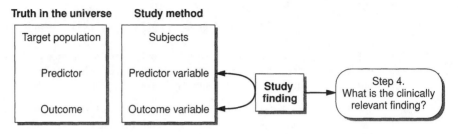

Truth in the universe　　**Study method**

Target population　　Subjects

Predictor　　Predictor variable

Outcome　　Outcome variable

Study finding

Step 4. What is the clinically relevant finding?

Figure 8–11. Schematic representation of step 4.

Studies of risk

Calculating Excess Risk. In studies of risk, the findings are most often presented in terms of **relative risk** or **odds ratio.** (For a more thorough description of these terms, see other texts.[16,17]) Remember that,

$$\text{Relative risk (RR)} = \frac{\text{incidence of disease in the exposed group (Iexp)}}{\text{incidence of disease in the unexposed group (Iunexp)}}$$

$$\text{Odds ratio (OR)} = \frac{\text{odds of disease in the exposed group}}{\text{odds of disease in the unexposed group}}$$

or

$$= \frac{\text{odds of exposure in the diseased group}}{\text{odds of exposure in the nondiseased group}}$$

The **incidence of an event** represents the number of subjects in whom an event occurs divided by the total number of subjects in a population at risk of the event over a given time period. The **odds of an event** represents the proportion of subjects with the event divided by the proportion of subjects without the event.

Although not intuitively obvious, in case-control studies when the disease is uncommon, the odds ratio approximates the relative risk (this is easy to demonstrate algebraically).[16] Note, however, that the incidence of disease can be derived only from cohort studies or the placebo group in experimental studies—*not* from case-control or cross-sectional studies.

A **relative risk** is a ratio that represents how much more or less likely it is that we will find disease in the exposed versus unexposed group. We may, however, have a better sense of the effect of the exposure by considering the **excess risk.** This is an estimate of the absolute risk that is attributable to the particular exposure.[30] This is represented as:

$$\text{Excess risk (ER)} = I_{exp} - I_{unexp}$$

For example, in male smokers aged 40–64 years, the incidence of a first coronary event has been found to be 13/1000 per year, whereas in the nonsmoking cohort, this incidence is 6.2/1000 per year.[31]

$$RR = \frac{13/1000}{6.2/1000} = 2.1$$

That is, the incidence of a first coronary event is 2.1 times as likely in smokers as it is in nonsmokers.

$$ER = 13/1000 - 6.2/1000 = 6.8/1000$$

That is, smoking increases the risk of first coronary events in male smokers aged 40–64 by 6.8/1000 per year.

Although the ER provides an intuitive sense of the impact of the exposure on the disease, it does not mean that intervening on the exposure can completely eliminate its effect. This task largely rests on the efficacy of the intervention. The potential impact of risk factor modification can, however, be estimated.[32]

Studies of intervention

When we are deciding with our patient whether to use a particular intervention, it is important to consider its overall costs and benefits, and well as to incorporate the principle of discounting.

Weighing costs & benefits. We may weigh costs and benefits either qualitatively or quantitatively. Most of us use a qualitative approach in our daily practice when we routinely discuss possible outcomes of interventions with our patients. We convey this information in terms of the likelihood of specific costs (eg, discomfort from a procedure, adverse reactions, financial costs) and benefits (eg, reduction in morbidity or mortality). If the overall cost of an intervention is small and its benefit great, our patient will more likely choose the intervention. Conversely, our patient will less likely choose the intervention if it has considerable risk and very small benefit.

There are many ways to present the study finding quantitatively. When you are assessing benefit from a study, it is important to note *how the finding is represented*. Studies of intervention often report the benefit of therapy in terms of its **relative risk reduction** (RRR). This representation, however, may not convey the true impact of the intervention on our patient population. A more effective way of representing benefit of an intervention is the **absolute risk reduction** (ARR) or the **number needed to treat** (NNT).[33]

Consider two studies with different patient populations. Both studies use the same intervention and follow-up for 5 years. Study A's intervention group has a 5% stroke rate, whereas its control group has a 10% stroke rate. Study B's intervention group has a 20% stroke rate, whereas its control group has a 40% stroke rate.

$$RRR = \frac{\text{incidence outcome control group} - \text{incidence of outcome study group}}{\text{incidence outcome control group}}$$

Note that for study A, the RRR = [10 − 5] ÷ 10 = 50% and for study B, the RRR = [40 − 20] ÷ 40 = 50%.

At first it may appear that the intervention has the same impact on study population A as it does on study population B. The **absolute risk reduction** (ARR), however, more clearly shows that the impact on each population is different.

$$ARR = \text{incidence of outcome control group} - \text{incidence of outcome study group}$$

For study A the ARR over 5 years = 10 − 5 = 5%, and for study B, the ARR = 40 − 20 = 20%. This means that for every 100 patients treated during the 5-year period, five strokes are prevented in study A and 20 strokes are prevented in study B.

The **number needed to treat** (NNT) represents the number of patients who we need to treat to prevent a single outcome event. This is simply the inverse of the ARR if ARR is in the form of a fraction or is 100 divided by ARR if ARR is displayed as a percentage.

$$NNT = 1/[ARR \text{ (fraction)}] \text{ or } 100/[ARR \text{ (\%)}]$$

Thus for study A, the NNT = 100/5 = 20, and for study B, the NNT = 100/20 = 5. That is, in study A, 20 patients are treated to prevent one stroke, whereas in study B, five patients are treated to prevent one stroke. The fewer patients who we have to treat to prevent a single event, the better. Clearly the impact of the intervention is greater in study population B than it is in study population A.

When the NNT is compared between multiple studies, it is important that the intervention be compared over similar lengths of time. The NNTs for the above example were calculated for the 5-year study period. If benefit accrues linearly over time, for study A, the NNT of 20 over 5 years is equivalent to treating 100 patients to prevent one stroke per year (ie, the NNT = 20/(1/5) = 100 per year). In general, the less the time of follow-up, the less the opportunity to see an effect. This often results in a smaller ARR and hence a larger NNT.

If the intervention results in harm instead of efficacy, we perform the same steps as above. The changes made are semantic. Instead of an ARR, we record an absolute risk increase (ARI). The inverse of ARI is known as the **number needed to harm** (NNH). This is the number of patients treated that results in a single adverse event.

With concomitant efficacy and harm of the intervention, we simply multiply the net proportion of subjects who experienced the adverse effect by the NNT.[4] For example, in study A, in which the NNT is 20, if nausea is experienced in 30% of those receiving the intervention versus in 10% of the control group, then:

$$\text{the number of nauseated patients per stroke prevented} = (0.3 - 0.1) \times 20 = 4$$

When you are calculating the NNT from a study, remember that the numerical value pertains to the *particular* study population. If our patient is either sicker or healthier than the average patient in the study, we need to make an adjustment to calculate the NNT for our particular patient. Such adjustment depends on the anticipated risk of the outcome in the absence of treatment for your patient. This number is divided by the risk of the outcome in the study's control group, thus providing a ratio "f." The NNT is then divided by f to yield the NNT for your patient.[33] For example, if the study's NNT is 28 and you estimate your patient's risk of the outcome without therapy to be twice that of the study's control group, f = 2 and the NNT for your patient is 28/2 = 14. Alternatively, if you estimate the risk of your untreated patient to be 0.4 and the risk of the event in the control group is 0.8, f = 0.4/0.8 = 0.5, which results in an NNT of 28/0.5 = 56. Another way to make this adjustment is to use a nomogram.[34]

Ultimately, when we use NNT to help us decide whether or not we will apply the intervention, we usually assess how few patients we need to treat to prevent the event. There is some threshold at which the NNT is low enough that we intuitively embrace the intervention. It is important to recognize that the threshold NNT varies for different diseases and therapies. The threshold is dependent on a number of factors, including the cost and benefit of the intervention. For very efficacious therapies with minimal adverse reactions, we are willing to treat more patients to prevent a single event. The threshold NNT would thus be higher than it would be for a less efficacious intervention associated with serious side effects. For those of you who have advanced quantitative aspirations, there is a formula that can help you calculate a threshold number needed to treat.[35]

The most rigorous but time-consuming quantitative approach to weigh cost and benefits is to incorporate them within the framework of the medical decision-making techniques described in Chapters 2–4. The probabilities of the various outcomes of a particular intervention and the outcome probabilities of no intervention (or an alternative intervention), in addition to measures of patient preference for the outcomes, are incorporated within the techniques of decision analysis, treatment thresholds, and cost-effectiveness analysis. Through a process of accounting, these methods help guide our choice to use a particular intervention.

Discounting. It is not enough that the benefit of an intervention simply outweighs its cost. Because most people value present life over future life, we must also incorporate a time perspective to consider when the costs and benefits are expected to occur. Another way of saying that present life is valued over future life is that future life is discounted relative to present life. Quantitative methods are available to calculate a patient's individual discount rate.[36,37] A 10% per year discount rate implies that a patient values the next year only 90% as much as the present year. The implication of this is that a patient may not want to take any risk today for the promise of a benefit in the future. Thus, even a relatively small risk of up-front morbidity or mortality for larger long-term gains may make an intervention undesirable. For example, a 1995 study evaluated the effect of carotid endarterectomy on stroke in patients with asymptomatic carotid artery stenosis.[18] The 2.7% up-front risk of perioperative stroke or death may eliminate the benefit of the 5.9% ARR in stroke at 5 years in patients who significantly discount their future life relative to their present life.

Studies of diagnostic tests

Calculating likelihood ratios. The following concepts are extensively discussed in Chapter 1 and are summarized here.

In studies of diagnostic tests, the test characteristics are often presented in the form of **sensitivity** and **specificity.** Although this representation may give us an intuitive sense about the strength of the test, it does not directly enable us to determine the likelihood of a particular disease in our patient. When the test characteristic is presented as a **likelihood ratio** (LR), however, it can be applied to our initial estimation of the probability of a particular disease (pretest probability) to provide a refined estimation of the probability of the disease (posttest probability).

If an article provides the sensitivity and specificity of a particular test, you may use the following approach to calculate the LR for a positive (+) or negative (−) result:

$$LR(+) = \frac{\text{sensitivity}}{1 - \text{specificity}} \quad \text{and} \quad LR(-) = \frac{1 - \text{sensitivity}}{\text{specificity}}$$

For example, in a study that reports a sensitivity of 70% and a specificity of 80%, the LR (+) = 70/20 = 3.5 and the LR (−) = 30/80 = 0.38.

Alternatively, if the study provides you with information regarding the number of patients with and without disease at different levels of test results, you can calculate the LR as follows:

$$LR = \frac{\text{The proportion of patients with a particular test result } \textit{with} \text{ disease}}{\text{The proportion of patients with the same test result } \textit{without} \text{ disease}}$$

Consider the test characteristics of serum ferritin in the diagnosis of iron-deficiency anemia. After an extensive literature review, the likelihood ratios for various cut-off points for ferritin were calculated.[38] Table 8–3 shows the raw data from which the likelihood ratios were calculated.

To demonstrate how the LR for the different ranges of serum ferritin are calculated, consider the range between 15 µg/L and 25 µg/L. Using the LR formula above:

The proportion of patients with a serum ferritin 15–25 µg/L *and* iron deficiency is 117/809
The proportion of patients with a serum ferritin 15–25 µg/L *without* iron deficiency is 29/1860

The LR for serum ferritin between 15 µg/L and 25 µg/L is thus $\dfrac{117/809}{29/1860} = 9.28$

Recall from Chapter 1 how we use these test characteristics to refine the estimated probability of disease. Suppose you have just discovered that your 45-year-old male patient has microcytic anemia on a screening blood count. You consider the differential diagnosis: iron deficiency, thalassemia, anemia of chronic disease, lead intoxication, and sideroblastic anemia.

TABLE 8–3. LIKELIHOOD RATIOS FOR RANGES OF SERUM FERRITIN.[38]

Serum Ferritin (µg/L)	No. Iron Deficient	No. Not Iron Deficient	LR*
> 100	48	1320	0.08
45 < 100	76	398	0.44
35 < 45	36	43	1.92
25 < 35	58	50	2.67
15 < 25	117	29	9.28
< 15	474	20	54.49
Total	809	1860	−

*LR = likelihood ratio. The article calculates slightly different LRs using a more sophisticated method.

On the basis of the history and physical examination, you estimate his probability of having iron deficiency to be 30%. You order a serum ferritin measurement and use the approach below to refine this pretest probability.

> Pretest probability   Posttest probability
> ↓   ↑
> Pretest odds × Likelihood ratio = Posttest odds

(1) The estimated pretest probability is converted to a pretest odds of disease.

$$\text{odds} = \frac{\text{probability}}{1 - \text{probability}}$$

The patient's estimated pretest probability of 30%, or 0.3, represents a pretest odds of 0.43, ie, $0.3/(1 - 0.3)$.

(2) The pretest odds is then multiplied by the LR for the given test result to provide a posttest odds of the disease.

The serum ferritin measurement result for your patient is 20 µg/L. From Table 8–3, you note that this corresponds to an LR of 9.28. Thus, the posttest odds = $0.43 \times 9.28 = 3.99$.

(3) The posttest odds is converted to a posttest probability of disease.

$$\text{probability} = \frac{\text{odds}}{\text{odds} + 1}$$

The posttest probability of iron deficiency thus = $3.99/(3.99 + 1) = 0.8$, or 80%.

Thus in your patient, the serum ferritin measurement of 20 µg/L has refined your initial estimate of iron deficiency from 30% to 80%.

Studies of prognosis

Studies of prognosis may be analytic, descriptive, or both. They are analytic when they evaluate the association between prognostic factors and morbidity or mortality. As in studies of risk, the association is often reported in terms of a relative risk. Analogous to studies of risk, the clinically relevant result in an analytic study of prognosis is the "excess risk" of the outcome associated with the prognostic variable. For example, if the presence of factor X is associated with an RR of 3 for mortality at 5 years, and the baseline mortality without factor X is 1/1000, then factor X increases the mortality by 2/1000 at 5 years (3/1000 – 1/1000).

Prognostic studies, however, are particularly informative when they are **descriptive** (see pages 177–180), ie, when they describe the variable of mortality or morbidity over a period in time in a particular population. The clinically relevant result derived from these studies is described below.

Calculating disease-specific mortality to determine your patient's life expectancy. Patients who have been diagnosed with a specific disease may ask you to provide them with an estimate of their life expectancy. This question is often stressful for both the patient and clinician; careful consideration as well as particular sensitivity is required when imparting the information.

Life expectancy (LE), the average future lifetime of a person, may be calculated from survival curves from the descriptive component of a prognostic study using the **declining exponential approximation of life expectancy** (DEALE). This method to approximate LE is presented in a two-part review by Beck, Kassirer, and Pauker where it compares favorably with the estimation provided by the more complex gold standard Gompertz approach.[39] The method is also summarized nicely in a text by Sox Jr and coworkers[23] and is briefly described below. Note, however, that although this method enables you to calculate the LE for your patient, it is in fact an *average* for a population of patients who are similar to your patient. Therefore, rather than telling the patient that they have the specific LE that you calculate, it is important to emphasize that the calculation is a way of arriving at a general estimate.

The DEALE assumes that survival decreases exponentially over time and with a constant mortality rate. Thus there is an inverse relationship between LE and the annual mortality rate (M):

$$LE = 1/M$$

In order to understand DEALE, we need to understand the terminology as it pertains to the different types of mortality rate:

- **Total mortality rate (m)**: The annual mortality rate due to all causes of death in a particular cohort characterized by its age distribution and sex and race
- **Age-specific mortality rate (asm)**: The annual mortality rate for a person of a particular age (and sex and race) that can be derived from the US Vital Statistics data[40]
- **Disease-specific mortality rate (dsm)**: The annual mortality rate attributed to a specific disease
- **Patient-specific mortality rate (psm)**: The annual mortality rate for a particular patient (which is what we ultimately want to determine)

The psm is simply:

$$psm = asm + dsm$$

If there is more than one disease process that may shorten the patient's LE, the psm is:

$$psm = asm + dsm1 + dsm2 + dsm3 + . . .$$

where dsm1, dsm2, and dsm3 are the disease-specific mortalities for individual diseases. Note that you can add the individual dsms only if they are independent of one another. In other words, the individual dsms should act in an additive rather than a synergistic fashion; one disease cannot influence the outcome of another disease.

The psm can be calculated using the following three steps.

(1) Calculate disease-specific mortality using the survival curve in the study.

This is done in one of two ways, depending on whether the study includes a survival curve of a control group who have not been diagnosed with the particular disease.

CONTROL GROUP PRESENT. The disease-specific mortality is the difference in the average annual mortality between the control group and the diseased cohort. It is the mortality that is specifically attributed to a particular disease.

The average annual mortality of a cohort may be calculated using the following formula:

$$m = (-1/t) \times \ln fs$$

where fs = the fraction of subjects surviving at time t and ln is the natural logarithm (base e).

To calculate the dsm in a study that includes a nondiseased control group, we use the formula to individually calculate the average annual mortality rates for the control group and for the diseased group. The dsm is the difference between these two mortality rates.

Figure 8–12 is a survival curve for disease X and a healthy control population. At 10 years of follow up, the fraction of patients surviving in the control group is 0.9 and that in the disease X group is 0.2. The average annual mortality rate in the control group is thus $(-1/10) \times \ln 0.9 = 0.01$ per year and that in the disease X group is $(-1/10) \times \ln 0.2 = 0.16$ per year. The dsm for disease X is thus $0.16 - 0.01 = 0.15$ per year.

CONTROL GROUP ABSENT. If there is no control group, we may use the life expectancy table published by the US National Center for Health Statistics to provide an approximation of the mortality rate for a "control population."[40] The table provides the LE by specific age, race, and sex. (For a reproduction of this table, see the Appendix at the end of this book.) Recall that the mortality rate is the inverse of the LE. We estimate the LE of our control population

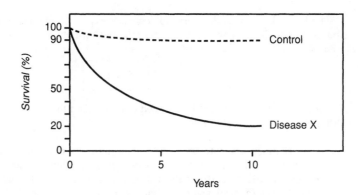

Figure 8–12. Survival curves for disease X and a control group.

using the average age of the diseased cohort. The inverse of this LE thus represents the average annual total mortality rate for our control population.

To calculate the m of the diseased group, we use the same formula as above: $(-1/t) \times \ln$ fs. As above, the dsm is the difference in mortality rates between the diseased and control groups.

Suppose a study presents the following survival curve for disease Y in a cohort whose average age is 70 years (Figure 8–13).

The fraction of patients surviving at 5 years is 0.3. Thus, the total average annual mortality for the cohort with disease Y = $(-1/t) \times \ln$ fs = $(-1/5) \times \ln 0.3) = 0.24$.

Next we calculate the mortality rate for the control population from the LE table using the average age in the diseased cohort. The LE for a cohort of 70-year-old subjects of all races and both sexes is 13.9 years (see the Appendix). The asm thus = $1/LE = 1/13.9 = 0.07$ per year.

For disease Y, the dsm equals the difference in mortality rates between the diseased and control population = $0.24 - 0.07 = 0.17$ per year.

There are two important issues to consider regarding the dsm calculated using the DEALE. First, if the specific disease is very common (eg, coronary artery disease), it will likely be present but not diagnosed in the control population, and this will result in an inaccurate estimate of the dsm. The second consideration involves the assumption that dsm is independent of age. Some diseases, however, may be more or less aggressive depending on the patient's age. Prostate cancer, for example, tends to be more aggressive in younger patients. When the aggressiveness of a disease is related to the age of a patient, the DEALE becomes a less accurate method for calculating LE.

You have just completed the difficult part of calculating your patient's LE. Steps 2 and 3 are quite easy!

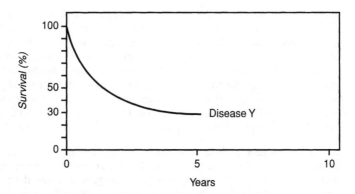

Figure 8–13. Survival curve for disease Y.

(2) Calculate the patient-specific mortality using the disease-specific mortality and the age-specific mortality for your patient.

Recall that psm = asm + dsm.

Now imagine that you have a patient with the above-mentioned disease X who is a black woman aged 65 years.

We have already calculated the dsm for disease X as being 0.15 per year.

To calculate the asm for your patient, we again turn to the LE table in the book's Appendix. The LE for a 65-year-old black female is 17.2 years. The asm is the inverse of LE and therefore = 1/17.2 = 0.06 per year.

Your 65-year-old-black female patient with disease X has a psm of 0.06 + 0.15 = 0.21 per year.

Now imagine that this same patient also has the above-mentioned disease Y and that disease Y did not change the aggressiveness of disease X (and visa versa). In this case, The psm = asm + dsm X + dsm Y = 0.06 + 0.15 + 0.17 = 0.38 per year.

(3) Calculate your patient's life expectancy by inverting the patient-specific mortality.

Throughout this discussion, we have been using the basic equation LE = 1/M, where M is any mortality rate. To calculate your patient's LE we thus simply invert the psm.

The LE for your 65-year-old black female patient with disease X is therefore 1/0.21 = 4.8 years. If your patient also had disease Y, her LE would be 1/0.38 = 2.6 years.

It is very important to identify the reference point for the LE that you have just calculated for your patient: that is the point at which the clock of LE starts ticking. To identify this point of reference, it is critical to note the inception point of the cohort—the point at which the subjects were enrolled in a particular study. For example, was the cohort assembled at the time of diagnosis or on referral to a particular clinic? If the inception point was at diagnosis and you have just diagnosed the patient with the disease, the LE will be that as calculated above. But what if the inception point was at the time of diagnosis and your patient is already 2 years out from diagnosis? A very crude way of determining your patient's LE today is to calculate your patient's LE when she was 2 years younger, at the time of diagnosis. That LE minus 2 years would be her LE today. (This crude approach tends to underestimate the LE.)

The final issue to consider when using the DEALE is that it works best for patients older than 50 years of age. For all patients, the DEALE is more accurate the higher the dsm.[39]

- If the dsm is greater than 0.1 per year, the error is less than 1 year regardless of patient age.
- If the dsm is between 0.05 and 0.1 per year, the DEALE underestimates the LE by approximately 2.0 years in 40-year-olds and even more in younger patients.
- If the dsm is less than 0.05 per year, the DEALE underestimates the LE by approximately 4 years in 40-year-olds and even more in younger patients.

Step 5. Will the study help me in caring for my patient?

(See Figure 8–14.)

A. Are the subjects adequately described and similar to my patient?

Recall from step 2 that we included in the outline the target population (defined by the inclusion and exclusion criteria), the subjects' temporal characteristics (including when the study took place and the duration of follow-up), the geographic characteristics (where the subjects were sampled from), and the subjects' demographics (usually presented in the first table of an article). Essentially, to determine whether the subjects are similar to our patient, we ask two questions: (1) Did the study adequately describe the subjects so that I can determine whether my patient is similar to these subjects? And (2) *is* my patient similar to these subjects?

Although the description of subjects is important for all study types, it is particularly critical for studies of prognosis. In this type of study, the subjects' point of inception into the study should be clearly defined (eg, are the subjects enrolled at the time of diagnosis or on referral to a particular clinic?). In addition, follow-up should be long enough so that we are able to place our patient on the survival curve.

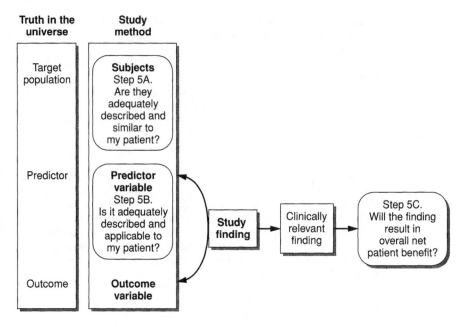

Figure 8–14. Schematic representation of step 5.

B. Is the predictor variable adequately described and applicable to my patient?

For a study of risk and prognosis, are the risk factor and prognostic factor well enough described for me to determine whether they would apply to my patient? If so, do they apply to my patient?

For a study of an intervention or a diagnostic test, are the details of the intervention (eg, dosage of medication) and the technique of the diagnostic test well enough described? Also, are there resources, local expertise, or both to implement the intervention or test?

C. Will the finding result in an overall net benefit for my patient?

Our first task in answering this final question is to summarize the above questions. On the basis of the questions in step 3, we may briefly comment on whether the finding was believable. If we can determine that the study subjects represent our patient and that the predictor can be applied to our patient, we assess whether the clinically relevant result leads to an overall net benefit for *our* patient.

As clinicians, we strive to benefit our patient by curing disease, prolonging life, preventing disease or disease progression, and facilitating quality of life. We attempt to achieve these outcomes by making diagnoses, outlining choices, and providing effective counseling using information derived from different types of studies. The processes of making a diagnosis, outlining choices, and providing counseling can be approached either qualitatively or quantitatively using the concepts and calculations presented in step 4 or using the medical decision-making techniques extensively discussed in Section 1 of this book.

In Chapter 1, we learned how to use information derived from studies of diagnostic tests (likelihood ratios) to refine our estimated probability of a disease. This technique thereby helps us establish a diagnosis. In step 4 we learned how to calculate numbers needed to treat from studies of intervention. Alternatively, in Chapters 2–4 we learned how to incorporate data derived from various studies into frameworks of decision analysis, thresholds, and cost-effectiveness analysis to help us make choices with our patient.

In step 4, we further discovered how to use studies of risk and prognosis to counsel our patient on the basis of calculations of excess risk and estimations of life expectancy.

In conclusion, using this guide, we have assessed the validity of the study, determined its clinically relevant finding, and ultimately considered whether the study can be applied to provide a net benefit for our patient. As intended, this process should provide us with a deeper insight and greater confidence when we analyze study findings to offer our patient diagnostic tests, make recommendations about interventions, or provide counseling.

Next, you will find a concise summary of the study guide. In Chapter 9, we offer examples demonstrating the guide's application to a study of a diagnostic test, an intervention, and a prognosis.

ANALYTIC STUDY GUIDE SUMMARY

(See Figure 8–15.)

Step 1. Do I want to evaluate the study? (INR) Is the research question interesting, novel, and relevant?

Step 2. Outline the study.

(See Figure 8–16.)

Step 3. Is the study finding believable?

   A. Do the study subjects and variables accurately represent the research question?

   B. Is the finding attributable to other factors?
   - Chance
   - Bias
   - Confounders

   C. Is the finding believable within the context of other knowledge?
   - Consistency with other literature
   - Biological plausibility
   - Analogy

Step 4. What is the clinically relevant finding?

Step 5. Will the study help me in caring for my patient?

   A. Are the subjects adequately described and similar to my patient?

   B. Is the predictor variable adequately described and applicable to my patient?

   C. Will the finding result in an overall net benefit for my patient?

GUIDE MODIFIED FOR DESCRIPTIVE STUDIES

As mentioned, descriptive studies describe single or multiple variables in a study, but unlike analytic studies, they do not evaluate the association between these variables. An example of a descriptive study is one that describes the prevalence of disease in a given population. Some types of studies may be descriptive or analytic or both. For example, studies of prognosis are analytic when they evaluate the association between a prognostic factor and mortality or morbidity. Prognostic studies, however, are considered descriptive when they describe the single variable of mortality or morbidity in a particular target population. Often, these studies contain both descriptive and analytic components.

Because descriptive studies do not evaluate associations between a predictor and outcome variable but only describe variables, our guide is modified slightly in some places. In particular, step 2, outlining the study, has been modified as shown in Figure 8–17.

Although the research question in the analytic study evaluated the association between a predictor and outcome in a target population, in a descriptive study it simply considers the description of an event (or events) in a target population. Thus, whereas analytic studies consider the association of "what" with "what" in "whom," descriptive studies simply consider "what" in "whom." In the outline, the research question in truth in the universe is divided into its key components: the event(s) and the target population. In the study method we note the subjects who represent the target population and the variable(s) that represent the event(s). In the outline, we also note the descriptive study finding, with its associated confidence interval.

Step 3B, which asks whether the finding can be attributed to other factors, modifies its approach with respect to bias and confounding.

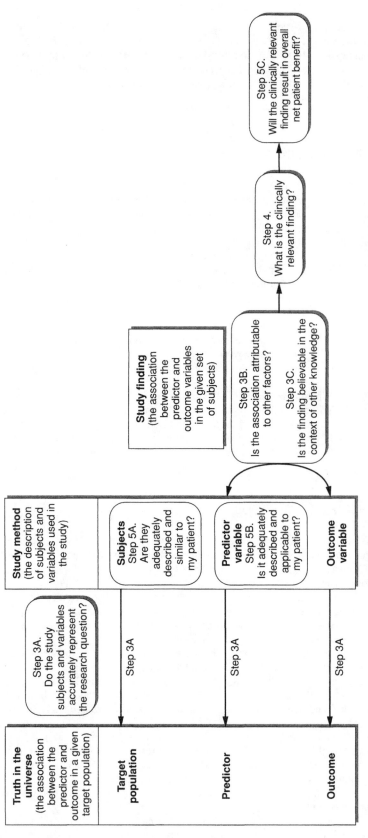

Figure 8–15. Schematic summary of the study guide showing step 2 (the outline); steps 3A, 3B, and 3C (determining whether the study finding is believable); step 4 (determining the clinically relevant finding); and steps 5A, 5B, and 5C (determining whether the study helps us in caring for our patient). Recall that step 1 was the consideration of whether you wanted to evaluate the study.

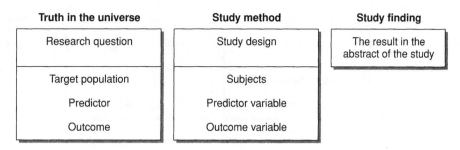

Figure 8–16. Outline of the study.

Because descriptive studies measure a variable rather than evaluate the association between a predictor and outcome variable, we need to modify slightly the components that may bias a study. Biases may occur in:

1. Selecting the study subjects
2. Following up on patients
3. Measuring the variable
4. Analyzing the data

You may note some redundancy in step 3A, which considers whether the variable accurately represents the event, and step 3B, which considers bias in measuring the variable. The former considers whether the definition is a qualitatively appropriate representation of the event, whereas the latter considers whether the variable is quantitatively precise in its measurement.

Regarding confounding, well, this is easy. Because descriptive studies only describe a variable (or variables) and do not consider issues of association, confounding does not play a role in explaining the finding.

In step 4, the clinically relevant result is dependent on the type of descriptive study. In studies of prevalence or incidence, the "relevant result" is simply determining which variable among many applies to the patient. For example, these studies may provide a finding that best helps determine the pretest probability of a disease or, alternatively, describes the probability of an adverse outcome that can be incorporated into a decision analysis. As discussed, studies of prognosis that describe mortality in a particular population provide us with an opportunity to calculate the disease-specific mortality using the DEALE. This allows us to calculate the life expectancy for our patient.

The final modification to step 5 is very subtle. Because descriptive studies do not contain a predictor, question 5B simply considers whether the "variable" is adequately described and applicable to my patient.

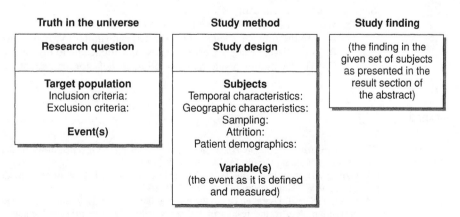

Figure 8–17. Outline modified for a descriptive study.

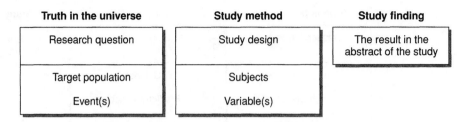

Figure 8–18. Modified outline for descriptive studies.

The benefit a patient derives from a descriptive study depends on the variable described. As mentioned above, survival data provided in a study of prognosis enable you to estimate the patient's life expectancy. Prevalence data may enable you to better estimate the patient's pretest probability of a disease, which enables you to more accurately make a diagnosis. The description of probability of an adverse reaction, when incorporated in a decision analysis, facilitates a patient's choice between strategies. Descriptive studies, however, often benefit patients indirectly. Consider a case series that describes the survival of a patient population undergoing a particular procedure. Although descriptive studies cannot evaluate the *association* between an intervention and mortality (and therefore cannot ascribe a benefit to the procedure) they may provide the stimulus to perform an analytic study to determine whether the procedure reduces mortality. The analytics study then may ultimately enable you to decide whether the procedure will result in an overall net benefit for your patient.

A summary of the guide as it applies to descriptive studies follows.

Descriptive study guide summary

Step 1. Do I want to evaluate the study? (INR) Is the research question interesting, novel, and relevant?

Step 2. Outline the study.
(See Figure 8–18.)

Step 3. Is the study finding believable?
   A. Do the study subjects and variables accurately represent the research question?
   B. Is the finding attributable to other factors?
      • Chance
      • Bias
   C. Is the finding believable within the context of other knowledge?
      • Consistency with other literature
      • Biological plausibility
      • Analogy

Step 4. What is the clinically relevant finding?

Step 5. Will the study help me in caring for my patient?
   A. Are the subjects adequately described and similar to my patient?
   B. Is the variable adequately described and applicable to my patient?
   C. Will the finding result in an overall net benefit for my patient?

REFERENCES

1. Evidence-based medicine. A new approach to teaching the practice of medicine. Evidence-Based Medicine Working Group. JAMA 1992;268:2420.
2. Oxman AD et al: Users' guides to the medical literature. I. How to get started. Evidence-Based Medicine Working Group. JAMA 1993;270:2093.
3. Guyatt GH et al: Users' guides to the medical literature. II. How to use an article about therapy or prevention. A. Are the results of the study valid? Evidence-Based Medicine Working Group. JAMA 1993;270:2598.

4. Guyatt GH et al: Users' guides to the medical literature. II. How to use an article about therapy or prevention. B. What were the results and will they help me in caring for my patients? Evidence-Based Medicine Working Group. JAMA 1994;271:59.

5. Jaeschke R et al: Users' guides to the medical literature. III. How to use an article about a diagnostic test. A. Are the results of the study valid? Evidence-Based Medicine Working Group. JAMA 1994;271:389.

6. Jaeschke R et al: Users' guides to the medical literature. III. How to use an article about a diagnostic test. B. What are the results and will they help me in caring for my patients? Evidence-Based Medicine Working Group. JAMA 1994;271:703.

7. Levine M et al: Users' guides to the medical literature. IV. How to use an article about harm. Evidence-Based Medicine Working Group. JAMA 1994;271:1615.

8. Laupacis A et al: Users' guides to the medical literature. V. How to use an article about prognosis. Evidence-Based Medicine Working Group. JAMA 1994;272:234.

9. Oxman AD et al: Users' guides to the medical literature. VI. How to use an overview. Evidence-Based Medicine Working Group. JAMA 1994;272:1367.

10. Richardson WS, Detsky AS. Users' guides to the medical literature. VII. How to use a clinical decision analysis. A. Are the results of the study valid? Evidence-Based Medicine Working Group. JAMA 1995;273:1292.

11. Richardson WS, Detsky AS. Users' guides to the medical literature. VII. How to use a clinical decision analysis. B. What are the results and will they help me in caring for my patients? Evidence-Based Medicine Working Group. JAMA 1995;273:1610.

12. Hayward RSA et al: Users' guides to the medical literature. VIII. How to use clinical practice guidelines. A. Are the recommendations valid? Evidence-Based Medicine Working Group. JAMA 1996;274:570.

13. Hayward RSA et al: Users' guides to the medical literature. VIII. How to use clinical practice guidelines. B. What are the recommendations and will they help you in caring for your patients? Evidence-Based Medicine Working Group. JAMA 1996;274:1630.

14. Drummond MF et al: Users' guides to the medical literature. XIII. How to use an article on economic analysis of clinical practice. A. Are the results of the study valid? Evidence-Based Medicine Working Group. JAMA 1997;277:1552.

15. Drummond MF et al: Users' guides to the medical literature. XIII. How to use an article on economic analysis of clinical practice. B. What are the results and will they help me in caring for my patients? Evidence-Based Medicine Working Group. JAMA 1997;277:1802.

16. Hulley SB, Cummings SR: *Designing Clinical Research: An Epidemiologic Approach.* Williams & Wilkins, 1988.

17. Gelbach SH: *Interpreting the Medical Literature,* 3rd ed. Macmillan, 1992.

18. Executive Committee for the Asymptomatic Carotid Atherosclerosis Study. Endarterectomy for asymptomatic carotid artery stenosis. JAMA 1995;273:1421.

19. Goodman SN, Berlin JA: The use of predicted confidence intervals when planning experiments and the misuse of power when interpreting results. Ann Intern Med 1994;121:200.

20. Browner WS, Newman TB: Are all significant P values created equal? JAMA 1987;257:2459.

21. Adapted by Sackett DL, from Murphy EA: *The Logic of Medicine.* Johns Hopkins University Press, 1976.

22. Sackett DL: Bias in analytic research. J Chron Dis 1979;32:51.

23. Sox HC Jr et al: *Medical Decision Making.* Butterworth-Heinemann, 1988.

24. Glantz SA. Biostatistics: How to detect, correct and prevent errors in the medical literature. Circulation 1980;61:1.

25. Borrowed, with permission, from Browner WS: Veterans Affairs Medical Center, San Francisco, 1997.

26. Adapted from Hill AB: Pages 288–296 in *A Short Textbook of Medical Statistics,* 10th ed. Lippincott, 1977.

27. Echt DS et al: Mortality and morbidity in patients receiving encainide, flecainide or placebo: The Cardiac Arrhythmia Suppression Trial. N Engl J Med 1991;324:781.

28. Brophy MB, Lawrence J: Placing trials in context using Bayesian analysis. GUSTO revisited by Reverend Bayes. JAMA 1995;273:871.

29. Wynder El et al: The epidemiology of lung cancer: Recent trends. JAMA 1970;213:2221.

30. Kelsey JL et al: *Methods in Observational Epidemiology.* Oxford University Press, 1986.

31. Pooling Project Research Group: Relationship of blood pressure, serum cholesterol, smoking habit, relative weight and EKG abnormalities to incidence of major coronary events: Final report of the pooling project. J Chron Dis 1978;31:201.

32. Browner WS: Estimating the effect of risk factor modification programs. Am J Epidemiol 1986;123:143.

33. Cook RJ, Sackett DL: The number needed to treat: A clinically useful measure of treatment effect. BMJ 1995;310:452.

34. Chattelier G:. The number needed to treat: A clinically useful nomogram in its proper context. BMJ 1996;312:426.

35. Guyatt GH: Users' guides to the medical literature. IX. A method for grading health care recommendations. JAMA 1995;274:1800.
36. Redelmeier DA et al: Probability judgment in medicine: Discounting unspecified possibilities. Med Decis Making 1995;15:227.
37. Johanneson M et al: A note on QALY's, time tradeoff, and discounting. Med Decis Making 1994;14:188.
38. Guyatt GH et al: Laboratory diagnosis of iron-deficiency anemia: An overview. J Gen Intern Med 1992;7:145.
39. Beck JR et al: A convenient approximation of life expectancy. Parts 1 and II. Am J Med 1982;73:883.
40. United States Department of Health and Human Services: Vital Statistics of the United States. Hyatsville, 1990. Life Tables, Part IIA, Table 6.3.

APPLICATION OF THE STUDY GUIDE

Daniel J. Friedland, MD • Peter E. Alperin, MD
Jeffrey A. Tice, MD • Philippe O. Szapary, MD

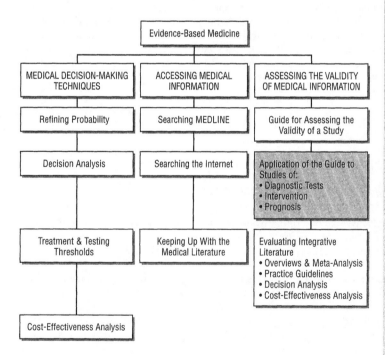

9.1 GUIDE APPLIED TO A STUDY OF A DIAGNOSTIC TEST

Peter E. Alperin, MD • Daniel J. Friedland, MD

THE PIOPED INVESTIGATORS:

Value of the ventilation/perfusion scan in acute pulmonary embolism: Results of the Prospective Investigation of Pulmonary Embolism Diagnosis (PIOPED). JAMA 1990; 263:2753.*

(See pp 188–194.)

Step 1. Do I want to evaluate the study? (INR)

Is the study:

Interesting? Yes, it is helpful to know what the result of a commonly used diagnostic test means.

Novel? Compared with previously published studies, PIOPED attempted to quantify the sensitivity and specificity (and, therefore, likelihood ratios) of ventilation-perfusion (V/Q) scans, as opposed to quantifying the positive predictive value, which is dependent on the prevalence of disease.

Relevant? Pulmonary embolism (PE) is associated with up to 5.4% of all deaths in the hospital setting,[1-3] with fewer than 15% of patients receiving treatment.[1] This statistic underscores the difficulty in making the diagnosis. In addition, the mortality rate of untreated PE ranges from 5% to 30%.[4,5] This study is designed to provide information regarding the test characteristics of a V/Q scan that will enable us to refine our estimation of a patient's probability of having PE.

Step 2. Outline the study

(See Figure 9.1–1.)

Step 3. Is the study finding believable?

A. Do the study subjects and variables accurately represent the research question?

Subjects: As far as we can determine from the study, the subjects fulfilled the inclusion and exclusion criteria and therefore are representative of patients with suspected acute PE.

Predictor variable: The methodology of the V/Q scan appears to be rigorous and is acceptable.

Outcome variable: The outcome of PE is measured by the variable pulmonary angiography. This variable is appropriate, as this test is considered the gold standard to diagnose PE.

For patients who did not undergo angiography or who had an uninterpretable angiogram, the study used the outcome variable of clinical follow-up to determine whether a patient had PE. This slightly modifies the research question to "What are the test characteristics of a V/Q scan to determine whether patients have had a *clinically significant* PE?"

B. Is the finding attributable to other factors?

?Chance. The 95% confidence interval around sensitivity and specificity is approximately ± 8%. The finding is thus reasonably precise.

---

* The PIOPED Investigators: Value of the ventilation/perfusion scan in acute pulmonary embolism. JAMA 1990;273:2753. Copyright 1990. American Medical Association. Printed with permission.

Truth in the universe	Study method
Research question What are the test characteristics of a V/Q scan for the evaluation of patients with suspected acute PE?	**Study design** Cohort
Target population Inclusion: Inpatients and outpatients > 18 years of age with symptoms of acute PE within 24 hours of onset Exclusion: Serum creatinine of > 2.9 mg/dL, allergy to contrast medium, pregnancy	**Subjects** Temporal characteristics: 1/85–9/86 Geographic characteristics: 6 centers Sampling: 5587 V/Q scan requests → 3016 eligible → 1493 consented → 933 randomized to enter → 931 scan completed → 755 patients had an angiogram. 150 patients had clinical follow-up (includes 14 patients with uninterpretable angiograms). Patient characteristics: see Table 3, page 2756 (JAMA article).
Predictor V/Q scan	**Predictor variable** V/Q scan methodology as described on pages 2754–2755
Outcome PE	**Outcome variable** Angiogram methodology as described on pages 2754–2755 Clinical follow-up at 1 year via telephone

Study finding

Abnormal scan (high, intermediate, low probability): sensitivity, 98%; specificity, 10%.
High-probability scan: sensitivity, 41%; specificity, 97%.
(95% confidence interval; approximately ± 8%)

Figure 9.1–1. Outline of the PIOPED study.

?Bias. BIASES IN SELECTING THE STUDY SUBJECTS In studies of diagnostic tests, the most important factor in subject selection is that an appropriate *spectrum* of subjects is represented. If the study's spectrum of patients differs from that in our patient population, the finding will be biased. Consider a study that selects subjects with disease whose illness is advanced and nondiseased patients who are very healthy. Because subjects with advanced disease are less likely to have false-negative test results and very healthy nondiseased subjects are less likely to have false-positive test results, such a spectrum of patients would overestimate the sensitivity and specificity of the test in a population with a broader spectrum of disease severity. The PIOPED study enrolled a broad spectrum of patients, which is appropriate because this selection represents the general population of patients who would be expected to be seen for consideration of PE. Thus, the finding in this study is unlikely to be attributable to spectrum bias.

BIASES IN FOLLOWING UP ON THE STUDY SUBJECTS. In studies of diagnostic tests, it is important that subjects who have negative test results are still evaluated with the gold standard. If these patients drop out of the study, the proportion of patients with both false-negative and true-negative results would be reduced and, therefore, the sensitivity of the test would be overestimated and the specificity of the test would be underestimated. This is known as **verification bias.** In the PIOPED investigation, had all the patients who did not receive an angiogram (mostly subjects with a normal or low-probability result) dropped out of the study, verification bias would have occurred. It appeared as if the researchers attempted to limit the effect of this bias by evaluating those patients who did not receive an angiogram with another "gold standard," clinical follow-up for 1 year. It seems, however, that the specificities that the researchers present do not include the subjects with uninterpretable or no angiograms who had clinical follow-up. The reported specificities are as follows: high-probability scan = 466/480 = 97%; high- or intermediate-probability scan = 249/480 = 52%; high-, intermediate-, or low-probability scan = 50/480 = 10% (see Tables 4 and 5 of the JAMA article, pages 2756 and 2757). If the 150 patients without angiographic correlation for low-probability or normal scans, who had no clinical evidence of PE at 1-year follow-up, had been included, these specificities would have been reported as 98% (616/630), 63% (399/630), and 20% (126/630), respectively. Thus, the reported specificities are underestimated and can be attributed to verification bias.

BIASES IN EXECUTING OR MEASURING THE PREDICTOR VARIABLE. Had the readers of the V/Q scan been knowledgeable of the result of angiography, the scan would more likely have been read as concordant with the angiogram. This would have overestimated both the sensitivity and specificity of the test. Although the PIOPED study does not specifically mention blinding, another article that evaluated this study ensured (through personal communication with the researchers) the interpretation of both the V/Q scan and angiogram was blinded.[6] The finding is thus not attributable to gold standard test review bias.

BIASES IN MEASURING THE OUTCOME VARIABLE. Similar to above, had the readers of the angiogram been knowledgeable of the V/Q scan result, the sensitivity and specificity of the finding would have been overestimated. Because readers of the angiogram were blinded from the V/Q scan result, the finding is not attributable to index test review bias.

BIASES IN ANALYZING THE DATA. The appropriate statistics were used in this study.

?Confounders. Confounders are not applicable to studies of diagnostic tests.

C. Is the finding believable within the context of other knowledge?

?Consistency with other literature. Yes, although there is a limited amount of previous data.

?Biological plausibility. Yes, it is plausible that the V/Q testing method should be able to diagnose PE.

?Analogy. There are no analogous tests comparable to a V/Q scan.

Step 4. What is the clinically relevant finding?

As described in Chapter 1, likelihood ratios (LRs) enable us to use the result of the test to refine the estimated probability of disease for our patient. From this study, we were able to calculate the LRs for the different V/Q scan results (Table 9.1–1).

Step 5. Will the study help me in caring for my patient?

A. Are the subjects adequately described and applicable to my patient?

The patient population is fairly well described: both inpatients and outpatients, 45% male, mean age of 56 years. The study population appears representative of the general population of patients who present for consideration of having PE.

TABLE 9.1–1. NUMBERS OF PATIENTS WITH SPECIFIC LEVELS OF V/Q SCAN RESULTS IN WHOM PE WAS EITHER PRESENT OR ABSENT AND THE CALCULATED LR.

V/Q Scan Result	PE Present	PE Absent	LR
High probability	102	14	18.3
Intermediate probability	105	217	1.2
Low probability	39	273	0.4
Normal/near normal	5	126	0.1
Total	251	630*	–

* Includes 150 patients with low-probability (74) or normal (76) scans who did not undergo angiography or had uninterpretable angiograms and who had no clinical evidence of PE at 1-year follow-up. The study does not mention the outcome of the 50 subjects with high- and intermediate-probability scans who had uninterpretable or no angiograms. They are thus not included in the analysis.

PE = pulmonary embolism; V/Q = ventilation-perfusion; LR = likelihood ratio.

B. Is the predictor variable adequately described and applicable to my patient?

Yes, V/Q scans are readily available at most hospitals, and the study describes in detail how to perform and interpret the test so that the test can be easily reproduced. Note, however, that if the established protocol at our institution differs from the method and interpretation of the V/Q scan in the study, our test characteristics may differ from those in the study.

C. Will the finding result in an overall net benefit for my patient?

Based on the preceding steps, the study finding is believable, with the exception of the effect of verification bias in underestimating the reported specificities. The clinically relevant finding that we determined includes most subjects who had clinical follow-up. Verification bias, therefore, does not play a significant role in explaining the LRs that we have calculated, so these values are likely valid.

We can now apply the likelihood ratios to the treatment threshold to determine the upper and lower testing thresholds (see Chapter 3). If the patient's pretest probability of having PE lies between the upper and lower testing thresholds for the V/Q scan, the test is performed to refine the probability of PE (see Chapter 1). We may then observe where the posttest probability lies relative to the treatment threshold to help us determine the preferred course of action.

REFERENCES

1. Stien PD, Henry JW: prevalence of acute pulmonary embolism among patients in a general hospital at autopsy. Chest 1995;108:978.
2. Rubenstein I et al: Fatal pulmonary embolism in hospitalized patients: An autopsy study. Arch Intern Med 1988;148:1425.
3. Goldhaber SZ et al: Factors associated with correct antemortem diagnosis of major pulmonary embolism. Am J Med 1982;73:822.
4. Stien PD et al: Untreated patients with pulmonary embolism. Chest 1995;107:931.
5. Barritt DW, Jordan SC: Anticoagulant drugs in the treatment of pulmonary embolism. Lancet 1960;1:1309.
6. Jaeschke R et al: Users' guides to the medical literature. III. How to use an article about a diagnostic test. A. Are the results of the study valid? Evidence-Based Medicine Working Group. JAMA 1994;271:389.

Original Contributions ▬▬▬▬▬▬

Value of the Ventilation/Perfusion Scan in Acute Pulmonary Embolism

Results of the Prospective Investigation of Pulmonary Embolism Diagnosis (PIOPED)

The PIOPED Investigators

To determine the sensitivities and specificities of ventilation/perfusion lung scans for acute pulmonary embolism, a random sample of 933 of 1493 patients was studied prospectively. Nine hundred thirty-one underwent scintigraphy and 755 underwent pulmonary angiography; 251 (33%) of 755 demonstrated pulmonary embolism. Almost all patients with pulmonary embolism had abnormal scans of high, intermediate, or low probability, but so did most without pulmonary embolism (sensitivity, 98%; specificity, 10%). Of 116 patients with high-probability scans and definitive angiograms, 102 (88%) had pulmonary embolism, but only a minority with pulmonary embolism had high-probability scans (sensitivity, 41%; specificity, 97%). Of 322 with intermediate-probability scans and definitive angiograms, 105 (33%) had pulmonary embolism. Follow-up and angiography together suggest pulmonary embolism occurred among 12% of patients with low-probability scans. Clinical assessment combined with the ventilation/perfusion scan established the diagnosis or exclusion of pulmonary embolism only for a minority of patients—those with clear and concordant clinical and ventilation/perfusion scan findings.

(JAMA. 1990;263:2753-2759)

PERFUSION lung scans have been reported to be sensitive in detecting pulmonary emboli, but many other condi-

For editorial comment see p 2794.

tions such as pneumonia or local bronchospasm cause perfusion defects.[1] Ventilation scans were added to perfusion scans with the idea that ventilation

Reprint requests to Division of Lung Diseases, National Heart, Lung, and Blood Institute, Westwood Bldg, Room 6A16, 5333 Westbard Ave, Bethesda, MD 20892 (Carol E. Vreim, PhD).

would be abnormal in areas of pneumonia or local hypoventilation, but that in pulmonary embolism ventilation would be normal.[2] A number of investigators have attempted to make ventilation/perfusion (V/Q) scans more useful for diagnosing pulmonary embolism by classifying them not just as normal or abnormal, but if abnormal, as indicating high probability, intermediate probability (indeterminate), or low probability of pulmonary embolism.[3] Under the auspices of the National Heart, Lung, and Blood Institute, the Prospective Investigation of Pulmonary Embolism Diag-

nosis (PIOPED) investigators have assessed the diagnostic usefulness of V/Q lung scans in acute pulmonary embolism. The project protocol and consent forms were approved by the institutional review boards of all participating centers. (Participating centers and investigators are listed at the end of the article.)

METHODS

Patient Enrollment

From January 1985 through September 1986 in each of six clinical centers, all patients for whom a request for a V/Q scan or a pulmonary angiogram was made were considered for study entry. The eligible study population consisted of patients, 18 years or older, inpatients and outpatients, in whom symptoms that suggested pulmonary embolism were present within 24 hours of study entry and without contraindications to angiography such as pregnancy, serum creatinine level greater than 260 μmol/L, or hypersensitivity to contrast material. Once approached for the study, patients with recurrences were not approached for recruitment a second time.

Recruitment

A total of 5587 requests for V/Q scans were recorded in the six PIOPED clinical centers from January 1985 through September 1986 (Figure). Although

Reprinted from JAMA® The Journal of the American Medical Association
May 23/30, 1990, Volume 263
Copyright 1990, American Medical Association

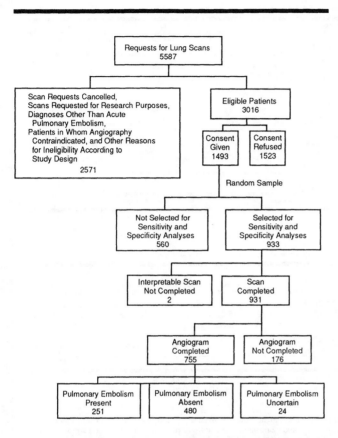

Requests for Lung Scans
5587

Scan Requests Cancelled,
Scans Requested for Research Purposes,
Diagnoses Other Than Acute
Pulmonary Embolism,
Patients in Whom Angiography
Contraindicated, and Other Reasons
for Ineligibility According to
Study Design
2571

Eligible Patients
3016

Consent
Given
1493

Consent
Refused
1523

Random Sample

Not Selected for
Sensitivity and
Specificity Analyses
560

Selected for
Sensitivity and
Specificity Analyses
933

Interpretable Scan
Not Completed
2

Scan
Completed
931

Angiogram
Completed
755

Angiogram
Not Completed
176

Pulmonary Embolism
Present
251

Pulmonary Embolism
Absent
480

Pulmonary Embolism
Uncertain
24

Flow chart illustrating the numbers of requests for lung scans, recruitment of patients, completion of lung scans, and results of angiography in the Prospective Investigation of Pulmonary Embolism Diagnosis.

some patients could not be thoroughly evaluated prior to completion of the V/Q scan, clinical investigators made every effort to record their individual clinical impressions as to the likelihood of pulmonary embolism prior to learning the results of V/Q scans and angiography. Impressions were based on an agreed on set of information—history, results of physical examination, arterial blood gas analyses, chest roentgenograms, and electrocardiograms—but without standardized diagnostic algorithms. The medical records of a random sample of patients who refused or were ineligible for study entry (refuser/ineligible patients) were evaluated retrospectively for comparison with study patients.

Lung Scan

The protocol directed ventilation and perfusion studies with the subject in the upright position, but other positions were acceptable. Ventilation studies were performed with 5.6×10^8 to 11.1×10^8 Bq of xenon 133 using a 20% symmetric window set over the 80-keV energy peak. They started with a 100 000-count, posterior-view, first-breath image and then posterior equilibrium (wash-in) images for two consecutive 120-second periods. Washout consisted of three serial 45-second posterior views, 45-second left and right posterior oblique views, and a final 45-second posterior view. Then, perfusion

scans were obtained with 1.5×10^8 Bq of technetium Tc 99m macroaggregated albumin that contained 100 000 to 700 000 particles using a 20% symmetric window set over the 140-keV energy peak. Particles were injected into an antecubital vein over 5 to 10 respiratory cycles, with the patient supine or at most semierect. The perfusion images consisted of anterior, posterior, both posterior oblique, and both anterior oblique views, with 750 000 counts per image for each. For the lateral view with the best perfusion, 500 000 counts per image were collected; the other lateral view was obtained for the same length of time. Scintillation cameras with a wide field of view (38.1 cm in diameter) were used with parallel-hole, low-energy, all-purpose collimators. Perfusion scans were satisfactory or better in 96% of cases, ventilation scans adequate or better in 95%.

Angiography

The femoral-vein Seldinger technique with a multiple side-holed, 6F to 8F pigtail catheter was used. Small amounts of contrast material (5 to 8 mL) were injected by hand, to check the patency of the inferior vena cava by fluoroscopy. The catheter was directed into the main pulmonary artery of the lung with the greatest V/Q scan abnormality. Initial filming was in the anteroposterior projection. Seventy-six percent iodinated contrast material was injected at a rate of 20 to 35 mL/s for a total of 40 to 50 mL (2-second injection). Film rates were three per second for 3 seconds, followed by one per second for 4 to 6 seconds. Depending on the size of the lungs, filming was not magnified or given a low magnification of 1.4. A 12:1 grid was used and roentgenographic factors were in the range of 70 to 80 kilovolts (peak) and 0.025 to 0.040 seconds at 1000 mA (large focal spot of 1.2 to 1.5 mm in diameter). If emboli were not identified, injections were repeated and magnification (1.8 to 2.0 times) oblique views were obtained of the areas suspicious for pulmonary embolism. Films were obtained with an air-gap technique (ie, no grid used). Roentgenographic factors were in the range of 78 to 88 kV(p) and 0.040 to 0.080 seconds at 160 mA (small focal spot of 0.3 to 0.6 mm in diameter). If no emboli were found in the first lung, or if bilateral angiography in the clinical center was routine, identical techniques were used for the second lung. Angiography was completed within 24 hours, and usually within 12 hours of V/Q scans. Pulmonary angiograms were adequate or better in 95% of cases.

Central Scan and Angiogram Interpretations

Two nuclear medicine readers, not from the center that performed the scan, independently interpreted the lung scans with chest roentgenograms according to preestablished study criteria (Table 1). Angiograms were likewise randomly assigned to pairs of angiographers from clinical centers other than the originating hospital. The angiogram readers interpreted the angiograms with lung scans as having acute pulmonary embolism present—which required the identification of an embolus obstructing a vessel or the outline of an embolus (filling defect) within a vessel—absent, or uncertain. If two readers disagreed, the interpretations were adjudicated by readers who were selected randomly from the remaining clinical centers. If adjudicating readers did not agree with either of the first two readers, scans or angiograms went to panels of nuclear medicine or angiography readers. The final adjudicated V/Q scan readings consisted of four categories—high probability, intermediate probability (indeterminate), low probability, and low/very low probability through normal (near normal/normal). The near-normal/normal category includes readings of very low probability by one reader and low probability by the other, very low probability by both, very low probability by one and normal by the other, and normal by both. Refuser/ineligible patients' scans were read in each clinical center by the clinical center's PIOPED nuclear medicine reader(s) and not reread.

Follow-up and Outcome Classification

Patients were contacted by telephone at 1, 3, 6, and 12 months after study entry. Deaths, new studies for pulmonary embolism, and major bleeding complications were reviewed by an outcome classification committee using all available information. Only 23 (2.5%) of the 931 patients had incomplete (16) or no (7) follow-up. Angiograms, follow-up data, and outcome classifications were used to determine pulmonary embolism status as positive for patients with angiograms that showed pulmonary emboli and for patients for whom outcome review established the presence of pulmonary emboli at the time of PIOPED recruitment. Pulmonary embolism status was determined as negative for patients with angiograms that did not show pulmonary emboli and no contrary outcome review and for patients who lacked a definitive angiogram reading who were discharged from the hospital without a prescription for anticoagu-

lants and in whom no outcome event suggested pulmonary embolism. Pulmonary embolism status could be determined as positive or negative for 902 patients. A clinical assessment of the likelihood of pulmonary embolism was available for 887 (98%) of these patients.

Statistical Methods

Probability values for the comparison of percentages and proportions and 95% confidence intervals (CIs) were calculated using standard z tests.[4] A χ^2 test for homogeneity of proportions was used to compare distributions.[5] *Sensitivity* is defined as the proportion of cases of pulmonary embolism correctly diagnosed and *specificity* as the proportion of diagnoses that pulmonary embolism is absent for patients without pulmonary embolism. Sensitivity, specificity, and percent agreement have been calculated according to standard methods for proportions.[6] Analyses were performed with the Statistical Package for the Social Sciences statistical software package.[7] Recruitment of

900 to 1000 patients in the random sample for PIOPED angiography was planned to obtain estimates of sensitivity and specificity with 95% CIs no wider than ±8%. To determine the sensitivity and specificity of V/Q lung scans without the biases associated with haphazard patient selection (ie, convenience sampling),[8,9] a 933-patient sample of the 1493 patients who consented to PIOPED participation was selected according to random sampling schedules created separately by the data and coordinating center for each clinical center. The PIOPED protocol required these 933 patients to undergo angiography if their scans were abnormal. Of the 933 patients selected for angiography, 1 patient died before the V/Q scan could be completed and 1 other patient's V/Q scan was determined to be uninterpretable. These 2 patients are not further reported herein.

RESULTS

Of the 3016 patients eligible for PIOPED, 1493 (50%) gave consent to

Table 1.—PIOPED Central Scan Interpretation Categories and Criteria*

High probability
- ≥2 Large (>75% of a segment) segmental perfusion defects without corresponding ventilation or roentgenographic abnormalities or substantially larger than either matching ventilation or chest roentgenogram abnormalities
- ≥2 Moderate segmental (≥25% and ≤75% of a segment) perfusion defects without matching ventilation or chest roentgenogram abnormalities and 1 large mismatched segmental defect
- ≥4 Moderate segmental perfusion defects without ventilation or chest roentgenogram abnormalities

Intermediate probability (indeterminate)
- Not falling into normal, very-low-, low-, or high-probability categories
- Borderline high or borderline low
- Difficult to categorize as low or high

Low probability
- Nonsegmental perfusion defects (eg, very small effusion causing blunting of the costophrenic angle, cardiomegaly, enlarged aorta, hila, and mediastinum, and elevated diaphragm)
- Single moderate mismatched segmental perfusion defect with normal chest roentgenogram
- Any perfusion defect with a substantially *larger* chest roentgenogram abnormality
- Large or moderate segmental perfusion defects involving no more than 4 segments in 1 lung and no more than 3 segments in 1 lung region with *matching* ventilation defects either equal to or larger in size and chest roentgenogram either normal or with abnormalities substantially smaller than perfusion defects
- >3 Small segmental perfusion defects (<25% of a segment) with a normal chest roentgenogram

Very low probability
- ≤3 Small segmental perfusion defects with a normal chest roentgenogram

Normal
- No perfusion defects present
- Perfusion outlines exactly the shape of the lungs as seen on the chest roentgenogram (hilar and aortic impressions may be seen, chest roentgenogram and/or ventilation study may be abnormal)

*PIOPED indicates Prospective Investigation of Pulmonary Embolism Diagnosis.

Table 2.—Recruitment of Patients and Completion of Angiography*

Clinical Center	% of Eligible Patients Recruited	No. of PIOPED Patients With Lung Scans Who Were Selected for Angiographic Pursuit	Angiograms Obtained, No. (%)
Duke University	46	137	115 (84)
Henry Ford Hospital	62	228	177 (78)
Massachusetts General Hospital	33	140	120 (86)
University of Michigan	52	102	65 (64)
University of Pennsylvania	70	168	134 (80)
Yale University	43	156	144 (92)
Total	50	931	755 (81)

*PIOPED indicates Prospective Investigation of Pulmonary Embolism Diagnosis.

Table 3.—Patient Characteristics*

	PIOPED (N = 931)	Refuser/ Ineligible (N = 326)
Age (mean), y	56.1	56.4
Male, %	45	44
Service, %		
Medical/CCU	40	36
Surgical	18	21
Emergency department/clinic	30	32
ICU	10	10
Other	1	1
Hospital mortality, %	9	10

*PIOPED indicates Prospective Investigation of Pulmonary Embolism Diagnosis; CCU, coronary care unit; and ICU, intensive care unit.

Table 4.—Comparison of Scan Category With Angiogram Findings

Scan Category	Pulmonary Embolism Present	Pulmonary Embolism Absent	Pulmonary Embolism Uncertain	No Angiogram	Total No.
High probability	102	14	1	7	124
Intermediate probability	105	217	9	33	364
Low probability	39	199	12	62	312
Near normal/normal	5	50	2	74	131
Total	251	480	24	176	931

Table 5.—Comparison of Scan Category With Angiogram Findings, Sensitivity and Specificity

Scan Category	Sensitivity, %	Specificity, %
High probability	41	97
High or intermediate probability	82	52
High, intermediate, or low probability	98	10

participate in PIOPED (Figure). The clinical centers varied in the percentage of eligible patients for whom consent could be obtained, from 33% to 70%, and in the percentage of patients for whom angiograms were obtained among those selected to determine the sensitivity and specificity of V/Q lung scans (PIOPED angiographic pursuit), from 64% to 92% (Table 2). The PIOPED patients resembled refuser/ineligible patients in a variety of clinical characteristics (Table 3). The PIOPED patients and refuser/ineligible patients were different, however, in their lung scan abnormalities (P<.01). Although they had similar frequencies of high-probability scans (13% among PIOPED patients and 11% among refuser/ineligible patients), the PIOPED patients had intermediate-probability scans almost twice as often as refuser/ineligible patients (39% vs 22%). The PIOPED study had a smaller proportion of patients with low-probability and near-normal/normal lung scans. Of the 931 patients who were selected for mandatory angiography in PIOPED, 755 (81.1%) completed angiography; 69 (7.4%) did not complete angiography because their V/Q scans were interpreted locally as normal; and 107 (11.5%) did not complete angiography in spite of the requirements of the protocol.

Reader Agreement

Agreement among scan readers was excellent for high-probability (95%), very-low-probability (92%), and normal (94%) scan categories. For intermediate-probability (indeterminate) and low-probability scan categories, the readers agreed less frequently (75% and 70%, respectively). In only 24 (2.6%) of 931 scans was panel adjudication necessary. Agreement among angiogram readers was excellent for the presence of pulmonary embolism (92%). For the absence of pulmonary embolism and pulmonary embolism uncertain, independent readers agreed on 83% and 89%

of angiograms, respectively. In only 13 (1.7%) of 755 angiograms was panel adjudication necessary.

Scan Findings

Most (676) of the 931 patients had intermediate- or low-probability V/Q scan readings (39% and 34%, respectively) (Table 4). Only 131 (14%) had near-normal/normal V/Q scans and 124 (13%) had high-probability scans. The 176 patients who did not undergo angiography, in spite of their selection for mandatory angiography, had less severe scan abnormalities than those who completed angiography (P<.01).

Angiogram and Outcome Findings

Among the 755 patients who completed angiography, 251 (33%) had thromboemboli seen on the angiogram, 480 (64%) had no thromboemboli seen, and 24 (3%) had angiograms in which the presence of thromboemboli was uncertain (Table 4). For the vast majority of patients, 1 year of follow-up revealed clinical courses entirely consistent with angiographically established diagnoses. The outcome classification committee disagreed with central angiography interpretations for 4 patients with pulmonary angiograms free of signs of acute embolism who had pulmonary embolism at autopsies performed 2 to 6 days after angiography. The scan interpretations were of low probability for 3 and of intermediate probability (indeterminate) for 1 of these 4 patients.

Scans Compared With Angiograms

One hundred two of 251 patients with angiograms that showed thromboemboli had high-probability V/Q scans. The sensitivity, therefore, was 41% (95% CI, 34% to 47%) (Tables 4 and 5). If the patient had either a high- or intermediate-probability V/Q scan, the sen-

sitivity for thromboemboli on angiography increased to 207 (82%) of 251 (95% CI, 78% to 87%). If the patient had either a high-, intermediate-, or low-probability V/Q scan, then 246 of 251 had thromboemboli on angiography, a sensitivity of 98% (95% CI, 96% to 100%).

Only 14 (3%) of 480 patients who did not have thromboemboli on angiography had high-probability V/Q scans. The specificity of a high-probability scan—ie, the percentage of patients with angiograms free of signs of acute embolism who had a scan that showed other than high probability—was 97% (466/480) (95% CI, 96% to 98%). For high- and intermediate-probability scans together, specificity was 52% (249/480 patients with angiograms free of signs of acute embolism) (95% CI, 47% to 56%). For high-, intermediate-, and low-probability scans together, specificity was 10% (50/480 patients with angiograms free of signs of acute embolism) (95% CI, 8% to 13%). The 36 sensitivities and specificities calculated by reproducing Table 5 for each clinical center varied about the studywide sensitivities and specificities—25 (69%) of 36 were within ±5% of the studywide estimates and 34 (94%) of 36 within ±10%.

Most patients with high-probability V/Q scans had angiographic evidence of pulmonary embolism (102/116 definitive studies, or a positive predictive value of 88%). Of the 60 patients with previous histories of pulmonary embolism, 20 were found to have pulmonary emboli on angiography. Of the 19 patients with histories of pulmonary embolism and a high-probability V/Q scan, only 14 were found to have acute pulmonary emboli on angiography. The positive predictive value of a high-probability V/Q scan in patients with histories of pulmonary

Table 6.—Pulmonary Embolism (PE) Status*

| Scan Category | Clinical Science Probability, % | | | | | | | |
| | 80-100 | | 20-79 | | 0-19 | | All Probabilities | |
	PE+/No. of Patients	%	PE+/No. of Patients	%	PE+/No. of Patients	%	PE+/No. of Patients	%
High probability	28/29	96	70/80	88	5/9	56	103/118	87
Intermediate probability	27/41	66	66/236	28	11/68	16	104/345	30
Low probability	6/15	40	30/191	16	4/90	4	40/296	14
Near normal/normal	0/5	0	4/62	6	1/61	2	5/128	4
Total	61/90	68	170/569	30	21/228	9	252/887	28

*PE+ indicates angiogram reading that shows pulmonary embolism or determination of pulmonary embolism by the outcome classification committee on review. Pulmonary embolism status is based on angiogram interpretation for 713 patients, on angiogram interpretation and outcome classification committee reassignment for 4 patients, and on clinical information alone (without definitive angiography) for 170 patients.

embolism was only 74% (14/19), compared with 91% (88/97) for those without a history of pulmonary embolism ($P<.05$). This difference in positive predictive values reflects a loss of specificity in the high-probability V/Q scan diagnosis for patients with histories of pulmonary embolism (88%) vs those with no prior pulmonary embolism (98%) ($P<.01$).

The percentage of patients whose angiograms showed thromboemboli was less in the intermediate-probability (indeterminate), low-probability, and near-normal/normal scan categories—33%, 16%, and 9%, respectively (Table 4). The frequency of angiographically demonstrable emboli among patients with low-probability scans (39 [16%] of 238) and near-normal/normal scans (5 [9%] of 55) is influenced by the relatively large numbers of patients (74 patients and 76 patients, respectively) for whom angiography was not completed or interpretations were uncertain in these scan categories (Table 4). Since none of these patients received anticoagulants and none developed clinically evident pulmonary embolism during follow-up, important pulmonary emboli did not occur in this group. If all 150 patients were regarded as not having had pulmonary emboli, then the frequency of clinically important pulmonary emboli in patients with low-probability scans could be no less than 39 (12%) of 312, and in patients with near-normal/normal scans, 5 (4%) of 131.

There were 21 patients whose V/Q scans were read centrally as normal on first reading by both readers. Three underwent angiography and none showed thromboemboli. None of the remaining 18 patients received anticoagulants and none had clinically evident pulmonary embolism on follow-up.

Clinical Assessment of the Likelihood of Pulmonary Embolism

The clinician's assessment of the likelihood of pulmonary embolism recorded before the scan was performed ("prior probability") was compared with pulmonary embolism status as determined by angiography and follow-up information (Table 6) for 887 patients with prior probability assessments and definite pulmonary embolism status. A clinical assessment of 80% to 100% likelihood of pulmonary embolism was made in 90 patients (10%) and was correct in 61 (68%) of 90. A clinical assessment of 0% to 19% likelihood of pulmonary embolism was made in 228 (26%) and was correct in 207 (91%) of 228. Clinical assessment, therefore, was more often correct in excluding pulmonary embolism than in identifying pulmonary embolism. In the majority of patients (569 [64%]), clinical assessments were noncommittal (20% to 79% likelihood of pulmonary embolism).

Combining clinical assessments with the V/Q scan interpretations improved the overall chance of reaching a correct diagnosis of acute pulmonary embolism (Table 6). Among patients in whom the clinical impression and the scan interpretation were both of high probability for pulmonary embolism, 28 (96%) of 29 had pulmonary embolism. If the high-probability scan interpretation was paired with an intermediate-likelihood clinical assessment or a low-likelihood clinical assessment, then the probability that the patient had pulmonary embolism fell to 70 (88%) of 80 and 5 (56%) of 9, respectively. The addition of the clinical evaluation also helped in the low-probability and in the near-normal/normal scan categories. A low-probability clinical assessment (0% to 19% likelihood of pulmonary embolism based on clinical judgment), when paired with a low-probability V/Q scan, correctly excluded the diagnosis of pulmonary embolism in 86 (96%) of 90 patients. The near-normal/normal V/Q scan category, when paired with a low-likelihood clinical assessment, correctly excluded pulmonary embolism in 60 (98%) of 61 patients.

COMMENT

The PIOPED study was conducted as a multicenter, prospective effort to estimate the sensitivity and specificity of the V/Q lung scan for the diagnosis of pulmonary embolism. Other retrospective and prospective studies have focused on positive predictive values, which are influenced by prevalence of pulmonary embolism and patient selection. Sensitivity and specificity, however, are fundamental characteristics of a diagnostic test and are not affected by the prevalence of disease.[10]

In PIOPED, almost all patients (98%) with clinically important pulmonary embolism had lung scans that fell into one of the three abnormal categories—high, intermediate (indeterminate), or low probability. If all three abnormal categories are combined into one, the lung scan is sensitive enough to serve as a screening test for the diagnosis of pulmonary embolism, but the specificity is limited. The high-probability scan lacked sensitivity in diagnosing pulmonary embolism, since it failed to identify 59% of patients with this disorder.

Only 14 (3%) of 480 patients who did not have evidence of acute pulmonary embolism on angiography had high-probability scans (Table 4). Therefore, the specificity of a high-probability scan was 97%. For patients with histories of pulmonary embolism, the specificity of the high-probability scan was reduced. This finding is consistent with other reports of previous pulmonary embolism as a cause of V/Q scan abnormality that may be confused with acute pulmonary embolism.[11,12] The specificity of scans of intermediate or low probability was much less than the specificity of the high-probability scan.

The PIOPED's study design included patient enumeration and recruitment prior to scan completion to avoid bias in patient selection. Nonetheless, patients who ultimately had high- and intermediate-probability scans were more often successfully recruited for PIOPED. If anything, this selection bias would suggest that PIOPED tends to overestimate V/Q scans' sensitivities and underestimate specificities.

Clinical decisions are often made on the basis of the predictive values, which depend not only on the test's sensitivity and specificity, but also on the prevalence of disease in the population studied. Based on angiogram results, the prevalence of pulmonary embolism in PIOPED was 33% (251/755) (Table 4); based on pulmonary embolism status—derived from angiogram evaluation and/or clinical evaluation—the prevalence was 28% (Table 6), similar to the prevalences described in previous reports.[13-21] In PIOPED, the positive predictive value of the high-probability scan was 88%, whereas the negative predictive value of a low-probability scan was 84%. The negative predictive value of the near-normal/normal scan category was better at 91%. Estimates of negative predictive values increased when analyses took into account patients who did not undergo angiography, did not receive anticoagulants, and had no evidence of pulmonary embolism occurring during 1 year of follow-up. Including these patients among those not having pulmonary embolism in the analysis improved the negative predictive value of the low-probability scan from 84% to 88% and of the near-normal/normal scan from 91% to 96%. Because some instances of acute pulmonary embolism may not have been detected among these patients, the true negative predictive values may be less than 88% for low-probability scans and 96% for near-normal/normal scans, but still ought to be closer to these latter values than to the 84% and 91%, which did not account for patients without angiography results.

Although pulmonary emboli did occur in patients with scans classified in the categories between low probability and normal, pulmonary embolism was documented in only 5 (4%) of 131 of such patients. The true proportion of patients with pulmonary embolism must be inferred with caution, because large numbers of patients with near-normal/normal scans were not successfully recruited for the study. Only 42% of the 131 PIOPED patients in this category completed angiography. Only 3 of the 21 patients with lung scans read as normal by both readers on the final reading completed angiography; all 3 had normal pulmonary angiograms. None of the remaining 18 had clinically evident pulmonary emboli on follow-up. This finding is consistent with the findings of Kipper et al.[22]

The value of combining clinical judg-ment with the interpretation of the scan is supported by the PIOPED study. The predictive value of the high- and low-probability lung scans improved when supported by similar clinical assessments. For 90 patients, the negative predictive value of the low-probability scan rose to 96% when accompanied by a clinical assessment of low likelihood. In 29 patients, the positive predictive value of a high-probability scan increased to 96% if supported by a high-likelihood clinical assessment. In the PIOPED experience, combining a lung scan interpretation with a strong clinical suspicion as to whether acute pulmonary embolism is present is a sound diagnostic strategy, as previously suggested by McNeil and colleagues,[20,21] but is sufficient for only a minority of patients (Table 6). For a substantial number of patients in the PIOPED study, angiography was required for a definitive diagnosis of pulmonary embolism.

The PIOPED study employed pulmonary angiography, which proved to be a safe and accurate method of diagnosing pulmonary embolism, although it is invasive. The four patients (0.5%) for whom the outcome classification committee disagreed with blinded angiogram interpretations that showed acute pulmonary embolism to be absent must be considered carefully in light of the angiographic criteria's design for acute pulmonary embolism, the variable time between angiographic evaluation and the patients' deaths, and the variability in pathophysiology and pathological interpretation of thromboemboli in evolution. In the PIOPED study, a normal angiogram almost excluded the possibility of pulmonary embolism, confirming the results of two previous studies.[14,15]

The PIOPED findings extend observations made by other investigators,[1-3,12-20] from whom the PIOPED investigators derived study criteria for angiogram and V/Q scan interpretation. Although predictive values for patients with high-probability scans and patients with low-probability scans in previous series are generally consistent with the PIOPED findings, the underrepresentation of patients with low-probability scans in previous studies has in the past led to an exaggerated impression of the sensitivity of the high-probability lung scan.

The findings of Hull and colleagues[17,18] in the Hamilton District Thromboembolism Programme are particularly interesting in comparison with the PIOPED results. Of the 305 patients with suspected pulmonary embolism and abnormal perfusion lung scans in their study, 173 (57%) had adequate ventilation scans and adequate pulmonary angio-grams. Ninety-five patients (31%) had pulmonary emboli demonstrated on angiography. The predictive values from their study are similar to PIOPED results in the high-probability and intermediate-probability (indeterminate) scan categories. The PIOPED study, likewise, found pulmonary emboli among patients with scans in the low-probability category, but fewer than the 25% for subsegmental matched lesions and 40% for subsegmental mismatched lesions found by Hull et al. Patient referral patterns or lung scan interpretation criteria may account for the differences between PIOPED results and the Hamilton study results. Since angiographic studies are not available and clinical follow-up has not been applied to determine pulmonary embolism status for the 110 patients without adequate angiography, for the 22 patients without adequate ventilation scans, and for the patients with normal scans in the Hamilton District Thromboembolism Programme, comparisons of estimates of sensitivity and specificity between the two studies are not possible.

The PIOPED results lead to a number of conclusions that settle controversies about the diagnostic value of the lung scan in pulmonary embolism.[23,24] A high-probability scan usually indicates pulmonary embolism, but only a minority of patients with pulmonary embolism have a high-probability scan. A history of pulmonary embolism decreases the accuracy of diagnoses based on high-probability scans. A low-probability scan with a strong clinical impression that pulmonary embolism is not likely makes the possibility of pulmonary embolism remote. Near-normal/normal lung scans make the diagnosis of acute pulmonary embolism very unlikely. An intermediate-probability (indeterminate) scan is not of help in establishing a diagnosis. In PIOPED, the scan combined with clinical assessment permitted a noninvasive diagnosis or exclusion of acute pulmonary embolism for a minority of patients.

This study was supported by contracts NO1-HR-34007, NO1-HR-34008, NO1-HR-34009, NO1-HR-34010, NO1-HR-34011, NO1-HR-34012, and NO1-HR-34013 from the National Heart, Lung, and Blood Institute, Bethesda, Md.

The secretarial assistance of JoAnne Decker has been greatly appreciated.

Steering Committee

The PIOPED investigators are as follows:

Herbert A. Saltzman, MD, chairman; Abass Alavi, MD, Richard H. Greenspan, MD, Charles A. Hales, MD, Paul D. Stein, MD, Michael Terrin, MD, MPH, Carol Vreim, PhD, John G. Weg, MD; alternates: Christos Athanasoulis. MD, Alexander Gottschalk. MD.

Clinical Centers

Duke University
Herbert A. Saltzman, MD, principal investigator; Russell Blinder, MD, R. Edward Coleman, MD, N. Reed Dunnick, MD, William J. Fulkerson, Jr, MD, Lee Mallatratt, RN, Carl E. Ravin, MD.

Henry Ford Hospital
Paul D. Stein, MD, principal investigator; Deborah Adams, RN, Matthew Burke, MD, Jerry W. Froelich, MD, Kenneth V. Leeper, MD, Barry A. Lesser, MD, John Popovich, Jr, MD, P. C. Shetty, MD, James Thrall, MD.

Massachusetts General Hospital
Charles A. Hales, MD, principal investigator; Christos Athanasoulis, MD, Stuart Geller, MD, Kenneth McKusick, MD, Deborah Quinn, RN, MS, B. Taylor Thompson, MD, Arthur C. Waltman, MD.

University of Michigan
John G. Weg, MD, principal investigator; Grace Ball, RN, Kyung J. Cho, MD, Charles A. Easton, MD, Andrew Flint, MD, Thomas A. Griggs, MD, Jack E. Juni, MD, Jerold Wallis, MD, David Williams, MD.

University of Pennsylvania
Abass Alavi, MD, principal investigator; Margaret Ahearn-Spera, RNC, MSN, Dana R. Burke, MD, Jeffrey Carson, MD, Mark A. Kelley, MD, Gordon K. McLean, MD, Steven G. Meranze, MD, Harold I. Palevsky, MD, Sanford Schwartz, MD.

Yale University
Richard H. Greenspan, MD, principal investigator; Donald F. Denny, Jr, MD, Alexander Gottschalk, MD, Lee H. Greenwood, MD, Jacob S. O. Loke, MD, Richard A. Matthay, MD, Steven S. Morse, MD, H. Dirk Sostman, MD, Felicia Tencza, MPH.

Data and Coordinating Center

Maryland Medical Research Institute: Michael L. Terrin, MD, MPH, principal investigator; Wilmot Ball, MD, Mary Burke, Martha Canner, MS, Paul Canner, PhD, Margie Carroll, Martin Goldman, MD, Carol Handy, Elizabeth Heinz, Thomas E. Hobbins, MD, Frank Hooper, ScD, Steven Kaufman, MD, Christian R. Klimt, MD, DrPH (principal investigator, September 1983 through September 1984), William F. Krol, PhD, Norman LaFrance, MD, Gerard J. Prud'homme, MA, Sharon Pruitt, Pauline Raiz, Bruce Thompson, PhD, Heidi Weissman, MD.

Project Office

National Heart, Lung, and Blood Institute: Carol E. Vreim, PhD, Margaret Wu, PhD.

Policy and Data Safety Monitoring Board

Myron Stein, MD, chairman; Daniel M. Biello, MD (deceased), Sarah Greene Burger, MPH, Robert Henkin, MD, Thomas Hyers, MD, Paul S. Levy, ScD, Franklin Miller, Jr, MD, Robert E. O'Mara, MD, Morris Simon, MD, Gerard Turino, MD, George W. Williams, PhD.

Outcome Classification Committee

Mark A. Kelley, MD, chairman; Jeffrey Carson, MD, William J. Fulkerson, MD, Thomas E. Hobbins, MD, Richard A. Matthay, MD, Harold Palevsky, MD, John Popovich, Jr, MD, B. Taylor Thompson, MD, John G. Weg, MD.

References

1. Wagner HN, Sabiston DC, Iio M, McAfee JG, Meyer JK, Langan JK. Regional pulmonary blood flow in man by radioisotope scanning. *JAMA.* 1964;187:601-603.
2. Wagner HN Jr, Lopez-Majano V, Langan JK, Joshi RC. Radioactive xenon in the differential diagnosis of pulmonary embolism. *Radiology.* 1968;91:1168-1184.
3. Biello DR, Mattar AG, McKnight RC, Siegel BA. Ventilation perfusion studies in suspected pulmonary embolism. *Am J Radiol.* 1979;133:1033-1037.
4. Snedecor JW, Cochran WG. *Statistical Methods.* 6th ed. Ames: Iowa State University Press; 1967.
5. Cochran WG. Some methods of strengthening the common χ^2 tests. *Biometrics.* 1954;10:417-451.
6. Fleiss JL. *Statistical Methods for Rates and Proportions.* 2nd ed. New York, NY: John Wiley & Sons Inc; 1981.
7. Nie NH, ed. *SPSS^x User's Guide.* New York, NY: McGraw-Hill International Book Co; 1983.
8. Hill AB. *Principles of Medical Statistics.* 9th ed. New York, NY: Oxford University Press Inc; 1971.
9. Murphy EA. *Probability in Medicine.* Baltimore, Md: The Johns Hopkins University Press; 1979.
10. Vecchio JJ. Predictive value of a single diagnostic test in unselected populations. *N Engl J Med.* 1966;274:1171-1175.
11. Li DK, Seltzer SG, McNeil BJ. V/Q mismatches unassociated with pulmonary embolism: case report and review of the literature. *J Nucl Med.* 1978;19:1331-1333.
12. Biello DR, Kumar B. Symmetrical perfusion defects without pulmonary embolism. *Eur J Nucl Med.* 1982;7:197-199.
13. Alderson PO, Martin EC. Pulmonary embolism: diagnosis with multiple imaging modalities. *Radiology.* 1987;164:297-312.
14. Cheely R, McCartney WH, Perry JR, et al. The role of noninvasive tests versus pulmonary angiography in the diagnosis of pulmonary embolism. *Am J Med.* 1981;70:17-22.
15. Novelline RA, Baitarowich OH, Athanasoulis CA, Waltman AC, Greenfield AJ, Mckusick KA. The clinical course of patients with suspected pulmonary embolism and a negative pulmonary arteriogram. *Radiology.* 1978;126:561-567.
16. Sasahara AA, Stein M, Simon M, Littmann D. Pulmonary angiography in the diagnosis of thromboembolic disease. *N Engl J Med.* 1964;270:1075-1081.
17. Hull RD, Hirsh J, Carter CJ, et al. Pulmonary angiography, ventilation lung scanning and venography for clinically suspected pulmonary embolism with abnormal perfusion lung scan. *Ann Intern Med.* 1983;98:891-899.
18. Hull RD, Hirsh J, Carter CJ, et al. Diagnostic value of ventilation-perfusion lung scanning in patients with suspected pulmonary embolism. *Chest.* 1985;88:819-828.
19. Poulose KP, Reba RC, Gilday DL, Deland FH, Wagner HN. Diagnosis of pulmonary embolism: a correlative study of the clinical, scan, and angiographic findings. *BMJ.* 1970;3:67-71.
20. McNeil BJ. Ventilation-perfusion studies and the diagnoses of pulmonary embolism: concise communication. *J Nucl Med.* 1980;21:319-323.
21. McNeil BJ, Hessel SJ, Branch WT, Bjork L, Adelstein SJ. Measures of clinical efficacy, III: the value of the lung scan in the evaluation of young patients with pleuritic chest pain. *J Nucl Med.* 1976;17:163-169.
22. Kipper MS, Moser KM, Kortman KE, Ashburn WL. Long-term follow-up of patients with suspected pulmonary embolism and a normal lung scan. *Chest.* 1982;82:411-415.
23. Robin ED. Over diagnosis and over treatment of pulmonary embolism: the emperor may have no clothes. *Ann Intern Med.* 1977;87:775-781.
24. Biello DR. Radiological (scintigraphic) evaluation of patients with suspected pulmonary thromboembolism. *JAMA.* 1987;257:3257-3259.

9.2 GUIDE APPLIED TO A STUDY OF AN INTERVENTION

Jeffrey A. Tice, MD • Daniel J. Friedland, MD

EXECUTIVE COMMITTEE FOR THE ASYMPTOMATIC CAROTID ATHEROSCLEROSIS STUDY:

Endarterectomy for asymptomatic carotid artery stenosis. JAMA 1995;273:1421.*
(See pp 200–207.)

Step 1. Do I want to evaluate the study? (INR)

Is the study:

Interesting? Yes, this study sheds light on the controversy surrounding the usefulness of carotid endarterectomy (CEA) in the treatment of asymptomatic carotid artery stenosis (CAS).

Novel? The effect of CEA on asymptomatic CAS has been evaluated in two previous randomized controlled trials. One study (CASANOVA) showed no benefit.[1] The other (Veterans Affairs Cooperative Study)[2] showed a significant benefit for the combined end points of ipsilateral stroke and transient ischemic attacks (TIAs), but not for ipsilateral stroke alone. The study we are reviewing, however, is the largest study of its kind to date and evaluates the end point of reduction in ipsilateral stroke in patients receiving CEA.

Relevant? Stroke is the third most common cause of death in the United States. A significant number of strokes are attributable to asymptomatic CAS. If CEA were shown to be beneficial in asymptomatic CAS, many strokes could be prevented. Stroke is clearly a relevant issue, but does the research question address a clinically relevant outcome? The end point that was used in this study—any ipsilateral stroke—is more relevant than the end point of ipsilateral TIA but is less relevant than the outcome of major ipsilateral stroke.

Step 2. Outline the study

(See Figure 9.2–1.)

Step 3. Is the study finding believable?

A. Do the study subjects and variables accurately represent the research question?

Subjects: The target population in the research question refers to asymptomatic patients with CAS of greater than 60%. Most subjects did have stenosis of greater than 60% (only 5% of subjects had CAS of < 60%). Many subjects, however, did not have their stenosis measured by angiography. During recruitment, CAS was measured by angiography in 39%; by carotid Doppler ultrasonography in 55%; and by ocular pneumoplethysmography in 6%. Nevertheless, we are reassured by the reported reliability of the latter two techniques. The researchers determined that the cut points used for Doppler ultrasonography and ocular pneumoplethysmography had a positive predictive value of 95% and 90%, respectively. Although most subjects had the appropriate degree of stenosis, it is debatable whether the subjects represent a truly *asymptomatic* population. Before enrollment in the study, 20% of

---

* Executive Committee for the Asymptomatic Carotid Atherosclerosis Study: Endarterectomy for asymptomatic carotid artery stenosis. JAMA 1995;273:1421. Copyright 1990. American Medical Association. Printed with permission.

Truth in the universe	Study method

Research question

Does addition of CEA to intensive medical management of patients with asymptomatic CAS ≥ 60% decrease the risk of ipsilateral stroke?

Study design

Randomized controlled trial

Target population

Inclusion:
Asymptomatic CAS ≥ 60%

Exclusion:
Previous ipsilateral or vertebrovascular CVA, contralateral CVA within the last 45 days, contraindication to aspirin, poor prognosis within the next 5 years, or poor surgical candidacy

Subjects

Temporal characteristics:
12/87–12/93
Intended follow-up, 5 years.

Geographic characteristics:
39 sites in the United States

Sampling:
42,000 screened (referrals from carotid Doppler labs, physicians noting carotid bruits or finding CAS on work-up of peripheral vascular disease or contralateral CEA). 1659 randomized.

Surgery:
n = 825.
101 did not receive CEA.
9 lost to follow-up.
5% of subjects had CAS < 60%.

Medicine:
n = 834.
45 received CEA.
11 lost to follow-up.

Patient characteristics:
see Table 1, page 1423, JAMA article

Predictor

Addition of CEA to intensive medical management

Predictor variable

Addition of CEA to medical treatment with 325 mg daily aspirin as well as counseling about stroke risk factors (hypertension, diabetes mellitus, lipids, alcohol and tobacco use)

Outcome

Ipsilateral stroke or perioperative death or stroke.

Outcome variable

Ipsilateral stroke is defined as a focal neurological deficit lasting > 24 hours (TIA is considered a deficit lasting between 30 seconds and 24 hours).

Stroke or death is considered perioperative if it occurred within 30 days of CEA. Stroke and death are also counted during an analogous "perioperative" period in the medical group, lasting 40 days after randomization.

Stroke outcome is diagnosed by physical examination, head CT, and confirmation by the blinded End Point Review Committee.

Study finding

Perioperative stroke or death or ipsilateral stroke projected over 5 years:
Medical (11%), Surgical (5.1%), RRR (53%).
Note that the study was stopped at a median of 2.7 years and the reported findings are Kaplan-Meier estimates predicting the event risk at 5 years of follow-up.

Figure 9.2–1. Outline of the endarterectomy for asymptomatic carotid artery stenosis study. CEA = carotid endarterectomy; CAS = carotid artery stenosis; CVA = cerebrovascular accident; TIA = transient ischemic attack; CT = computed tomography; RRR = relative risk reduction.

subjects had contralateral CEA, and 24% had contralateral TIA or stroke. Although the subjects are asymptomatic for ipsilateral events, they are fairly symptomatic for contralateral events; therefore, they may not be representative of what many physicians consider a truly asymptomatic state.

Predictor variables: The predictor variables (CEA, 325 mg of aspirin therapy, and risk factor reduction) accurately represent the predictors (CEA and intensive medical management) in the research question.

Outcome variable: In this study, the outcome of stroke is defined as a focal neurological deficit lasting more than 24 hours. Diagnosis is established through history, physical examination, computer tomography (CT) of the head and confirmation by the blinded End Point Review Committee. Thus, as defined and measured, the outcome variable appears to be an accurate representation of stroke.

B. Is the finding attributable to other factors?

?Chance. At $p = 0.004$, it is improbable that the finding is attributable to chance.

?Bias. BIASES IN SELECTING THE STUDY SUBJECTS   The randomization was successful, resulting in similar baseline characteristics in the medical and surgical groups (see Table 1 of the JAMA article, page 1423). Therefore, the outcomes are not attributable to a bias in subject selection.

BIASES IN FOLLOWING UP ON THE STUDY SUBJECTS. The relatively small number of subjects lost to follow-up (approximately 1% in each arm) should not affect the finding. However, approximately 12% of surgical subjects did not receive surgery, and 5% of the medical subjects underwent CEA—*this* potentially biases the finding. But be careful; if subjects in the surgical arm do not receive surgery while those in the medical arm do, the magnitude of the finding would be smaller (assuming, of course, that CEA is truly effective and subjects are not crossed over). Thus, the magnitude of the finding may have been even larger if this bias were not present. In other words, this bias strengthens rather than weakens the finding.

BIASES IN EXECUTING OR MEASURING THE PREDICTOR VARIABLE. Surgical and medical subjects obviously knew their treatment assignments. It is possible that the behavior of the surgical patients differed from that of the medical patients. For example, surgical patients may have been more compliant with aspirin therapy, which could have resulted in a decreased incidence of strokes in that arm. In addition, it is possible that one arm may have received more aggressive counseling on the reduction of risk factors. Although compliance rates on medication and success of risk factor reduction are not explicitly discussed, the relatively smaller incidence of cardiac mortality in the surgical group (see Table 4 of the JAMA article, page 1425) supports the possibility of greater compliance of aspirin or more effective risk factor reduction compared with the medical group.

BIASES IN MEASURING THE OUTCOME VARIABLE. It is difficult to ensure that the determination of the outcome is blind to the intervention. For example, subjects without a surgical scar (ie, the medical group) may have been more likely to be sent for outcome review if they reported subtle neurological symptoms. If so, this would bias toward increased efficacy of CEA.

BIASES IN ANALYZING THE DATA. The use of intention-to-treat analysis is appropriate, as it preserves the equality of baseline characteristics between the surgical and medical groups generated through randomization.

Although it may be ethical to terminate a study early when a certain level of statistical significance has been reached, estimating the results at the intended completion of the study can introduce bias. Using the data at the median 2.7 years of follow-up, the investigators apply Kaplan-Meier statistics to estimate the findings at 5 years. Not knowing the assumptions used in their model, it is difficult to predict whether the technique overestimates or underestimates the true efficacy of CEA.

?Confounders. Table 1 of the JAMA article suggests that the randomization was successful; therefore, both known and unknown confounders should be distributed equally between the medical and surgical groups. Thus it is unlikely that the finding is attributable to confounding.

C. Is the finding believable within the context of other knowledge?

?Consistency with other literature. Yes, both case series compared with historical control subjects and one previous randomized controlled trial suggest benefit.[1]

?Biological plausibility. It is plausible that if the potential source responsible for a stroke (ie, carotid atherosclerotic plaque) were removed, the risk of stroke would decrease.

?Analogy. If CEA reduces the risk of stroke in symptomatic patients,[3] it may also reduce the risk of stroke in asymptomatic patients.

Step 4. What is the clinically relevant finding?

Weighing costs & benefits. The principal cost of CEA is perioperative stroke or death. The principal benefit of CEA is a reduction in ipsilateral stroke or death. One way of weighing these costs and benefits is using numbers needed to treat (NNT).

Recall from Chapter 5: The **absolute risk reduction** (ARR) = risk of event in the control group − risk of event in the study group. The NNT to prevent a single event = 1/ARR (when risk is expressed as a fraction) or 100/ARR (when risk is expressed as a percentage).

With reference to the study findings in the Table 9.2–1, it is easy to calculate the NNT to prevent a single event in this study.

The ARR to prevent *any ipsilateral stroke or any perioperative stroke or death* = 11% − 5.1% = 5.9%. Therefore, the NNT to prevent any ipsilateral stroke or any perioperative stroke or death = 17.

Table 9.2–1 also shows the findings for the more clinically relevant end point of *major ipsilateral stroke or any perioperative stroke or death*. Although CEA did lead to a small ARR of 2.6% for this outcome, this did not reach statistical significance (p = 0.12), and therefore we cannot calculate the NNT to prevent this outcome.

Discounting. Patients usually value their present life over their future life. Because surgery and angiography are themselves risk factors for stroke, it takes about 1 year for the survival curve of *ipsilateral stroke or any perioperative stroke or death* to cross (see Figure in the JAMA article on page 1425). A patient who significantly values present life over future life may be reluctant to take this up-front risk of stroke or death associated with surgery for the relatively small benefit of stroke reduction in the future.

Step 5. Will the study help me in caring for my patient?

A. Are the subjects adequately described and applicable to my patient?

The authors of the study give an adequate description of the cohort: 95% are white, 66% are male, and the mean age is 67 years. In addition, 20% had previous contralateral CEA and 24% had previous contralateral TIA or stroke. Does this represent your *asymptomatic* patient population?

TABLE 9.2–1. PRINCIPLE STUDY FINDINGS.

Event Type	Medical 5-Year Event Risk (%)	Surgical 5-Year Event Risk (%)
Ipsilateral stroke or any perioperative stroke or death	11.0	5.1
Major ipsilateral stroke or any perioperative stroke or death	6.0	3.4

B. Is the predictor variable adequately described and applicable to my patient?

The predictor variables are adequately described, but is a perioperative CEA event rate of 2.7% realistic for your center? Recent reviews document perioperative morbidity and mortality event rates ranging from 1% to 18%.[4,5] An analysis of Medicare data,[6] considering perioperative mortality alone, reported a 2.5% risk of death compared with 1% in most clinical trials and 0.36% in the study published in JAMA we are reviewing. The authors of the Medicare analysis conclude "this difference in community practice may limit the applicability of clinical trials."[6]

C. Will the finding result in an overall net benefit for my patient?

There may be some concern about the difficulty in blinding surgical and medical patients that could lead to differential compliance rates with medical management and possibly diagnosis of stroke. In addition, using Kaplan-Meier statistics to estimate the results at 5 years may have introduced some degree of bias. Despite these potential limitations, the study appears valid and believable within the context of other knowledge.

This article is a good example of a study that was performed well but in which the result that favors the intervention is of questionable benefit for our patient. Although the study finding is believable, its applicability and magnitude of benefit for your patient population may lead you to reject the intervention. Because the study population is fairly symptomatic for contralateral events, the magnitude of benefit may not be as great if your patient is truly asymptomatic. Furthermore, if your center cannot duplicate the study's relatively impressive surgical complication rate, CEA at your institution may be less beneficial or even harmful. Even if your patient is representative of this *asymptomatic* population and your center's surgical complication rate is low, your patient may be unimpressed by the relatively small absolute risk reduction in *major* as well as minor strokes. Furthermore, because patients discount their future life relative to their present life, they probably would not want to take an up-front surgical risk for only a modest benefit thereafter. What would *your* patient do if you told them that they had an 89% chance of not having *any* ipsilateral stroke over the next 5 years, but if they underwent CEA, the chance of no event would be 94.9%? What would they say if you then told them that 2.7% of the CEA risk is up-front in the form of perioperative stroke or death?

Although beyond the scope of this chapter, if you are particularly ambitious, it is possible to quantitatively evaluate the effect of patient discounting and the surgical complication rate on the choice to perform CEA. You may incorporate data from the study into a decision analysis (preferably a Markov model) and use sensitivity analysis to determine the discount and surgical complication rate thresholds at which the medical benefit outweighs the surgical benefit.

REFERENCES

1. CASANOVA Study Group: Carotid surgery versus medical therapy in asymptomatic carotid stenosis. Stroke 1991;22:1229.
2. Hobson RW II et al, for the Veterans Affairs Cooperative Study Group: Efficacy of carotid endarterectomy for asymptomatic carotid stenosis. N Engl J Med 1993;328:221.
3. North American Symptomatic Carotid Endarterectomy Trial Collaborators: Beneficial effect of carotid endarterectomy in symptomatic patients with high-grade stenosis. N Engl J Med 1991;325:445.
4. Chassin MR: *The Appropriateness of Selected Medical and Surgical Procedures: Relationship to Geographical Variations*. Rand, 1989.
5. Moore WS: Carotid endarterectomy for prevention of stroke. West J Med 1993;159:37.
6. Hsia DC et al: Epidemiology of carotid endarterectomy among Medicare beneficiaries. Stroke 1996;27:266.

Original Contributions

Endarterectomy for Asymptomatic Carotid Artery Stenosis

Executive Committee for the Asymptomatic Carotid Atherosclerosis Study

Objective.—To determine whether the addition of carotid endarterectomy to aggressive medical management can reduce the incidence of cerebral infarction in patients with asymptomatic carotid artery stenosis.

Design.—Prospective, randomized, multicenter trial.

Setting.—Thirty-nine clinical sites across the United States and Canada.

Patients.—Between December 1987 and December 1993, a total of 1662 patients with asymptomatic carotid artery stenosis of 60% or greater reduction in diameter were randomized; follow-up data are available on 1659. At baseline, recognized risk factors for stroke were similar between the two treatment groups.

Intervention.—Daily aspirin administration and medical risk factor management for all patients; carotid endarterectomy for patients randomized to receive surgery.

Main Outcome Measures.—Initially, transient ischemic attack or cerebral infarction occurring in the distribution of the study artery and any transient ischemic attack, stroke, or death occurring in the perioperative period. In March 1993, the primary outcome measures were changed to cerebral infarction occurring in the distribution of the study artery or any stroke or death occurring in the perioperative period.

Results.—After a median follow-up of 2.7 years, with 4657 patient-years of observation, the aggregate risk over 5 years for ipsilateral stroke and any perioperative stroke or death was estimated to be 5.1% for surgical patients and 11.0% for patients treated medically (aggregate risk reduction of 53% [95% confidence interval, 22% to 72%]).

Conclusion.—Patients with asymptomatic carotid artery stenosis of 60% or greater reduction in diameter and whose general health makes them good candidates for elective surgery will have a reduced 5-year risk of ipsilateral stroke if carotid endarterectomy performed with less than 3% perioperative morbidity and mortality is added to aggressive management of modifiable risk factors.

(JAMA. 1995;273:1421-1428)

MORE THAN 500 000 new strokes occur annually in the United States, and it has been estimated that carotid artery disease may be responsible for 20% to 30% of them.[1] The annual stroke event rate for asymptomatic patients with hemodynamically significant carotid artery stenosis ranges from 2% to 5%.[2-5] Carotid artery stenosis usually is identified after transient ischemic attack (TIA), but for many patients, cerebral infarction caused by artery-to-artery embolism or carotid occlusion is the initial event. Progression of asymptomatic carotid artery stenosis to occlusion is unpredictable and can be disastrous; at the time of occlusion, dis-

abling stroke may occur in 20% of patients, and thereafter in 1.5% to 5% annually.[6-8] On the other hand, the 30-day major morbidity and mortality for patients who undergo surgery for asymptomatic stenosis ranges from 0.0% to 3.8%, and that for patients with symptomatic stenosis may be 6%.[9] Because the role of carotid endarterectomy (CEA) for asymptomatic carotid artery stenosis had not been proved,[10-12] the Asymptomatic Carotid Atherosclerosis Study (ACAS) was initiated in 1987.[13] The ACAS is an investigator-initiated randomized trial designed to test whether CEA should be a component of management for selected patients with asymptomatic stenosis of the common carotid bulb, the internal carotid sinus, or both. The question addressed was: Will CEA added to aggressive reduction of modifiable risk factors and administration of aspirin reduce the 5-year risk of ipsilateral cerebral infarc-

tion in individuals with asymptomatic hemodynamically significant carotid artery stenosis?

For editorial comment see p 1459.

Secondary objectives were to determine the surgical success in lesion removal and the incidence of recurrent carotid stenosis, the rate of progression or regression of carotid atherosclerosis in the medically treated comparison group, and the incidence of all other vascular events, such as TIA, myocardial infarction, and death related to vascular disease during follow-up.

METHODS

The design and organization of the ACAS are detailed elsewhere.[13] Thirty-nine clinical centers were chosen from an applicant pool of 55. All obtained institutional review board approval of the study protocol.

Recruitment

Study participants were recruited from ultrasound vascular laboratories, practitioners who auscultated carotid bruits, and physicians who found carotid stenosis during evaluation for peripheral vascular surgery or contralateral CEA.

Inclusion criteria were age between 40 and 79 years; compatible history and findings on physical and neurological examinations; performance of required laboratory and electrocardiographic examinations no earlier than 3 months before randomization; patient accessibility and willingness to be followed for 5 years; and valid informed consent.

Exclusion criteria were cerebrovascular events in the distribution of the study carotid artery or in that of the vertebrobasilar arterial system; symptoms referable to the contralateral cerebral hemisphere within the previous 45 days; contraindication to aspirin therapy; a disorder that could seriously complicate surgery; or a condition that could prevent continuing participation or was likely to produce disability or death within 5 years. (Detailed information regarding eligibil-

A complete list of the collaborators in the Asymptomatic Carotid Atherosclerosis Study appears at the end of this article.

Reprint requests to Stroke Center and Department of Neurology, Bowman Gray School of Medicine of Wake Forest University, Medical Center Blvd, Winston-Salem, NC 27157-1068 (James F. Toole, MD).

Reprinted from JAMA ® The Journal of the American Medical Association
May 10, 1995 Volume 273
Copyright 1995, American Medical Association

ity and exclusion is available on request from the corresponding author.)

The ACAS definition of hemodynamically significant carotid stenosis required that at least one of three criteria was met: arteriography within the previous 60 days indicating stenosis of at least 60% reduction in diameter (if the arteriogram was performed 61 to 364 days before randomization, Doppler ultrasonography was required to verify that the artery had not occluded); Doppler examination within the preceding 60 days showing a frequency or velocity greater than the instrument-specific cut point with 95% positive predictive value (PPV); or Doppler examination showing a frequency or velocity greater than the instrument-specific 90% PPV cut point confirmed by ocular pneumoplethysmographic (OPG-Gee) examination performed within the previous 60 days.

A patient could enter the study with unilaterally or bilaterally asymptomatic, hemodynamically significant stenosis, but only one artery was the study artery. If two arteries were eligible, the one with the greater stenosis was selected. If the stenoses were identical, the left carotid artery was chosen. Patients randomized to surgery on the basis of Doppler or Doppler with OPG-Gee were required to have an arteriogram prior to CEA. If a postrandomization arteriogram revealed the contralateral artery to have the greater stenosis, it then became the study artery. The nonstudy artery was managed medically unless a cerebrovascular event occurred, at which time CEA could be considered.

Arteriographic Measurements

The minimal residual lumen (MRL) and the distal lumen (DL) were measured on the same radiograph. The MRL was the smallest lumen diameter at the site of the stenotic lesion. The DL was the diameter at the first point distal to the MRL at which the arterial walls became parallel. Percentage of stenosis was calculated as $100 \times (1-[MRL/DL])$.

Ultrasound Measurements

Because of the heterogeneity among ultrasound devices and techniques, we established a cut point for each by comparing Doppler ultrasonography with arteriograms performed within 42 days of each other. Doppler cut points were computed for peak systolic frequency or, if indeterminant, end diastolic frequency, based on data from 50 consecutive patients.[14]

Randomization

An ACAS neurologist and an ACAS surgeon gave joint approval for entering patients. Once the eligibility criteria had been confirmed and after informed consent was obtained, the patient was randomized using the permuted block method with at least three different block sizes determined randomly, stratified by center, gender, number of eligible arteries, and previous contralateral CEA. The assignment category was communicated to each clinical center by the statistical coordinating center through an individualized computer program arranged so that the clinical center could neither predict nor reject an assignment.

Medical Treatment

All patients received 325 mg of regular or enteric-coated aspirin daily (provided by Sterling Health USA, New York, NY). Stroke risk factors and their modification were reviewed with all patients at the time of randomization and again during subsequent interviews and telephone follow-up. This included discussion of diastolic and systolic hypertension, diabetes mellitus, abnormal lipid levels, excessive consumption of ethanol, and tobacco use. Whenever possible, the recommendations of the ACAS Risk Factor Reduction Committee were followed (available on request from the corresponding author).

Surgical Treatment

In addition to 325 mg of aspirin daily and risk factor modification counseling, patients randomized to the surgical arm received the normal evaluation and care of a surgical patient. They were scheduled to undergo CEA within 2 weeks of randomization. If an arteriogram or cranial computed tomogram (CCT) had not been performed, the patient underwent the procedure(s) before CEA. The arteriogram must have demonstrated a stenosis of 60% or greater. Patients with a postrandomization, presurgery arteriogram demonstrating less than 60% stenosis or a distal abnormality such as an eurysm, arteriovenous malformation, or siphon stenosis exceeding the proximal stenosis did not undergo surgery but were retained in the surgical arm for comparison analyses. Asymptomatic cerebral infarction demonstrated by CCT was not an exclusion for surgery.[15] No attempt was made to standardize or control anesthesia or surgical techniques used by the 117 ACAS-credentialed surgeons.[16]

The surgeon, the ACAS neurologist, and the ACAS patient coordinator examined each patient 24 hours after CEA. All deficits occurring through the 30-day perioperative period required the administration of the end point review process (described below).

Follow-up

Follow-up evaluations were conducted at 1 month and thereafter every 3 months, alternating between clinic visits and telephone contacts. During the clinic visit, patients completed a medical history questionnaire and TIA/stroke questionnaire and underwent physical and neurological examinations and a Mini-Mental State Examination.[17] Risk reduction management was reviewed and aspirin adherence was determined by pill count.

Doppler ultrasound studies were repeated at the 3-month follow-up, every 6 months thereafter during the first 24 months, then yearly, and at potential or verified end point or at exit from the study after 5 years; CCT was repeated at potential end point or exit. Electrocardiogram was repeated when clinically indicated and at exit.

Patients were instructed to notify the coordinator if symptoms suggesting possible TIA or stroke occurred. The coordinator scheduled urgent evaluations by the ACAS neurologist and surgeon, and activated the end point verification system.

In addition to identification of events from clinic visits and telephone contacts, hospital discharge diagnoses and death certificates were reviewed for coronary events and strokes.

End Point Definition and Verification

A TIA was defined as a focal ischemic neurological deficit of abrupt onset lasting at least 30 seconds and resolving completely within 24 hours. Deficits persisting longer than 24 hours were classified as stroke.[18] All strokes or deaths occurring within 30 days after randomization in the surgical and 42 days in the medical groups were included as end points to reflect operative morbidity and mortality. The difference in times reflected an average 12-day interval between randomization and surgery.

Initial review was conducted under a stringent timetable involving one external expert masked for local diagnosis, treatment assignment, clinical center, and temporal relationship to surgery (if done). In addition, every potential event was abstracted, masked, and reviewed together by all six experts on the End Point Review Committee. Our analyses are based on their diagnoses.

Secondary analyses considered any stroke and perioperative death; any stroke and any death; and any ipsilateral TIA and stroke and any perioperative TIA, stroke, or death. The ACAS used categories 2 through 5 of the Glasgow scale to determine a major stroke, defined as a stroke resulting in moderate or severe disability, persistent vegetative state, or death.[19]

Statistical Analyses

Initially, the primary end points for evaluation of the two treatments were

Table 1.—Baseline Characteristics of Randomized Patients by Treatment Assignment, in Percentages*

Baseline Characteristic	Treatment Assignment	
	Surgical (n=825)	Medical (n=834)
Age, y		
40-49	2	2
50-59	13	15
60-69	50	46
70-79	36	38
Race		
White	94	95
Black	3	3
Other	3	2
Sex		
M	66	66
F	34	34
History		
Coronary artery disease†	69	69
Hypertension‡	64	64
Cancer	12	10
Diabetes mellitus	25	21
Lung disease at entry	6	5
Current cigarette smoker	28	24
Bilaterally eligible arteries	10	9
Previous contralateral		
Endarterectomy	20	19
TIA or stroke§	22	27
EC-IC bypass	<1	0
Subclavian bypass	<1	<1
Bruits in neck‖		
Ipsilateral	76	74
Contralateral	44	42
Infarct on CT scan¶		
Any location	22	24
Ipsilateral silent	8	9
Contralateral occlusion by Doppler	10	9

*TIA indicates transient ischemic attack; EC-IC, external carotid–internal carotid; and CT, computed tomographic.
†Defined as positive history of angina, coronary artery bypass, previous myocardial infarction, or abnormal electrocardiogram.
‡Positive response to "Has your doctor ever told you that you had high blood pressure or were hypertensive?"
§Significant difference between groups at .05 level (unadjusted for multiple comparisons).
‖Bruit question not evaluated for 51 surgical and 52 medical patients. Ipsilateral/contralateral refers to randomized artery.
¶CT scan was not available on 71 surgical and 60 medical patients.

Table 2.—Arteriographic Stenosis of the Ipsilateral Carotid Artery

% Stenosis	Prerandomization Arteriogram			Postrandomization Presurgery Arteriogram
	Medical	Surgical	Total (%)	
0-59	Not applicable	NA	NA	32 (8)
60-69	131	137	268 (42)	139 (34)
70-79	94	93	187 (29)	110 (26)
80-89	75	79	154 (24)	107 (26)
90-99	13	20	33 (5)	24 (6)
Total	313	329	642*	412†

*Two patients were missing, one in each group.
†Two patients were missing.

ther resolved the issue of whether CEA prevents unheralded cerebral infarction. Therefore, in March 1993, the ACAS Executive Committee and the Data and Safety Monitoring Committee voted to restrict the primary end point to stroke and perioperative complications or death.

For baseline comparisons, we used two-tailed t tests for comparing the means of continuous variables and χ^2 for comparing distributions of categorical variables, with no adjustment for multiple comparisons. Kaplan-Meier estimates of 5-year aggregate risk were compared between treatment groups using either Greenwood's formula for variances, for a large-sample test ignoring randomization stratification,[22] or randomization tests, respecting randomization strata.[23] In the initial years of treatment comparison, 1991 through 1993, the tests were for 2-, 3-, or 4-year aggregate risk. The randomization test was the primary method for interim treatment comparisons (see below). By the time of study closure P values from the two methods agreed within .002, so that all test results and confidence intervals (CIs) reported are based on large-sample tests unless otherwise noted.

Semiannual treatment comparison analyses were used to advise the Data Safety and Monitoring Committee whether a significance boundary had been crossed. The stopping rule was a modified O'Brien-Fleming[24] rule for maintaining the desired overall significance level despite repeated testing. The modification was for testing at selected intervals rather than predetermined numbers of events. The five analyses originally planned were changed to 10, because recruitment lagged and TIA was deleted as a primary end point. The critical value for the test statistic was 6.00 at the first test and 2.07 for the 10th, as compared with 1.96 for a single test at the significance level .05. The study was stopped after the eighth test, when the critical value was 2.38, corresponding to a nominal significance level of .017.

Treatment comparisons are reported herein in terms of relative risk reduction, the 5-year risk reduction due to surgery as a proportion of risk in the medical group.[25] Absolute treatment group–specific risk levels are also provided for calculation of absolute risk reduction. For the primary event the number of patients treated to prevent one event over 5 years was calculated as the inverse of the absolute risk reduction.[25]

Intention-to-treat analyses were used for all comparisons unless otherwise indicated, regardless of postrandomization ineligibility or crossover. End points for medical patients who received CEA after verified ipsilateral end point were categorized as perioperative if they occurred within 30 days of CEA. All tests were two tailed.

COHORT CHARACTERISTICS

During the 6 years of the study, more than 42 000 patients were screened and 1662 patients were randomized. Twenty-four centers contributed more than 30 patients each, and 13 contributed more than 50 patients. The average number of patients recruited per center was 43.

From March 1988 through October 1993, 12 080 CEAs were performed at the sites. Six percent (683) were performed on "likely eligible nonrandomized" patients of ACAS physicians, 6% (758) were performed on already randomized ACAS patients, and the rest were performed on symptomatic patients, ineligible patients, or patients of surgeons not collaborating in the ACAS.

Patient characteristics are presented in Table 1. Of the 1662 randomized patients, three in the surgery group were lost to follow-up after randomization and are excluded from analysis, leaving 1659. The 825 surgical and 834 medical patients were compared for 189 baseline characteristics, with only six tests yielding nominal statistically significant differences at the .05 level. Two thirds of the patients were men, 95% were white, and 48% were aged 60 through 69 years. Mean age was 67 years; mean weight, 81 kg for men and 67 kg for women; mean systolic blood pressure, 146 mm Hg; mean diastolic blood pressure, 78 mm Hg; and mean total cholesterol concentration, 5.90 mmol/L (228 mg/dL). Approximately 75% of patients had a bruit associated with the study artery, and in 43%, a contralateral carotid bruit was heard; 21% had a previous myo-

ipsilateral TIA, stroke, or any perioperative TIA, stroke, or death. The primary analysis is the comparison of the 5-year risk of cerebrovascular events in the two groups. Because both treatments were in wide use, a two-sided test of the null hypothesis ($\alpha=.05$) was chosen. Power calculations included all randomized patients according to original treatment assignments (intention-to-treat analysis). Assuming an annual event rate in the worse-outcome group of 3% for TIA and 1% for cerebral infarction, these calculations indicated that 750 patients were needed in each treatment arm for 90% power to detect a 35% difference in 5-year event rates, allowing for as much as 20% loss to follow-up.

The results of the Veterans Affairs trial[20] demonstrated that CEA is preferable to medical management for preventing TIA in asymptomatic carotid stenosis, and the North American Symptomatic Carotid Endarterectomy Trial[21] demonstrated that infarction following TIA is better managed surgically. Nei-

Table 3.—Number of Observed Events in Median 2.7-Year Follow-up, Estimated Number and Percentage of Events in 5 Years, Reduction Due to Surgery in 5-Year Risk as a Proportion of Risk in the Medical Group (95% CI), and Large-Sample P Value for Treatment Group Difference, by Event Type*

Event Type	Medical (n=834)		Surgical (n=825)		Reduction Due to Surgery in 5-y Risk as a Proportion of Risk in Medical Group (95% CI)	P
	Observed No. of Events in Median 2.7-y Follow-up	Kaplan-Meier Estimate of 5-y Event Risk, No. (%)	Observed No. of Events in Median 2.7-y Follow-up	Kaplan-Meier Estimate of 5-y Event Risk, No. (%)		
Ipsilateral stroke or any perioperative stroke or death	52	92 (11.0)	33	42 (5.1)	0.53 (0.22 to 0.72)	.004
Major ipsilateral stroke or any perioperative major stroke or death	24	50 (6.0)	21	28 (3.4)	0.43 (−0.17 to 0.72)	.12
Ipsilateral TIA or stroke or any perioperative TIA or stroke or death	102	160 (19.2)	55	67 (8.2)	0.57 (0.39 to 0.70)	<.001
Any stroke or any perioperative death	86	146 (17.5)	60	102 (12.4)	0.29 (−0.05 to 0.52)	.09
Any major stroke or perioperative death	40	76 (9.1)	28	53 (6.4)	0.30 (−0.30 to 0.62)	.26
Any stroke or death	155	266 (31.9)	127	211 (25.6)	0.20 (−0.02 to 0.37)	.08
Any major stroke or death	116	213 (25.5)	100	171 (20.7)	0.19 (−0.08 to 0.39)	.16

*CI indicates confidence interval; and TIA, transient ischemic attack.

cardial infarction, and 21% a previous coronary artery bypass. Sixty-four percent had hypertension, 26% were cigarette smokers, and 23% had diabetes mellitus.

Four hundred seven patients (25%) had had a previous hemispheric event contralateral to the study artery, and 1155 (70%) were asymptomatic in the distribution of both arteries.

Thirty-nine percent of patients were randomized on the basis of an arteriogram showing at least 60% stenosis of the carotid artery. Fifty-five percent were randomized with a Doppler PPV cut point of at least 95%, and 6% with a Doppler cut point of at least 90% confirmed by OPG-Gee. The positive predictive value of Doppler, estimated from the postrandomization presurgery angiogram, was 93%.

Table 2 shows the distribution of percentage of stenosis for prerandomization and postrandomization arteriograms before CEA. Because the health status of patients who received prerandomization arteriograms may differ from that of those who did not, a weighted estimate based on both categories is included. Five percent of patients had stenosis of the randomized artery less than 60%; 39%, 60% to 69% stenosis; 28%, 70% to 79% stenosis; 25%, 80% to 89% stenosis; and 5%, 90% to 99% stenosis, for a mean percentage of stenosis of 73%.

The Central Reading Center classified 536 baseline CCTs[15] as showing cerebral infarction. If an infarct was present, it was further classified by age, size, distribution, and volume. Local and central readers agreed on 89% of the cases. Using the Central Reading Center as the standard, the sensitivity of local reading was 71% and the specificity was 94%.

RESULTS

Of the 825 surgical patients, 101 did not have ipsilateral arteriography or CEA, 45 because of patient refusal despite prior agreement to accept either treatment. Twelve patients were rejected for sur-

gery because of severe cardiac disease. Three had a stroke or died before arteriography or surgery was performed. Arteriograms found 33 patients to be ineligible, six because of intracranial abnormalities and 27 because of less than 60% carotid artery stenosis. Eight patients did not have surgery for various other reasons. Of the 834 patients randomized to medical treatment, 45 received CEA without a verified ipsilateral TIA or stroke. Thus, 146 (9%) patients did not receive the assigned treatment. Eleven patients dropped out from follow-up in the medical and nine in the surgical group.

During the perioperative period, 19 surgical patients (2.3%) had a stroke or died. Two patients had a stroke, one died prior to hospitalization, and five had a cerebral infarction as a direct result of arteriography, one of whom died. There were 10 nonfatal strokes and one fatal myocardial infarction during the 30-day postsurgery period. In the comparable perioperative period for the medical group, three patients (0.4%) had a cerebral infarction (two patients) or died (one patient). For the surgical group, the risk in the perioperative period was 2.3% (95% CI, 1.28% to 3.32%), whereas for the medical group it was 0.4% (95% CI, 0.0% to 0.8%).

All patients randomized to the surgical group were required to have arteriography. Of the 414 patients who underwent arteriography prior to CEA, five experienced a cerebral infarction, for an arteriographic complication rate of 1.2%. It is estimated that if all 724 patients receiving CEA had undergone arteriography as a part of the ACAS, 8.7 arteriographic cerebral infarctions would have occurred in addition to the 11 primary events in the 30 days following surgery, for an overall rate of 2.7% for cerebral infarction or death from the procedure.

Sixteen fatalities, potentially due to strokes, were reviewed by the Cerebrovascular End Point Review Committee. In no case was there a difference between the End Point Review Com-

mittee diagnosis and the local physician diagnosis. These events included six hemorrhagic strokes, two cerebral infarctions in the distribution of the randomized artery, three cerebral infarctions in the nonrandomized distribution, and five deaths not due to stroke.

Treatment Comparisons

The study achieved its significance boundary after a median of 2.7 years of follow-up, with 9% of patients having completed 5 years; 26%, 4; 44%, 3; 68%, 2; and 87%, 1 year of follow-up. Because surgical patients were at greatest risk during the first month after endarterectomy, whereas the risk for medical patients was distributed throughout 5 years, comparisons near term greatly understated the differences expected after 5 years. Table 3 presents the observed number of events and also the Kaplan-Meier estimates predicted if all patients had been followed for 5 years. The estimated 5-year risk of ipsilateral stroke and any perioperative stroke or death was 11.0% for the medical group and 5.1% for the surgical group. The reduction in 5-year ipsilateral stroke risk in the surgical group was 53% of the estimated 5-year risk in the medical group (95% CI, 22% to 72%). The P value for the test of the difference between the treatment groups in 5-year risk of primary event was .004 by the large-sample test and the randomization test. For the primary end point of ipsilateral stroke and any perioperative stroke or death, the survival curves in the Figure cross near 10 months and become significantly reduced in the surgical group by 3 years ($P<.05$).

The results for secondary end points are in the same direction although not always statistically significant (Table 3 and Figure). Ipsilateral TIA or stroke or any perioperative TIA, stroke, or death—the original primary end point for the ACAS—showed a 57% reduction in 5-year risk for the surgery group (95% CI, 39% to 70%). In terms of any stroke or death,

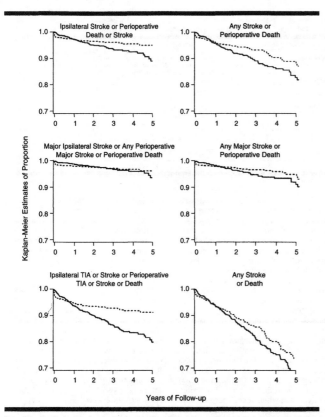

Kaplan-Meier Estimates of Proportion

Ipsilateral Stroke or Perioperative Death or Stroke

Any Stroke or Perioperative Death

Major Ipsilateral Stroke or Any Perioperative Major Stroke or Perioperative Death

Any Major Stroke or Perioperative Death

Ipsilateral TIA or Stroke or Perioperative TIA or Stroke or Death

Any Stroke or Death

Years of Follow-up

Proportion of patients without end point at a given time during follow-up, by treatment group, using Kaplan-Meier estimation method. Solid line indicates medical patients; broken line, surgical patients; and TIA, transient ischemic attack.

Table 4.—Number of Deaths, Overall and by Treatment Group, in the ACAS, December 1987 Through December 31, 1994*

Cause of Death	Treatment Group	
	Surgical	Medical
Perioperative only	3	1
Ipsilateral stroke	2	3
Stroke on contralateral side or posterior circulation	1	2
Cerebral hemorrhage	3	4
Acute myocardial infarction	21	24
Other cardiac disease	15	24
Other vascular disorder	1	2
Respiratory failure	10	9
Cancer	15	13
Tuberculosis	1	0
Renal failure	4	2
Gastrointestinal system disease	4	3
Nervous system disease	1	0
Trauma	2	0
Unknown	0	2†
Total Deaths	**83**	**89**
Deaths per 100 person-years of follow-up	3.5	3.8

*ACAS indicates Asymptomatic Carotid Atherosclerosis Study.

†One patient died at home, the other at a non-ACAS facility. The patient coordinators were unable to obtain information as to the causes of deaths.

all had an arteriogram performed before randomization, so the risk of stroke from undergoing an arteriogram was not included in the calculations. If a 1.2% arteriogram risk were added to the surgery groups at the three stenosis levels, the risk reductions become 0.35, 0.49, and 0.13, respectively, which are consistent with the overall results of the ACAS.

COMMENT

The ACAS was designed to test the efficacy of CEA for preventing ipsilateral stroke during a 5-year period. Even though this report includes patients followed up for a median of only 2.7 years, with 9% having completed 5 years of follow-up, the data demonstrate a statistically significant ($P=.004$) difference between the estimated 5-year ipsilateral stroke rates of 11.0% for the medical and 5.1% for the surgical group. Moreover, the results are in the same direction for all subgroups considered, including deciles of stenosis (although not statistically significant because of small sample size), and for various secondary cerebrovascular end points. Furthermore, the results are virtually the same when restricted to all patients receiving the assigned treatment, and are almost identical for patients without previous contralateral symptoms or endarterectomy.

Approximately 70% of our medical and surgical patients had arteriographic stenoses less than 80%. Even so, the estimated 5-year ipsilateral stroke rate in the ACAS medical group was 11.0% (about 2.3% annually). The stroke rate in the medically managed group decreased to the lower end of the previously reported range, perhaps as a re-

the surgery group had a 20% reduction in events (95% CI, −2% to 37%). The reduction due to CEA in major ipsilateral stroke or perioperative death was 43% (95% CI, −17% to 72%). Table 4 shows the causes of death were similar for the two groups, except for death not proved to result from myocardial infarction.

Table 5 summarizes results for ipsilateral stroke or any perioperative stroke or death by patient subgroups. In men, CEA reduced the 5-year event rate by 66% (95% CI, 36% to 82%); in women, the event rate was reduced by 17% (95% CI, −96% to 65%). However, the difference between genders was not statistically significant ($P=.10$). The proportion of women with perioperative complications was 3.6%, compared with 1.7% for men ($P=.12$). However, among patients who had no perioperative event, 5-year risk was reduced by 56% for women (95% CI, −50% to 87%), compared with a reduction of 79% for men (95% CI, 52% to 91%) (data

not shown). Table 5 shows a larger risk reduction due to CEA for younger patients, but the difference is not statistically significant ($P=.50$).

Reanalysis excluding the 146 crossovers, ie, restricted to those patients who received the assigned treatment, shows that surgery reduced 5-year stroke risk by 55% (95% CI, 23% to 74%). Alternatively, for the 1155 patients who had no contralateral TIA, stroke, or endarterectomy prior to randomization, surgery reduced the 5-year stroke risk by 46% (95% CI, 0% to 71%) (Table 5).

The percentage of stenosis for the 642 patients who received an arteriogram within 6 months preceding randomization is shown in Table 5. Throughout the three groups, ie, for patients with 60% to 69%, 70% to 79%, and 80% to 99% stenosis, there was no statistically significant gradation in reduction of 5-year risk of primary event, but sample sizes were small. The patients for this comparison

Table 5.—Number and Percentage of Perioperative Strokes or Deaths, Number of Observed Events in Median 2.7-Year Follow-up, Estimated Number and Percentage of 5-Year Ipsilateral Strokes or Perioperative Strokes or Deaths, and Reduction Due to Surgery in 5-Year Risk as a Proportion of Risk in the Medical Group, With 95% CI, by Subgroup*

| Patient Group | Treatment Group | No. at Risk | Total Events | | | Reduction Due to Surgery in 5-y Risk as Proportion of Risk in the Medical Group | |
			Perioperative Events, No. (%)	No. of Events Observed in Median 2.7-y Follow-up	Estimated Events† for 5-y Follow-up, No. (%)	Estimate	95% CI
All	Surgical	825	19 (2.3)	33	42 (5.1)	0.53	0.22 to 0.72
	Medical	834	3 (0.4)	52	92 (11.0)	...	...
Men	Surgical	544	9 (1.7)	18	22 (4.1)	0.66	0.36 to 0.82
	Medical	547	3 (0.5)	38	66 (12.1)	...	...
Women	Surgical	281	10 (3.6)	15	20 (7.3)	0.17	−0.96 to 0.65
	Medical	287	0 (0.0)	14	25 (8.7)	...	...
Age <68 y	Surgical	408	6 (1.5)	13	19 (4.7)	0.60	0.11 to 0.82
	Medical	394	2 (0.5)	23	47 (11.8)	...	...
Age ≥68 y	Surgical	417	13 (3.1)	20	23 (5.5)	0.43	−0.07 to 0.70
	Medical	440	1 (0.2)	29	43 (9.7)	...	...
Bilaterally asymptomatic	Surgical	585	12 (2.1)	24	32 (5.5)	0.46	0.00 to 0.71
	Medical	570	3 (0.5)	34	58 (10.2)	...	...
Previous contralateral endarterectomy or previous TIA or stroke	Surgical	240	7 (2.9)	9	11 (4.5)	0.65	0.13 to 0.86
	Medical	264	0 (0.0)	18	33 (12.6)	...	...
Patients receiving assigned treatment	Surgical	724	16 (2.2)	28	37 (5.1)	0.55	0.23 to 0.74
	Medical	789	3 (0.4)	50	91 (11.5)	...	...
% Stenosis‡ 60.0-69.9	Surgical	137	4 (2.9)	7	9 (6.3)	0.45	−0.70 to 0.82
	Medical	131	0 (0.0)	8	15 (11.4)	...	...
% Stenosis‡ 70.0-79.9	Surgical	93	1 (1.1)	2	2 (2.2)	0.67	−0.65 to 0.94
	Medical	94	0 (0.0)	5	6 (6.7)	...	...
% Stenosis‡ 80.0-99.9	Surgical	99	1 (1.0)	2	2 (2.0)	0.45	−2.19 to 0.91
	Medical	88	0 (0.0)	3	3 (3.7)	...	...

*CI indicates confidence interval; and TIA, transient ischemic attack.
†Using Kaplan-Meier estimation.
‡Percentage of stenosis of randomized artery at baseline, for patients with prerandomization angiogram within 6 months of randomization.

sult of vigorous risk factor management and exclusion of high-risk patients.

There were no significant differences in primary event rates between patient groups with and without symptoms or previous CEA of the contralateral carotid artery. With an annual mortality rate of 3.7%, approximately 89% of patients survived long enough to benefit from the protective effect of the operation, because the crossover in favor of surgery occurred within the first year.

Four other randomized prospective studies of CEA for asymptomatic carotid artery stenosis have been reported. One did not include stenosis exceeding 90%,[26] another was terminated early because of excess cardiac events,[27] and a third, the European Asymptomatic Carotid Surgery Trial, is ongoing.[28] The fourth, the Veterans Affairs Cooperative Trial, randomized 444 patients and published results based on a mean follow-up of 47.9 months. The Veterans Affairs study differed from the ACAS in that only men were studied and all patients had an arteriogram.[20] Like the Veterans Affairs trial, the ACAS showed an advantage for CEA in preventing TIAs, cerebral infarctions, and death in men. In addition, the ACAS showed an advantage in reducing the risk of ipsilateral stroke alone. Our results are

consistent with others that established that symptomatic patients with carotid stenosis greater than 70% were best treated by CEA.[21,29]

Because a 10% difference in lumen diameter on arteriogram is approximately 0.5 mm, and the lumen area stenosis difference is only 6%, this cannot be measured accurately, and when miniaturized images are used, these differences cannot be discerned. Therefore, we believe that stenoses with 60% and 70% reductions in diameter are both hemodynamically significant, and that putative difference by decile is within the range of observer variability.[30-32]

It has been suggested that arteriography should have been required for all ACAS patients to ensure that only those with greater than 60% stenosis were entered. However, it was the judgment of the ACAS group that the hazards and costs of arteriography were not warranted for patients in our medical group. This was borne out by the 1.2% stroke rate from arteriography. Our Doppler criteria were established to maintain a PPV of 95%.[14] Retrospective analysis of all postrandomization, presurgery arteriograms demonstrated that our actual PPV was 93%. This indicates that our medical patients did indeed have significant carotid artery stenosis, with fewer than 5% hav-

ing less than the required 60%.

If all patients who underwent surgery had received arteriography as part of the surgical treatment, the absolute risk reduction would have been from 11.0% to 5.6%. Using ACAS eligibility requirements, 19 CEAs would be necessary to prevent one stroke over 5 years.[25] This ratio would be less if patient subsets at higher risk for stroke could be identified.

A CEA can be performed with a low complication rate even in elderly patients. In selected instances, some ACAS surgeons now operate without arteriography on the basis of noninvasive studies[33,34] and sometimes discharge patients 24 hours following surgery.[35] These and other measures may reduce costs if proved generally feasible.

CONCLUSIONS

The ACAS has demonstrated that the incidence of cerebral infarction can be reduced by CEA and that stringent quality control measures can reduce surgical morbidity and mortality. A major reason was the 30-day morbidity and mortality of ACAS patients, estimated to have been 2.7% if all surgery patients had undergone arteriography as part of the study. This includes arteriographic complications of 1.2%. These results may be improved further by reducing risk associated with contrast arteriography. The ACAS has established that men with a good life expectancy who have asymptomatic carotid artery stenosis with at least 60% reduction in diameter are protected from stroke by CEA, whereas the results for women are less certain. Following CEA, the relative stroke risk reduction for men and women combined is 53%, with an absolute 5-year risk reduction from 11.0% to 5.1%. The 5-year reduction in stroke risk among men was 66% and among women 17%, perhaps because of the higher perioperative complication rate in women. Excluding arteriographic and perioperative complications, the risk reduction was 79% for men and 56% for women.

The Asymptomatic Carotid Atherosclerosis Study clinical trial was supported by an investigator-initiated research grant (ROI NS22611) from the US Public Health Service National Institute of Neurological Disorders and Stroke.

The authors acknowledge the volunteerism of all patients in the Asymptomatic Carotid Atherosclerosis Study.

Funding Agency.—National Institute of Neurological Disorders and Stroke, Bethesda, Md: Michael D. Walker, MD; John R. Marler, MD; Murray Goldstein, DO; Patricia A. Grady, PhD.

Executive Committee.—James F. Toole, MD, chair; William H. Baker, MD; John E. Castaldo, MD; Lloyd E. Chambless, PhD; Wesley S. Moore, MD; James T. Robertson, MD; Byron Young, MD; Virginia J. Howard, MSPH (ex officio).

Executive Committee Liaison.—John R. Marler, MD.

Operations Center.—Bowman Gray School of Medicine of Wake Forest University, Winston-Salem, NC: James F. Toole, MD; Virginia J. Howard, MSPH; Suzanne Purvis; Dee Dee Vernon; Kelley Needham; Pam Beck; Marty Dozier; David S. Lefkowitz, MD; George Howard, DrPh; John R. Crouse III, MD; David M. Herrington, MD; Curt D. Furberg, MD, PhD; Karla Essick; Ralph M. Hicks, Jr, MA, MEd.

Statistical Coordinating Center.—University of North Carolina at Chapel Hill: Lloyd E. Chambless, PhD; J. J. Nelson, MSPH; Will Ball; Ernestine Bland; Sean Condon, MS; Thomas Elliott, MS (deceased); James E. Grizzle, PhD; Dick Hayes, MCJ; Scott Henley; Jeffrey Johnson, MSPH; James Locklear, MS; Margaret S. Misch, MS; Catherine C. Paton, MSPH; Skai Schwartz, MA; Climmon Walker; O. Dale Williams, PhD.

Data and Safety Monitoring Committee.—J. Donald Easton, MD, chair; Jerry Goldstone, MD; John M. Hallenbeck, MD; Julian T. Hoff, MD; Herbert R. Karp, MD; Richard A. Kronmal, PhD.

Cranial Computerized Tomography Reading Center.—University of Cincinnati (Ohio): Thomas G. Brott, MD; Thomas A. Tomsick, MD; Joseph Broderick, MD; Laura Sauerbeck, RN; Christine Blum, RN.

Cerebrovascular End Point Review Committee.—Mark Dyken, MD, chair; John C. M. Brust, MD; Arthur R. Dick, MD; Robert A. Gotshall, MD; Albert Heyman, MD; Phillip D. Swanson, MD.

Publications Committee.—James F. Toole, MD, chair; Harold P. Adams, Jr, MD; Lloyd E. Chambless, PhD; Robert Dempsey, MD; Calvin B. Ernst, MD; John Rothrock, MD (with special appreciation to Stanley N. Cohen, MD, for desk editing).

Participating Centers (in order of number of patients randomized, number of patients in brackets, and personnel listed in the following order: Principal Investigator, Co-Investigator, Coordinator, and Other Key Personnel, Current and Past)

Lehigh Valley Hospital, Allentown, Pa [142]: John Castaldo, MD; Gary Nicholas, MD; Joan Longenecker; Peter Barbour, MD; Alan Berger,

MD; Victor J. Celani; Nancy Eckert, RN; James Goodreau, MD; Judith Hutchinson, RN; Donna Jenny, RN; Zwu-Shin Lin, MD; Alice Madden, RN; James L. McCullough, MD; Kenneth McDonald, MD; William Pistone, MD; Alexander D. Rae-Grant, MD; James Redenbaugh, MD; James Rex, MD; Christopher J. Wohlberg, MD.

Marshfield Clinic, Wisconsin [121]: Percy Karanjia, MD; Mark Swanson, MD; Sandra Lobner, LPN; R. Lee Kolts, MD; Marvin E. Kuehner, MD; Bradley C. Hiner, MD; Kenneth P. Madden, MD; Robert D. Carlson, MD; J. Steven Davis, MD; Thomas Gallant, MD; John J. Warner, MD; Ann Faust, RVT; Nancy Fryza, RVT; John Hasenauer, RVT; Mary Regner, RVT; Linette Ronkin, RVT; Sharon Schaefer, RVT; Dawn Strack, RVT; Lynn C. Turner, RVT; Ann Walgenbach, RVT; Julie Graves; Sara Michalski; Linda Schuette.

Columbia University, New York, NY [91]: J. P. Mohr, MD; Donald Quest, MD; Annette Cruz; Ralph Sacco, MD; T. K. Tatemichi, MD; Randolph Marshall, MD; Henning Mast, MD; Oscar Ramos, MD; James Correll, MD; Richard Libman, MD; George Petty, MD; Anilda Cabrere, MD; Lorraine Oropeza, RN, RVT; Tina Gonzalez.

University of Kentucky Chandler Medical Center, Lexington [88]: Byron Young, MD; Creed Pettigrew, MD; Ruthie Sadler, RN; Robert Dempsey, MD; Eric Endean, MD; Jerry Sherrow, RVT; Marcie Hauer, RN; Charles Lee, MD; Jane Norton; Michael McQuillen, MD; Sally Mattingly, MD; Steven Dekosky, MD; Andrew Massey, MD.

Hôpital de l'Enfant Jesus, Québec City, Quebec [86]: Denis Simard, MD; Jean-François Turcotte, MD; Charlotte Benguigui, RN; Jacques Côte, MD (deceased); Jean-Marie Bouchard, MD; Claude Roberge, MD; Denis Brunet, MD; Fernand Bédard; Réginald Langelier, MD; Marcel Lajeunesse; Jean Marc Bigaouette; Jasmin Parent.

University of California at San Diego [78]: Patrick Lyden, MD; Robert Hye, MD; Stacy Lewis, RN; Gerry Cali, RN; Traci Babcock, RN; Barbara Taft-Alvarez, RN; John Rothrock, MD; Mark Brody, MD; Richard Zweifler, MD; Mark Sedwitz, MD; Bruce Stabile, MD; Julie A. Freischlag, MD; Yehuda G Wolf, MD; James Sivo; John Forsythe; Melody Adame.

Loyola University Medical Center, Maywood, Ill [77]: William H. Baker, MD; Sudha Gupta, MD; Katy Burke; Howard P. Greisler, MD; Fred N. Littooy, MD; Michael A. Kelly, MD.

University of Tennessee, Memphis [74]: James T. Robertson, MD; William Pulsinelli, MD; Judith A. Campbell, RN, BSN; John Crockarell, MD; Clarence Watridge, MD; J. Acker, MD; Samard Erkulwater, MD; Michael Jacewicz, MD; Gail Walker; Patrick O'Sullivan, MD; Curtis Sauer, MD; Ken Vasu, MD; Kenneth Gaines, MD; Bijan Bakhitian, MD; Tulio E. Bertorini, MD; Susan Bennett, PA-C; Terrye Thomas, BSN; Nan Stahl, RN; Connie Taylor, RN; Mary Ann Giampapa; Joan Connell; Judy Riley; Angeleah Bradley; Jeanette Davis, RN; Kathy Newman; Rebecca Manning; Marcella McCrea.

University Hospital, London, Ontario [63]: Vladimir Hachinski, MD; Gary Ferguson, MD; Cheryl Mayer, RN; Henry J. M. Barnett, MD; S. J. Peerless, MD; A. M. Buchan, MD; Howard Reichman, MD; Andrew Kertesz, MD; Stephen Lownie, MD; Carole White, RN; Allan Fox, MD; Richard Rankin, MD.

Victoria Hospital, London, Ontario [61]: J. David Spence, MD; H. W. K. Barr, MD; Leslie Paddock-Eliasziw, RN; L. J. P. Assis, MD; J. H. W. Pexman, MD; Maria DiCicco, RVT; Barb Tate, RN; Caroline James, RVT.

Virginia Mason Clinic, Seattle, Wash [57]: Edmond Raker, MD; James Coatsworth, MD; Sandy Harris, RN; Hugh Beebe, MD; Richard Birchfield, MD; Kathy Butler-Levy; Robert Crane, MD; David Fryer, MD; James MacLean, MD; Laird Patterson, MD; Terence Quigley, MD; John Ravits, MD; Lynne Taylor, MD; Stacy Pullen, RDMS; Shannon Boswell, RDMS; Karen Kenny, RDMS, RVT.

University of Cincinnati Ohio [55]: Thomas Brott, MD; Joseph Broderick, MD; Thomas Tomsick, MD;

Laura Sauerbeck, RN; L. R. Roedersheimer, MD; Richard Fowl, MD; John Tew, MD; Richard Kempczinski, MD; Robert Reed, MD; Richard Welling, MD; Christine Blum, RN; Bill Schomaker, RN.

Bowman Gray School of Medicine of Wake Forest University, Winston-Salem, NC [52]: David Lefkowitz, MD; J. Michael McWhorter, MD; Charles L. Branch, MD; Jean Satterfield; Robert Cordell, MD; Richard Dean, MD; George Plonk, MD; Gary Harpold, MD; James F. Toole, MD; Francis Walker, MD; Cathy Nunn, RN RVT; Larry Myers, MBA, RDMS, RVT; Charles Tegeler, MD; Sharon Hardin, RVT, RCMS; Dana Meads, RT-R, RVT.

University of Iowa Hospital and Clinics, Iowa City [49]: Harold P. Adams, Jr, MD; Christopher M. Loftus, MD; Lynn A. Vining, RN; Birgette H. Bendixen, MD, PhD; José Biller, MD; John D. Corson, MD; Patricia H. Davis, MD; John C. Godersky, MD; David L. Gordon, MD; Michael R. Jacoby, MD; Laurens J. Kappelle, MD; Timothy F. Kresowik, MD; E. Eugene Marsh III, MD; Betsy B. Love, MD; Asad R. Shamma, MD; Karla J. Grimsman, RN; Dawn M. Karboski, RN; Ed V. Miller, RVT.

Johns Hopkins Bayview Medical Center, Baltimore, Md [46]: Constance Johnson, MD; Calvin Jones, MD; Brenda Stone, CRNP; Mairi Pat Maguire, RN; Christopher Earley, MD; Peter Kaplan, MD; John Cavaluzzi, MD; Gerald Waters, PA-C; Betty Chachich, RN.

St John's Mercy Medical Center, St Louis, Mo [44]: Arthur Auer, MD; William Logan, MD; Mary Wilcox, RN, BSN; Barbara Green, MD; Joseph Hurley, MD; Richard Pennell, MD; John Woods, MD; Richard Levine, MD; James Nepute, MD; Jeffrey Thomasson, MD; Claire Blackburn, RN, RVT; Marcia Foldes, BSN, RVT; Kathy Klemp, RN, RVT; Becky Nappier, RT, RVT; Karen Rutherford, BSN, RVT; Sally Schroer, RN, BSN; Jena Hogan, RN, RVT; Lynne Thorpe, RN, RVT.

University of Arizona Health Sciences Center, Tucson [42]: William M. Feinberg, MD; Glenn C. Hunter, MD; Denise C. Bruck, AAS; Victor M. Bernhard, MD; Kenneth E. McIntyre, MD; L. Philip Carter, MD; Scott S. Berman, MD; Joseph L. R. Mills, MD; Enrique L. Labadie, MD; Darry S. Johnson, MD; Constantine G. Moschonas, MD; Robert H. Hamilton, MD; Scott C. Forrer, MD; Joachim F. Seeger, MD; Raymond F. Carmody, MD; Brenda K. Vold, RN, BSN; Richard L. Carlson; Joan E. Laguna; John P. Krikawa; Jenifer J. Devine, RN, BSN, RVT; Amalia M. Castrillo; Sheryl L. Kistler, RN, RVT; Betty Ledbetter; Kathleen (Sue) Dorr.

University of Mississippi Medical Center, Jackson [39]: Robert R. Smith, MD; Armin F. Haerer, MD; Robin L. Brown, RN, BSN; William Russell, MD; Edward Rigdon, MD; Robert Rhodes, MD; Evelyn Smith, RVT; Michael Graeber, MD; David Doorenbos, MD; S. H. Subramony, MD; David L. Gordon, MD.

Milton S. Hershey Medical Center, Hershey, Pa [35]: Robert G. Atnip, MD; Robert W. Brennan, MD; Diane Friedman, RN, MSN; Marsha M. Neumyer, RVT; Brian L. Thiele, MD; Florence Smith, RN; John D. Barr, MD; R. Bradford Duckrow, MD; Cindy Janesky, MD; Jon W. Meilstrup, MD; Kevin P. McNamara, MD; Lawrence D. Rodichok, MD; Leslie Stewart, MD; Maureen Sullivan, MD; Mark Wengrovitz, MD.

University of Texas Southwestern Medical Center, Dallas [35]: G. Patrick Clagett, MD; Hal Unwin, MD; Wilson Bryan, MD; Chris Matkins; Carolyn Patterson; Candy Alway, RDMS; Patty Boyd; Mary Inman, RN; Christie Albiston; Eva Scoggins; John Swilling.

University of California at Los Angeles [35]: Wesley S. Moore, MD; Stanley N. Cohen, MD; Kathleen G. Walden, RN; Samuel S. Ahn, MD; Edwin C. Amos, MD; J. Dennis Baker, MD; Bruce H. Dobkin, MD; Carlos E. Donayre, MD; Julie A. Freischlag, MD; Hugh A. Gelabert, MD; Sheldon E. Jordan, MD; Herbert I. Machleder, MD; William J. Quinones-Baldrich, MD; Jeffrey L. Saver, MD; Suzie M. El-Saden, MD; Richard C. Holgate, MD; Bradley A. Jabour, MD; J. Bruce Jacobs, MD; Theresa M. Abraham, RN; Candace L. Vescera,

RN; Jeanine A. von Rajcs, RN; Vicki L. Carter, RN, RVT; Dale T. Carter, RVT; De Ette Dix-Goss, RVT; Eugene C. Hernandez, RVT.

Oregon Health Sciences University, Portland [34]: Lloyd Taylor, MD; Bruce Coull, MD; Letha Loboa, RN, RVT; Gregory Moneta, MD; John Porter, MD; Richard Yeager, MD; Lucy Whittaker, RN.

Yale University, New Haven, Conn [34]: Lawrence M. Brass, MD; Richard J. Gusberg, MD; Anne M. Lovejoy, PA-C; Pierre B. Fayad, MD; Bauer Sumpio, MD, PhD; George H. Meier, MD; Vicky M. Chang, ANP, MSN; Karen Marzitelli, ANP, MSN; Douglas Chyatte, MD; Lynwood Hammers, DO; Fran Lepore, RDMS, RT; Frank J. Pavalkis, PA-C; Jill Mele; Donna Kisiel, PA-C.

University of Arkansas for Medical Sciences, Little Rock [32]: Robert W. Barnes, MD; Michael Z. Chesser, MD; R. Lee Archer, MD; Bernard W. Thompson, MD; Colette MacDonald; Gary W. Barone, MD; John F. Eidt, MD; David Harshfield, MD; David McFarland, MD; Jess R. Nickols, MD; E. Carol Howard, BSN, RN, RVT; M. Lee Nix, BSN, RN, RVT; Judy Kaye Overstreet, RN, RVT; Rhonda Troillett, RDMS, RVT.

Medical College of Virginia (Virginia Commonwealth University), Richmond [27]: John Taylor, MD; H. M. Lee, MD; Patricia Akins; John W. Harbison, MD; Rhonda M. Pridgeon, MD; Warren L. Felton, MD; Marc Posner, MD; M. Sobel, MD; Guy Clifton, MD; Chris Conway; Anne Cockrell; Warren Stringer, MD; Jean Wingo; Brenda Nichols; Wendy Smoker, MD; Ruth Fisher.

Barrow Neurological Institute at St Joseph's Hospital and Medical Center, Phoenix, Ariz [26]: Robert F. Spetzler, MD; James L. Frey, MD; Joseph M. Zabramski, MD; Sonna Lea Hunsley, RN; Heidi Jahnke, BSN; Kathryn L. Plenge, RN; Rosemary Holland, RVT; Roberta Turner, RVT; Duane Strava, RVT; Susan Stumpff, RVT; John Hodak, MD; Richard A. Flom, MD; Bruce L. Dean, MD; Richard A. Thompson, MD.

Oschner Clinic, New Orleans, La [21]: Richard Hughes, MD; Bruce Lepler, MD; John Bowen, MD; Cheryl Benoit, CCRC; Larry Hollier, MD; John Ochsner, MD; Richard Strub, MD; Vickie Lang; Vicki Cahanin.

University of Medicine and Dentistry of New Jersey, Newark [20]: Robert W. Hobson II, MD; Fred Weisbrot, MD; Stephen Kamin, MD; Tom Back; Zafar Jamil, MD; Carolyn Rogers; Bea Lainson; Larry Hart.

New England Medical Center, Boston, Mass [19]: Louis Caplan, MD; Thomas O'Donnell, MD; Loretta Barron, RN; Michael Pessin, MD; Dana DeWitt, MD; William Mackey, MD; Michael Belkin, MD; Robert McGlaughlin, RVT; Paula Heggerick, RVT.

Henry Ford Hospital, Detroit, Mich [17]: Calvin B. Ernst, MD; K. M. A. Welch, MD; Judith Wilczewski, RN; Wendy Robertson, PA-C; Sheila Daley, RN; Joseph P. Elliot, Jr, MD; Daniel J. Reddy, MD; Alexander D. Shephard, MD; Roger F. Smith, MD; Steven Levine, MD; Nabih Ramadan, MD; Gretchen Tietjen, MD; Panaytios Mitsias, MD; Mark Gorman, MD; Michalene McPharlin, RN; Suresh Patel, MD; Rajeev Deveshwar, MD; Nora Lee, MD; James Kokkinos, MD.

University of New Mexico, Albuquerque [13]: Askiel Bruno, MD; Eric Weinstein, MD; James Kunkel, MD (deceased); Anna Kratochvil, MD; Edie Johnson, RN, MSN, FNP; Susan Steel, RN.

Sunnybrook Health Science Centre, University of Toronto, North York, Ontario [11]: John Norris, MD; David Rowed, MD; Beverley Bowyer, RN; Marek Gawel, MD; Perry W. Cooper, MD; Dianne Brodie, RVT.

Harbin Clinic, Rome, Ga [10]: John S. Kirkland, MD, PhD; Jay A. Schecter, MD; Nell W. Farrar, PA-C; Raymond Capps, MD; E. Leeon Rhodes, MD; D. Michael Rogers, MD; Jeffrey T. Glass, MD; Robert Naguszewski, MD; William Naguszewski, MD; Bobbie Maddox; Bobbie Dollison; Lynda Moulton; Polly Cole; Paul Kinsella; Alisa Ansley; Noell Britz.

Roanoke Neurological Associates, Virginia [10]: Don H. Bivins, MD; Edwin L. Williams II, MD; Jesse T. Davidson III, MD; William Elias, MD;

Donna Atkins, RN; Phyllis B. Turner, RN, RVT; J. Gordon Burch, MD; Donald B. Nolan, MD; Renee Speese; Candace D. Foley, RN.

Singing River Hospital, Pascagoula, Miss [6]: Terrence J. Millette, MD; Dewey H. Lane, MD; Cynthia Almond, RN, RVT; Roland J. Mestayer III, MD.

California Pacific Medical Center, San Francisco [4]: Phillip Calanchini, MD; Robert Szarnicki, MD; Pat Radosevich; Linda Elias; Peggy McCormick; Charles Gould, MD; Forbes Norris, MD; Eric Denys, MD; Robert Bernstein, MD; Donna Dubono; Keith Atkinson; Mark Peters.

Northwestern University Medical School, Chicago, Ill [4]: Bruce Cohen, MD; James Yao, MD; Susan Roston, RN; Donna Blackburn, RN; José Biller, MD; Jeffrey Saver, MD; Linda Chadwick, RN; Douglas Chyatte, MD; Walter McCarthy, MD; William Pearce, MD; Jeff Frank, MD; Ernesto Fernandez-Beer, MD; James Patrick, MD.

University of Rochester, New York [3]: Richard Green, MD; Richard Satran, MD; John Ricotta, MD; James DeWeese, MD; Joshua Hollander, MD; Mollie O'Brien, RN; JoAnne McNamara, RN; Sandra Rose, RT, RDMS; Dahne Cohen, MD.

Cleveland Clinic, Ohio [1]: Anthony Furlan, MD; John Little, MD; Bernadine Bryerton, RN; Cathy Sila, MD; Isam Awad, MD; Marc Chimowitz, MD; Sylvia Robertson, ARRT, RDMS; Cindy Becker, ARRT, RDMS; David Paushter, MD.

Arteriogram Quality Control.—Bruce L. Dean, MD; Daniel H. O'Leary, MD.

Doppler and OPG-Gee Quality Control.—Anne M. Jones, BSN, RVT, RDMS; John J. Ricotta, MD; William Gee, MD; Nancy Shebel, BSN, RN, RVT.

Pathology.—Mark J. Fisher, MD; Eric A. Schenk, MD.

TIA/Stroke Validation.—Anthony J. Furlan, MD; Nancy N. Futrell, MD; Michael Kelly, MD; Clark H. Millikan, MD.

General Consultants.—H. C. Diener, MD; William S. Fields, MD; Marshall F. Folstein, MD; Jean-Claude Gautier, MD; Michael J. G. Harrison, MD; William K. Hass, MD; Michael G. Hennerici, MD; Richard Satran, MD; Merrill P. Spencer, MD; Gerhard M. von-Reutern, MD.

References

1. Timsit SG, Sacco RL, Mohr JP, et al. Early clinical differentiation of cerebral infarction from severe atherosclerotic stenosis and cardioembolism. *Stroke.* 1992;23:486-491.

2. Hennerici M, Hülsbömer H-B, Hefter H, Lammerts D, Rautenberg W. Natural history of asymptomatic extracranial arterial disease. *Brain.* 1987; 110:777-791.

3. Autret A, Saudeau D, Bertrand PH, Pourcelot L, Marchal C, DeBoisvilliers S. Stroke risk in patients with carotid stenosis. *Lancet.* 1987;1:888-890.

4. O'Hollerhan LW, Kennelly MM, McClurken M, Johnson JM. Natural history of asymptomatic carotid plaque. *Am J Surg.* 1987;154:659-662.

5. Norris JW, Zhu CZ, Bornstein NM, Chambers BR. Vascular risks of asymptomatic carotid stenosis. *Stroke.* 1991;22:1485-1490.

6. Jorgensen L, Torvik A. Ischaemic cerebrovascular diseases in an autopsy series, 2. *J Neurol Sci.* 1969;9:285-320.

7. Cote R, Barnett HJM, Taylor DW. Internal carotid occlusion. *Stroke.* 1983;14:898-902.

8. Nicholls SC, Kohler TR, Bergelin RO, Primozich JF, Lawrence RL, Strandness DE Jr. Carotid artery occlusion. *J Vasc Surg.* 1986;4:479-485.

9. Moore WS, Barnet HJM, Beebe HG, et al. Guidelines for carotid endarterectomy. *Stroke.* 1995;26:188-201.

10. Riles TS, Adelman MA, Gibstein LA. Incidence of premonitory transient ischemic attacks before ischemic strokes. In: Veith FJ, ed. *Current Critical Problems in Vascular Surgery.* St Louis, Mo: Quality Medical Publishing Inc; 1994;6:264-268.

11. Till JS, Toole JF, Howard VJ, Ford CS, Williams D. Declining morbidity and mortality of carotid endarterectomy. *Stroke.* 1987;18:823-829.

12. Wilson SE, Mayberg MR, Yatsu FM. Defining

the indications for carotid endarterectomy. *Surgery.* 1988;104:932-933.

13. The Asymptomatic Carotid Atherosclerosis Study Group. Study design for randomized prospective trial of carotid endarterectomy for asymptomatic atherosclerosis. *Stroke.* 1989;20:844-849.

14. Howard G, Chambless LE, Baker WH, et al. A multicenter validation study of Doppler ultrasound versus angiogram. *J Stroke Cerebrovasc Dis.* 1991; 1:166-173.

15. Brott T, Tomsick T, Feinberg W, et al, for the Asymptomatic Carotid Atherosclerosis Study Investigators. Baseline silent cerebral infarction in the Asymptomatic Carotid Atherosclerosis Study. *Stroke.* 1994;25:1122-1129.

16. Moore WS, Vescera CL, Robertson JT, Baker WH, Howard VJ, Toole JF. Selection process for surgeons in the Asymptomatic Carotid Atherosclerosis Study. *Stroke.* 1991;22:1353-1357.

17. Folstein MF, Folstein SE, McHugh PR. 'Mini-Mental State': a practical method for grading the cognitive state of patients for the clinician. *J Psychiatr Res.* 1975;12:189-198.

18. Lefkowitz DS, Brust JC, Goldman L, et al. A pilot study of the end point verification system in the Asymptomatic Carotid Atherosclerosis Study. *J Stroke Cerebrovasc Dis.* 1992;2:92-99.

19. Jennett B, Bond M. Assessment of outcome after severe brain damage: a practical scale. *Lancet.* 1975;1:480-484.

20. Hobson RW II, Weiss DG, Fields WS, et al, for the Veterans Affairs Cooperative Study Group. Efficacy of carotid endarterectomy for asymptomatic carotid stenosis. *N Engl J Med.* 1993;328:221-227.

21. North American Symptomatic Carotid Endarterectomy Trial Collaborators. Beneficial effect of carotid endarterectomy in symptomatic patients with high-grade stenosis. *N Engl J Med.* 1991;325:445-453.

22. Kalbfleisch JD, Prentice RL. *The Statistical Analysis of Failure Time Data.* New York, NY: John Wiley & Sons Inc; 1980:14.

23. Lachin JM. Statistical properties of randomization in clinical trials. *Control Clin Trials.* 1988; 9:289-311.

24. O'Brien PC, Fleming TR. A multiple testing procedure for clinical trials. *Biometrics.* 1979;35:549-556.

25. Laupacis A, Naylor CD, Sackett DL. How should the results of clinical trials be presented to clinicians? *ACP J Club.* May/June 1992:A12-A14.

26. CASANOVA Study Group. Carotid surgery versus medical therapy in asymptomatic carotid stenosis. *Stroke.* 1991;22:1229-1235.

27. Mayo Asymptomatic Carotid Endarterectomy Study Group. Results of a randomized controlled trial of carotid endarterectomy for asymptomatic carotid stenosis. *Mayo Clin Proc.* 1992;67:513-518.

28. Halliday AW, Thomas D, Mansfield A. The Asymptomatic Carotid Surgery Trial (ACST): rationale and design. *Eur J Vasc Surg.* 1994;8:703-710.

29. European Carotid Surgery Trialists' Collaborative Group. European Carotid Surgery Trial: interim results for symptomatic patients with severe (70-99%) or with mild (0-29%) carotid stenosis. *Lancet.* 1991;337:1235-1243.

30. Toole JF, Castaldo JE. Accurate measurement of carotid stenosis: chaos in methodology. *J Neuroimaging.* 1994;4:222-230.

31. Rothwell PM, Gibson RJ, Slattery J, Sellar RJ, Warlow CP, for the European Carotid Surgery Trialists' Collaborative Group. Equivalence of measurements of carotid stenosis. *Stroke.* 1994;25:2435-2439.

32. Alexandrov AV, Bladin CF, Magissano R, Norris JW. Measuring carotid stenosis: time for a reappraisal. *Stroke.* 1993;24:1292-1296.

33. Horn M, Michelini M, Greisler HP, Littooy FN, Baker WH. Carotid endarterectomy without arteriography. *Ann Vasc Surg.* 1994;8:221-224.

34. Chervu A, Moore WS. Carotid endarterectomy without arteriography. *Ann Vasc Surg.* 1994;8:296-302.

35. Morasch MD, Hodgett D, Burke K, Baker WH. Selective use of the intensive care unit following carotid endarterectomy. *Ann Vasc Surg.* In press.

9.3 GUIDE APPLIED TO A STUDY OF PROGNOSIS

Philippe O. Szapary, MD • Daniel J. Friedland, MD

ALBERTSEN PC ET AL:

Long-term survival among men with conservatively treated localized prostate cancer. JAMA 1995;274:626.*
(See pp 215–220.)

Step 1. Do I want to evaluate the study? (INR)

Is the study:

Interesting? Yes, this study attempts to quantitate the much-debated excess mortality associated with prostate cancer in elderly men. It provides useful prognostic information to help guide our patients with localized disease in making difficult treatment decisions.

Novel? This study adds to six previous studies on the natural history of conservatively treated localized prostate cancer. The two studies that have received the most attention are a European cohort of 223 Scandinavian men[1] who are older than those in this study's cohort and a pooled analysis of six nonrandomized studies.[2] The study reviewed here is population-based, measures the important predictors of tumor histology and patient comorbidities, and provides the longest follow-up to date.

Relevant? Prostate cancer is the most commonly diagnosed cancer in men, surpassing lung cancer. Prostate cancer accounts for 36% of all cancer diagnoses in men. In 1996, there were an estimated 318,000 new cases, reflecting a 48% increased incidence over the last 3 years.[3] (Serologic screening of asymptomatic men using prostate-specific antigen is most likely responsible for this increase.) In addition to dealing with such an important disease, this study is relevant because it both elucidates the most important prognostic factors for prostate cancer and provides information about life expectancy.

Step 2. Outline the study in the following format

(See Figure 9.3–1.)

Step 3. Is the study finding believable?

A. Do the study subjects and variables accurately represent the research question?

Subjects: A number of subjects probably did not have localized disease, because tumor staging was incomplete for many patients. Most patients did not undergo bone scans (80%) or metastatic surveys (81%), and the percentage of patients undergoing pelvic CT was not provided.

Predictor variables: The predictor variables that were used are valid representations of the predictor phenomena. The Gleason score was rigorously obtained by expert pathologists, and the index of co-existing disease (ICED) has been validated in previous studies as a useful measure of comorbidity. Chart review is an acceptable way of obtaining basic patient characteristics.

Outcome Variables: Death resulting from prostate cancer was measured using the Connecticut Tumor Registry (CTR). Although the reliability of the CTR as a measure for prostate cancer mortality was not explicitly stated, by inference it appears to be a fairly accurate representation of prostate cancer mortality. The CTR is the oldest state cancer registry

---

* Albertsen PC et al: Long-term survival among men with conservatively treated localized prostate cancer. JAMA 1995;274:626. Copyright 1990. American Medical Association. Printed with permission.

Truth in the universe	Study method
Research question	**Study design**
1. What is the long-term survival of men diagnosed with localized prostate cancer? 2. What are the most important prognostic factors that predict survival in CaP?	Retrospective cohort study with descriptive and analytic components (see research questions 1 and 2, respectively)
Target population	**Subjects**

Inclusion:
  Men aged 65–75 diagnosed with localized prostate cancer.
 	
Exclusion:
  Known metastatic disease, treatment with curative intent (radiation therapy or surgery), diagnosis at autopsy or incidentally found during cystectomy, incomplete or missing records
	Temporal characteristics:
	  1971–1976. Mean follow-up of 15.5 years.
	
	Geographic characteristics:
	  Connecticut
	
	Sampling:
	  CTR database; 991 cases of prostate cancer were identified.
	  Exclusion criteria were present in 54%, and thus the final cohort included 451 men. Those excluded were not significantly different from those included.
	
	Demographics:
	  Mean age of 71. 94% white. 49% tumors palpable. 45% of case patients received hormonal therapy within 3 months of diagnosis.

Predictor	**Predictor variables**
1. Histologic grade 2. Severity of comorbid disease 3. Race 4. Age at diagnosis 5. Year of diagnosis 6. Indication for test leading to diagnosis of prostate cancer 7. Method used in diagnosing prostate cancer 8. Clinical stage 9. Percentage of tumor involvement of the prostate	1. Gleason score as determined by a referee genitourinary pathologist blinded to case status while reviewing the original specimen. A sample of the cases were sent to an outside genitourinary pathologist to test inter-rater variability. 2. ICED: A validated score to adjust for comorbid disease. 3–7. Race, age, year of diagnosis, indication for diagnostic test, and method used in diagnosis: abstracted from the medical record. 8. National Cancer Institute approved staging. 9. Percentage tumor burden: Defined as greater or less than 5% tumor involvement of the prostate.
Outcome	**Outcome variable**
Survival: Overall and prostate cancer-specific	Probability of survival measured from the time of diagnosis using information in the CTR database. Death in the cohort was compared with that in the general population using Connecticut life tables from 1986.

Study finding

Descriptive: After a mean of 15.5 years of follow-up, age adjusted overall survival in men with localized CaP and a low Gleason score (2–4) was similar to that of men in the general population.

Analytic: With use of a proportional hazards model, both Gleason and ICED scores were the most powerful independent predictors of survival in men with localized CaP ($p < 0.001$). The other statistically significant predictor variables were clinical stage, indication for diagnosis, percentage tumor involvement of pathologic specimen, and method of diagnosis.

Figure 9.3–1. Outline of the long-term survival among men with conservatively treated localized prostate cancer study. CaP = prostate cancer; CTR = Connecticut Tumor Registry; ICED = index of co-existent disease.

and has been one of the 11 National Cancer Institute's Surveillance, Epidemiology, and End Results program sites since 1973. In addition, the CTR is frequently updated with tumor registries from individual hospitals and with files from the Health Care Financing Administration, the National Death Index, and the Department of Motor Vehicles databases. The CTR even has reciprocal agreements with surrounding states and Florida, in which many male residents of Connecticut reside during the winter. Although the cohort follow-up to measure mortality appears rigorous, the method to determine the cause of mortality may be less reliable. Prostate cancer is listed as a cause of death if it was listed as one of the three antecedent causes of death on the death certificate. Although an autopsy-based cause of death is more reliable, the use of death certificates is far more feasible, and under the circumstances of tracking a large cohort, it is probably the most reasonable method.

B. Is the finding attributable to other factors?

?Chance. Six of the nine predictor variables were statistically significant in their association with survival, but only Gleason score and ICED score are reported in the article, with $p < 0.001$. It is thus very unlikely that the association between Gleason or ICED score and survival can be explained by chance.

?Bias. BIASES IN SELECTING THE STUDY SUBJECTS. A major source of bias in this study is that the assembled cohort is likely contaminated with patients whose prostate cancer has metastasized. Because only a small number of patients had adequate metastatic surveys, the study sample probably includes patients with nonlocalized disease. This, however, would strengthen the authors' conclusion that localized low-grade disease has a favorable prognosis with watchful waiting. Similarly, life expectancy estimates that we calculate using this data would be more pessimistic than it would be using data from a population who truly had only localized disease.

BIASES IN FOLLOWING UP ON THE STUDY SUBJECTS. The study does not mention the number of subjects who are lost to follow up after being registered to the cohort with prostate neoplasia. However, as mentioned, we are reassured by the Connecticut Tumor Registry's efforts to follow up its subjects. There is some concern that reported prostate cancer mortality would have changed had 29% of those eligible not been excluded on the basis of incomplete data. Nevertheless, we are encouraged by the similar age and overall mortality of those excluded on this basis compared with those included.

BIASES IN EXECUTING OR MEASURING THE PREDICTOR VARIABLE. The authors did a rigorous job of blinding the pathologists and data abstractors to the patient outcome when reviewing Gleason scores, comorbidities, and other predictor variables gleaned from the medical record. The finding is thus unlikely to be attributed to measurement bias.

BIASES IN MEASURING THE OUTCOME VARIABLE. As mentioned, prostate cancer mortality was established as the cause of death if it was recorded as one of the three antecedent causes of mortality on the death certificate. Consider patients with high-, moderate-, and low-grade prostate cancer all dying under similar clinical circumstances. It is possible that physicians, knowing that higher-grade disease has a worse prognosis, would have been more likely to record prostate cancer as a cause of death on the death certificate for patients with high-grade disease. However, if in reality all grades of cancer were equally responsible for prostate cancer mortality, this supposed bias would have resulted in other cause mortality being higher for patients with low-grade disease. Because it is not, we may assume that the increased prostate cancer mortality in patients with high-grade disease is not due to a bias in recording the cause of death. Furthermore, because the data were evaluated retrospectively, follow-up appears rigorous, and mortality as it is recorded in the database does not lend itself to subjective interpretation, the researchers' documentation of the outcome variable should not be biased by knowledge of the predictor variable. (The study does not specifically mention whether determination of the outcome variable was blind to the predictor variable.)

BIASES IN ANALYZING THE DATA. For the descriptive part of the study that evaluates the single variable of survival, the authors used Kaplan-Meier survival curves to measure overall and prostate cancer mortalities (see Figure 1 in the JAMA article, page 628). Kaplan-Meier curves are considered an effective approach to estimate cohort survival by adjusting for varying follow-up times and dropouts. Life expectancy is calculated using a proportional hazards Gompertz model. The Gompertz distribution used in their model is considered the "gold standard" method used in determining survival.[4]

For the analytic component of the study, the authors evaluated the association between a number of prognostic factors and survival, appropriately using a stepwise proportional hazards model based on the Gompertz distribution.

?Confounders. The effect of confounding by the measured predictors is adjusted for in the proportional hazards model. The model, however, cannot correct for unmeasured confounders. Can you think of an unmeasured variable that is associated with the grade of prostatic neoplasia (ie, Gleason score) *and* that independently affects prostate cancer survival? It is hard to come up with any confounders that are not in the causal pathway that includes histologic tumor grade and eventual death resulting from prostate cancer.

C. Is the finding believable within the context of other knowledge?

?Consistency with other literature. Both descriptive and analytic studies have shown similar mortality rates and prognostic features. We have known through several previous studies that truly localized low-grade prostate cancer has an excellent prognosis and that less favorable histology and comorbid conditions decrease survival.[1,2,5,6]

?Biological plausibility. Yes, because less differentiated tumors grow more rapidly and metastasize, it is plausible that this would lead to decreased survival.

?Analogy. In many other cancers, less differentiated malignant processes are associated with a worse prognosis (eg, uterine cancer).

Step 4. What is the clinically relevant finding?

Analytic component

CALCULATING EXCESS RATE: The analytic component of the study analyzes the association between a host of prognostic factors and survival. The association is usually represented by a relative risk or hazard ratio. Although a relative risks is a ratio of risk (ie, the proportion of subjects with events in a population with the prognostic factor divided by the proportion with events in a control population), a hazard ratio is a ratio of rates (ie, the proportion of subjects with events per unit time in a population with the prognostic factor divided by the proportion with events per unit time in a control population). The clinically relevant result considers the excess risk or excess rate of an event in a population with a particular prognostic factor. The excess risk or rate uses absolute terms to describe how much more likely the outcome occurs in a patient with a given prognostic factor. For the study by Albertsen and coworkers, which reports hazard ratios over ranges of Gleason or ICED scores, we want to identify the excess rate of death with the respective prognostic factor.

Consider a 70-year-old man with high-grade prostate cancer. The study reports a hazard ratio of 3.3 for this grade of cancer. This means that the patient is 3.3 times more likely to die per year compared with the general population of 70-year-old Connecticut men (1986 life tables from this population were used to calculate the baseline rate of death). But what does this mean in absolute terms? We are told that the life expectancy for the general population of 70-year-old Connecticut men is 12.7 years. Assuming that life expectancy is the inverse of mortality, the mortality rate for this "baseline" population is approximately 8% per year (1/12.7). Therefore, the mortality rate in 70-year-old men with high-grade prostate cancer is approximately 26% per year (8 × 3.3). The excess rate of death attributable to high-grade prostate cancer is thus 18% per year (26 − 8).

DESCRIPTIVE COMPONENT. The descriptive component of the study describes a single variable in a population. Prognostic studies usually describe mortality in a population using survival curves. In this article, survival curves are presented for the general population and for populations with low-, moderate-, and high-grade localized prostate cancer. The clinically relevant result that is calculated from survival curves is the disease-specific mortality (dsm), ie, the mortality attributed *only* to the disease. This value enables us to use the DEALE,[4,7] presented in Chapter 8, to easily estimate an individual patient's mortality and ultimately, life expectancy (LE). In this particular article, however, LE data are already calculated using the gold standard Gompertz distribution (see Tables 2 and 3 of the JAMA article, page 631). Because the Gompertz distribution is too complex for routine use, and because most studies of prognosis present only survival curves and not LE data, we will practice calculating the LE using the less complicated DEALE approach. In this section, we will calculate the dsm using the survival curves in the study. In step 5 below, we will use the dsm to calculate the LE for our particular patient.

The survival curves for low-, moderate-, and high-grade localized prostate cancer are presented in Figure 2 of the JAMA article. Because the curves also display survival for the general population (ie, a control group is present), the dsm can be calculated using the approach presented on page 173 of Chapter 8.

Recall that the dsm is the difference in average annual mortality between the diseased cohort (m [disease]) and the nondiseased control cohort (m [control]). This represents the average annual mortality that is attributable to the disease itself. Also recall that the average annual mortality,

$$m = (-1/t) \ln fs,$$

where fs is the fractional survival at time t and ln is the natural logarithm (base e).

Referring to Figure 2 in the JAMA article (page 629) to calculate the dsm for moderate- and high-grade localized prostate cancer, we note that the probability of survival at 10 years for the control cohort is approximately 0.58; for the moderate-grade cohort (top right panel), it is approximately 0.34; and for high-grade cohort (bottom left panel), it is approximately 0.16.

As mentioned above, dsm = m (disease) − m (control). Therefore using the formula $m = (-1/t) \ln fs$:

$$\text{dsm (moderate grade)} = (-1/10) \ln 0.34 - (-1/10) \ln 0.58 = 0.053/\text{year}$$

and,

$$\text{dsm (high-grade)} = (-1/10) \ln 0.16 - (-1/10) \ln 0.58 = 0.129/\text{year}.$$

(Note that because there is no difference in mortality between the control and the low-grade cohort in the top left panel, the dsm for this grade of malignancy = 0.)

Step 5. Will the study help me in caring for my patient?

A. Are the subjects adequately described and similar to my patient?

The inception into the cohort is at the time of diagnosis. The mean age of the cohort was 71 years and 94% of the patients were white. Note that African-American and Latino patients, whose tumors may have a different natural history, are poorly represented. Even if our patient falls within these demographics, the study will probably not perfectly generalize to the present time for two reasons. First, 45% of the cohort initially received some form of hormonal therapy consisting of estrogens, bilateral orchiectomy, or antiandrogens. Subsequently it was shown that although hormonal therapy in early disease decreased prostate cancer–specific mortality, it increased cardiovascular mortality.[8] As a result, current practice dictates watchful waiting rather than hormonal therapy in the nonsurgical treatment of localized prostate cancer. Second, no patient underwent prostate-specific antigen (PSA) testing, and only a relatively small number received bone scans or metastatic surveys. This probably will result in the study cohort having more advanced disease than has our patient population.

B. Is the predictor variable adequately described and applicable to my patient?

We consider this question with respect to the analytic component of the study. Most pathology labs report Gleason scores when provided with tissue to diagnose prostate cancer. In this study, a Gleason score of 2–4 represents low-grade; 5–7, moderate-grade; and 8–10, high-grade tumors. ICED scores are more cumbersome to use. Most physicians are unfamiliar with this method to score morbidity, and because the method was not described in the study, we would have to obtain the index to evaluate our patient.

C. Will the findings result in an overall net benefit for my patient?

Except for the unlikely effect of an unmeasured confounder, and the unavoidable limitation of deriving cause of mortality data from death certificates, this study appears valid and is believable within the context of other knowledge.

The main limitation of this study probably lies in its generalizability. Is your patient hormonally treated and diagnosed in a manner similar to that in the study? Although hormonal treatment may lead to improved prostate cancer–specific mortality, the lack of PSA testing or metastatic evaluation in the study cohort probably means the cohort has a less favorable prognosis than our PSA tested patient population who have received a thorough evaluation for metastatic disease. However, even if the study cohort does not generalize to our patients, it can still be useful if we explain to our patients that the life expectancy information that we are providing probably underestimates the true value.

Let's use a real-life example to demonstrate how we can use the dsm derived from this study to provide our patient with life expectancy information.

A 75-year-old white man whom you have taken care of for many years comes to your clinic. He is very distraught over a recent diagnosis of prostate cancer, discovered incidentally by a urologist on a routine rectal examination during an evaluation for a worsening hydrocele. You review the pathology report in the medical record, which describes prostate cancer with a Gleason score of 6. You also note that the urologist's workup showed no evidence of metastatic disease. Your patient is understandably anxious, not knowing the implications of the diagnosis. He specifically asks you to provide an estimate of his life expectancy so that he can "get his affairs in order." You arrange follow-up in 1 week and assure him that you will review the literature to provide the best possible estimate that may further help him consider possible therapeutic actions. After retrieving the Albertsen and colleagues' JAMA article and having assessed its validity, you review pages 172–175 in Chapter 8 to determine your patient's life expectancy.

Recall that the process involves three steps.

First, calculate the disease-specific mortality using the survival curves in the study. The dsm for *moderate-grade* (ie, Gleason score = 6) prostate cancer as calculated in step 4 above is 0.053/year.

Second, calculate the patient-specific mortality (psm) by adding the dsm to the age specific mortality (asm) for your patient. The asm is derived from the Life Expectancy Table for the general population (see the Appendix to this book). According to this table, a 75-year-old white male has an LE = 9.4 years. Recall that the average annual mortality is the inverse of LE. Therefore, asm = 1/9.4 = 0.106/year.

Thus, *for your patient* the psm = asm (for 75-year-old white men) + dsm (for moderate-grade prostate) = 0.106 + 0.053 = 0.159/year.

Note that if your patient has more than one disease, you may retrieve the appropriate article for each disease and calculate the individual dsms from the respective survival curves, as in step 4. You would then sum these dsms, and add this value to the asm to calculate your patient's psm. However, in order to add the dsms together, the individual diseases must act independently of each other. In other words, one disease cannot accelerate the progression of another disease.

Third, calculate the life expectancy for your patient by inverting the psm. Thus, for the patient age, LE = 1/psm = 1/0.159 = 6.3 years.

His moderate-grade prostate cancer decreases his LE by 3.1 years (9.4 − 6.3). Assuming surgery is curative (and there is much debate about this), our patient must take into account the 0.1–2% up-front risk of death,[5] the daunting 30–60% risk of impotence,[5,9] and 34% risk of bothersome urinary incontinence.[9] Depending on your patient's discount rate and his quality-of-life assessment, he may decide to forgo the potential mortality benefit in the future to avoid the high risk of impotence or incontinence now.

A final word of caution. Remember that the DEALE is only an *approximation* of LE. If you compare the LE of 75-year-old white men with moderate-grade prostate cancer as calculated using the DEALE above (6.3 years) with that calculated using the gold standard Gompertz function in the study (6.7 years as seen in Table 2 of the JAMA article), you will note that the LE is underestimated by only 0.4 years. Similarly, if you use DEALE to calculate the LE of 75-year-old white men with high-grade prostate cancer, the approach is quite accurate, underestimating the LE by only 0.1 year. However, if you do the calculations for 70-year-old white men with moderate- and high-grade prostate cancer, the DEALE underestimates the LE by 1.4 and 1.2 years, respectively. If you perform the calculations for 65-year-old white men, you will see that the DEALE underestimates the LE by an even greater extent, by 2.9 years for moderate-grade cancers and by 2.8 years for high-grade cancers. These discrepancies are even greater than predicted by Beck and colleagues in their validation of the DEALE.[4] Thus, in addition to the fact that your cohort of patients will most likely have less advanced disease than the study cohort, you will want to emphasize to your patient that the calculations that you have made using the DEALE provide a pessimistic *approximation* of his LE, most likely representing a minimum estimate.

REFERENCES

1. Johansson JE et al: High 10-year survival rate in patients with early, untreated prostatic cancer. JAMA 1992;267:2191.
2. Chodak GW et al: Results of conservative management of clinically localized prostate cancer. N Engl J Med 1994;330:242.
3. Garnick MB, Fair WR: Prostate cancer: Emerging concepts. Part I. Ann Intern Med 1996;125:118.
4. Beck JR et al: A convenient approximation of life expectancy (the "DEALE"). I. Validation of the method. Am J Med 1982;73:883.
5. Catalona WJ: Management of cancer of the prostate. N Engl J Med 1994;331:996.
6. Whitmore W Jr: Conservative approaches to the management of localized prostatic cancer. Cancer 1993;71:970.
7. Beck JR et al: A convenient approximation of life expectancy (the "DEALE"). II. Use in medical decision-making. Am J Med 1982;73:889.
8. Scott WW et al: Hormonal therapy of prostatic cancer. Cancer 1980;45:1929.
9. Jonler M et al: Sequelae of radical prostatectomy. Br J Urol 1994;74:352.

Reprinted from JAMA ® The Journal of the American Medical Association   August 23/30, 1995 Volume 274   Copyright 1995, American Medical Association

Long-term Survival Among Men With Conservatively Treated Localized Prostate Cancer

Peter C. Albertsen, MD; Dennis G. Fryback, PhD; Barry E. Storer, PhD; Thomas F. Kolon, MD; Judith Fine

Objective.—To determine age-specific, all-cause mortality, disease-specific mortality, and life expectancy for men aged 65 to 75 years who are treated only with immediate or delayed hormonal therapy for newly diagnosed, clinically localized prostate cancer.

Design.—A population-based, retrospective cohort study.

Setting.—Patient records were abstracted from 37 acute care hospitals and two Veterans Affairs medical centers in Connecticut. Original pathology slides were sent to a referee pathologist who was blinded to case outcomes.

Subjects.—All men identified by the Connecticut Tumor Registry with clinically localized prostate cancer diagnosed in 1971 to 1976 who were aged 65 to 75 years at the time of diagnosis and were untreated or treated with immediate or delayed hormonal therapy.

Main Outcome Measures.—Parametric proportional hazards models incorporating tumor histologic findings, comorbidity, and age at the time of diagnosis to compare cohort survival with that of men in the general population.

Results.—After a mean follow-up of 15.5 years, the age-adjusted survival for men with Gleason score 2 to 4 tumors was not significantly different from that of the general population. Maximum estimated lost life expectancy for men with Gleason score 5 to 7 tumors was 4 to 5 years and for men with Gleason score 8 to 10 tumors was 6 to 8 years. Tumor histologic findings and patient comorbidities were powerful independent predictors of survival.

Conclusions.—Compared with the general population, men aged 65 to 75 years with conservatively treated low-grade prostate cancer incur no loss of life expectancy. Men with higher-grade tumors (Gleason scores 5 to 10) experience a progressively increasing loss of life expectancy. Case series reports of survival/mortality experienced by men with clinically localized prostate cancer that fail to control for age, tumor histologic features, and comorbidities risk significant bias.

(*JAMA*. 1995;274:626-631)

CONSIDERABLE controversy surrounds prostate cancer screening and the treatment of localized disease.[1] Many physicians and medical organizations recommend screening because prostate cancer claimed more than 38000 lives in 1994.[2] The belief that early diagnosis and treatment leads to improved survival has led to increasing rates of radiation therapy and radical surgery.[3,4] Unfortunately, no trials of sufficient power are available (of which we are aware) to document the therapeutic benefit of either of these therapies for men aged 65 to 75 years compared with the more conservative alternative, immediate or delayed hormonal therapy.[5] Recently published analyses of treatment and screening decisions have questioned whether the magnitude of benefit is sufficient to warrant the associated morbidity and cost.[6,7]

The arguments for and against widespread screening and treatment among men aged 65 to 75 years turn critically on inferences about the natural history of conservatively managed localized prostate cancer. Specifically, the discussion centers around the average number of years of life lost to the disease. To date, two studies have provided the main source of data for these inferences: a population-based study of conservatively treated men assembled from a Swedish cancer registry[8] and a meta-analysis that includes several case series of patients treated conservatively.[9] The study by Johanssen et al[8] is often criticized because it includes a large number of men with low-grade tumors, relies on findings from aspiration cytology rather than histologic material for many patients, and is based on an observed sample of men who are older than those typically encountered in current US practice. The study by Chodak et al[9] suffers from potential unknown selection biases, as only 60% of the studies identified with potential cases for analysis were included in the final analysis, and most of the studies included were neither randomized nor population based.

Our objective was to estimate long-term survival of men aged 65 to 75 years with conservatively treated newly diagnosed localized prostate cancer in a manner that minimizes susceptibility to bias from sources affecting earlier studies. We took advantage of the observation that during the 1970s, immediate or delayed hormonal therapy was the most common treatment of localized prostate cancer among older men. Retrospective data from men diagnosed and treated during this era can be used to estimate long-term survival, provided the data meet several criteria: (1) data collection must be population based to avoid selection biases inherent to case series; (2) data collection must be standardized with use of validated instruments to measure significant confounders, such as patient comorbidities and tumor histologic findings; and (3) the data must be sufficiently comprehensive to include long-term survival status collected in a consistent fashion. Our study attempts to meet these criteria.

From the Division of Urology, Department of Surgery, University of Connecticut Health Center, Farmington (Drs Albertsen and Kolon); the Departments of Preventive Medicine and Biostatistics, University of Wisconsin–Madison (Drs Fryback and Storer); and the Yale Cancer Center, Yale University, New Haven, Conn (Ms Fine).

Reprint requests to the Division of Urology, Department of Surgery, University of Connecticut Health Center, 263 Farmington Ave, Farmington, CT 06030-3955 (Dr Albertsen).

Conservatively Treated Prostate Cancer—Albertsen et al

SUBJECTS AND METHODS

Cohort Identification and Data Collection

Identifying information, hospital of diagnosis and treatment, and case disposition as of March 1993 were obtained from the Connecticut Tumor Registry (CTR) for all men in Connecticut meeting the following criteria: (1) diagnosed as having prostate cancer from 1971 to 1976, (2) aged 65 to 75 years at the time of diagnosis, and (3) prostate cancer putatively localized to the prostate at the time of diagnosis. Hospital records for each of the patients identified by the CTR were abstracted on location at each of the 37 hospitals and two Veterans Affairs medical centers where patients had been diagnosed. Study personnel, who were blinded to the case status as recorded by the CTR, abstracted hospital records using a standard form designed specifically for this project. A referee genitourinary pathologist, who was also blinded to the case status, reviewed the original pathology slides of 431 cases. Test-retest reliability of Gleason grading was ascertained by sending a sample of 83 cases to two other nationally prominent genitourinary pathologists (interclass correlation coefficient, 0.91; κ statistic, 0.70).

Data Elements

Data collected from the hospital record included the initial indication for surgery that resulted in case finding (benign prostatic hyperplasia or palpable lesion), the method by which the cancer was diagnosed (transurethral resection, open prostatectomy, needle biopsy, or other method), results of metastatic evaluation (acid phosphatase, bone scan, metastatic survey, or lymph node dissection) if completed, and initial treatment within 3 months of diagnosis. Data collected for patients treated at multiple hospitals were combined in a single, patient-specific abstract form.

Severity of comorbid disease is reported herein using the Index of Co-Existent Disease (ICED),[10] developed by Sheldon Greenfield, MD. During chart abstraction, we used three indexes to score comorbid disease: the ICED, an index introduced by Kaplan and Feinstein,[11] and an index presented by Charlson et al.[12] These indexes have been used successfully in published studies to adjust mortality rates, length-of-stay data, and complication rates in patients with major medical and surgical interventions. The latter two indexes have been used to adjust mortality rates following prostatectomy.[13] Because the scores of the three indexes were highly correlated in our sample, for simplicity we

report only ICED results, as this index accounted for somewhat more variation in survival than did the other two indexes.

The CTR provided the patients' birth date and date of diagnosis (both confirmed during chart abstraction), the date of last contact for follow-up, and the date and cause of death (from death certificates) for deceased patients. We recorded cause of death as secondary to prostate cancer if any one of three antecedent causes of death listed on the death certificate mentioned prostate cancer. The CTR is the oldest state cancer registry and has functioned as one of the 11 sites of the National Cancer Institute's Surveillance, Epidemiology, and End Results program since 1973. The CTR uses a variety of sources to obtain follow-up data for registered patients, including hospital tumor registrars who rely on hospital records and physician and patient contact. There are several reciprocal reporting agreements with surrounding states, as well as with Florida, where many Connecticut men reside during the winter. Every year, the CTR matches the files of the Health Care Financing Administration to determine the vital status of those men older than 65 years and, if alive, the date of their last medical claim. The National Death Index is linked every 2 years, while the Connecticut Department of Motor Vehicles files are linked twice each year.

The Connecticut Department of Public Health and Addiction Services provided the most recent (1986) abridged life tables reported by 5-year ages for Connecticut men.

Exclusions

The CTR provided the names of 991 men meeting our entry criteria. These men represent the entire population of incident cases of putatively localized prostate cancer in Connecticut fitting the age and date requirements to the level of ascertainment provided by the CTR and Surveillance, Epidemiology, and End Results methods. Unfortunately, included among these 991 individuals were men whose prostate cancer was diagnosed at autopsy or as an incidental finding during cystectomy. These cases are not informative for clinicians wishing to know the

natural history of this disease. Furthermore, review of primary source data failed to confirm the prostate cancer diagnosis in some cases, while in others identified patients with clinically advanced disease by modern staging criteria. We chose to exclude such cases to ensure a population cohort relevant to modern decision making. Criteria used to exclude cases were as follows:

- an acid phosphatase level, bone scan, or metastatic survey suggesting metastatic disease, or obvious extracapsular disease extension identified on review of original pathology slides (n=146);
- review of original pathology slides showed no evidence of prostate cancer (n=32);
- diagnosis made at autopsy (n=58);
- diagnosis was incidental to treatment of bladder cancer (n=5);
- patient was treated initially with either radical prostatectomy or definitive radiation therapy (n=111).

Of the remaining 639 eligible cases, 188 (29%) incomplete or missing charts led to the following exclusions:

- none of the patient records could be located (n=159);
- treatment provided to the patient could not be determined (n=3);
- neither a pathology report nor original pathology slide was available to confirm the diagnosis of prostate cancer (n=19);
- insufficient clinical information was available to compute a comorbidity index score (n=7).

The analyzed cohort of 451 men had a mean age of 70.9 years at the time of diagnosis. Based on our retrospective review of chart and pathologic data, we classified 63 cases (14%) as stage TA1 (tumor nonpalpable and involves <5% of specimen), 108 (24%) as TA2 (tumor nonpalpable and involves ≥5% of specimen), and 222 (49%) as TBx (tumor palpable) using the staging system approved by the Organ Systems Coordinating Center of the National Cancer Institute.[14] We classified the remaining 58 cases (13%) simply as stage TAx (tumor nonpalpable), because pathologic material was unavailable to permit further staging (Table 1). Hormonal treatment was initiated immediately for 202

Table 1.—Distribution of Cases by Tumor Stage and Gleason Score

Tumor Stage*	Gleason Score				All
	Gleason 2-4	Gleason 5-7	Gleason 8-10	No Histologic Detail	
TAx	0	0	0	58	58
TA1	24	34	5	0	63
TA2	14	51	43	0	108
TBx	6	75	82	59	222
All	44	160	130	117	451

*See text for explanation of tumor stages.

Conservatively Treated Prostate Cancer—Albertsen et al **627**

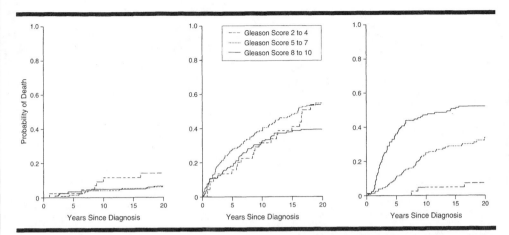

Figure 1.—Cumulative mortality since diagnosis of prostate cancer given tumor grade, displayed by cause of death (left, unknown cause [n=36]; center, cause other than prostate cancer [n=221]; and right, prostate cancer [n=154]). Cumulative mortality curves differ significantly by tumor grade for men dying of prostate cancer. Cumulative mortality curves for deaths due to causes other than prostate cancer are not statistically significantly different.

men, while the remaining 249 men received no therapy during the first 3 months following diagnosis.

Men excluded because of missing information did not differ statistically in year of entry into the CTR or in the number of years between entry in the registry and date of death or of last contact. Men excluded because of missing data were 0.54 year (95% confidence interval, 0.01 to 1.07) younger at the time of entry into the registry than were men who were included in the analysis (P=.05). Among excluded men, 8.5% were still alive at last contact, while among those included in the analysis, 8.9% were alive at last contact (P=.88). Men who were excluded were much more likely to have an undetermined cause of death than were those included in the analysis (84.6% vs 8.0%).

Statistical Analysis

We modeled survival using a parametric proportional hazards model based on the Gompertz distribution. From the Connecticut life tables, a reference background hazard rate $\lambda_o(t)$ was established for all-cause male mortality at age (t): log $\lambda_o(t)$ =A+Bt. The parameters A and B were estimated via least-squares procedures for the age range 65 to 85 years[15] and provided an excellent fit to the data (R^2=.999), with A being equal to −9.121 and B being equal to 0.08169. These were treated as fixed constants in the subsequent analyses. Based on an examination of complete US life tables to age 105 years, we estimated that this model would hold approximately to age 95 years but not necessarily beyond. Consequently, we considered survival times beyond age 95 years to be censored at age 95 years.

Given this baseline hazard function to account for age, we used a proportional hazards model with a forward stepwise selection procedure to examine the contributions of other independent variables.

Kaplan-Meier survival curves following diagnosis were computed for subgroups of men defined by their tumor histologic findings and comorbidity index value. An age-specific survival curve based on the baseline hazard model was also calculated for each man in the sample. The choice of the most applicable life table for this cohort can be debated, because the observed portions of their lives vary over a 20-year period. We selected the most recent life table available to ensure that any bias in baseline computations was toward longer survivals.

RESULTS

After a mean follow-up of 15.5 years, 40 men (9%) were alive at last contact, 154 (34%) had died of prostate cancer, 221 (49%) had died of other causes listed on the death certificate, and 36 (8%) are known dead but the cause of death could not be ascertained. Of the 40 men alive at last contact, the median time to last contact from diagnosis was 18 years. Only seven patients were unavailable for follow-up in less than 10 years.

Figure 1 shows the cumulative mortality rate from each of these causes as a function of histologic grade. Forty-six percent of men diagnosed as having high-grade prostate cancer (Gleason score 8 to 10) had died of their disease within 10 years, and 51% had died within 15 years; the corresponding percentages for men with moderate-grade disease (Gleason score 5 to 7) were 24% and 28%, respec-

tively. Men with low-grade prostate cancer (Gleason score 2 to 4) demonstrated no prostate cancer mortality before 7 years of follow-up. Their 10- and 15-year cumulative mortality from prostate cancer was 9%.

In contrast, the cumulative mortality from causes of death other than prostate cancer was no different between histologic groups. Men diagnosed as having prostate cancer between the ages of 65 and 75 years had a cumulative mortality of 35% at 10 years and 43% at 15 years from causes other than prostate cancer. Deaths could not be attributed to a specific cause for 5% of men at 10- and 15-year follow-up times.

The most powerful predictor of survival, above the baseline population age-specific, all-cause survival model, was the Gleason score of the tumor ($\chi^2_{(9)}$=60.4; P<.001). Figure 2 shows the cohort survival stratified by histologic group compared with the population survival model. The cohort Kaplan-Meier curve shows approximately a 5-year loss in median survival time for men aged 65 to 75 years with conservatively treated localized prostate cancer compared with the population curve based on 1986 life tables for Connecticut men. The survival curve for those cases for which Gleason scores were unavailable was similar to the average of the survival curve for cases with assigned Gleason scores.

Demographic factors, such as race, age at the time of diagnosis, and year of diagnosis, had no significant association with survival following diagnosis when considered individually. The remaining variables considered in the proportional hazards model, including clinical stage, initial in-

Conservatively Treated Prostate Cancer—Albertsen et al

dication for diagnostic procedure, percentage of tumor involvement of pathologic specimen, and method of diagnosis, were significantly associated with survival. Race was not predictive in this cohort, possibly because of low statistical power, as only 26 (5.8%) of the 451 men were nonwhite. Connecticut census data for 1970 show 4763 nonwhites (6.0%) among 79 347 resident men aged 65 to 75 years, indicating that our sample is representative of the state's racial mix at that time.

In stepwise models building on the baseline population age-specific, all-cause hazard, Gleason score of the tumor (as shown in Figure 2) was the first and most powerful predictor of the entire equation ($\chi^2_{(3)}=50.8; P<.001$), followed by the ICED comorbidity score ($\chi^2_{(3)}=43.0; P<.001$). Figure 3 shows the cohort survival stratified by ICED comorbidity score compared with the population survival model. Information concerning clinical stage or any of the other factors considered provided minimal additional predictive information. There was no statistically significant interaction between the Gleason score and ICED comorbidity ($\chi^2_{(8)}=11.7$), although the small sample size for some combinations of two variables limits the power to detect this. These two factors were assumed to act independently within the proportional hazard model, forming the basis of the calculations presented below.

Tables 2 and 3 present hazard ratios and life expectancies derived from the proportional hazards Gompertz model. The hazard (mortality rate) ratios are relative to the background rates from Connecticut men in 1986. For comparison, life expectancies for the 1986 Connecticut male population were 15.8 years, 12.7 years, and 10.0 years at ages 65, 70, and 75 years, respectively.

COMMENT

To our knowledge, these data present the first population-based survival analysis of conservatively treated prostate cancer in the United States. We believe that they overcome the potential biases noted in previously published results and provide quantitative estimates of life expectancy of 65- to 75-year-old men with conservatively treated clinically localized prostate cancer.

Our data differ from those of previous reports in several important ways. First, we collected population-based data to avoid the many biases associated with case series. Second, we used original pathologic specimens whenever possible to grade tumor histologic features and used an experienced genitourinary pathologist who was blinded to case results. Third, we reviewed original hospital records to obtain a consistent score for patient comorbidities. Although our

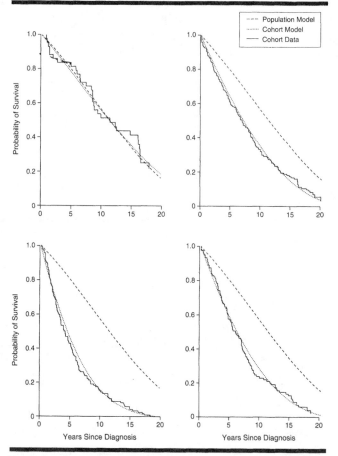

Figure 2.—Age-adjusted survival curves for low-, moderate-, and high-grade tumors. Observed cohort data are shown as Kaplan-Meier curves. Smooth curves are age-adjusted survival predicted for each group by the bivariate hazard model and by the general population model. Top left graph is for Gleason score 2 to 4 tumors (n=44); top right, Gleason score 5 to 7 tumors (n=160); bottom left, Gleason score 8 to 10 tumors (n=130); and bottom right, Gleason score unknown (n=117).

standards for data collection resulted in the exclusion of 29% of the potentially eligible cases, no differences were noted in demographic data or mortality rates between the excluded and included cases. Furthermore, this fraction is lower than the number of excluded or missing cases identified by Chodak et al[9] in their recently published meta-analysis of case series data.

Our data demonstrate two important findings: (1) tumor histologic features are highly predictive of survival for men aged 65 to 75 years and (2) patient comorbidities are nearly as potent a predictor of survival as tumor histologic findings among these men. Our findings are quali-

tatively concordant with those of previously published reports concerning conservative management of prostate cancer. Our methods, however, have yielded quantitative estimates that can be generalized to white American men.

Men aged 65 to 75 years diagnosed as having low-grade (Gleason score 2 to 4) prostate cancer face no apparent loss in life expectancy compared with a relevant general population. Most of these tumors were noted to be incidental to transurethral resection for benign prostatic hyperplasia, but 45% of these cases carried sufficient tumor burden to be classified as stage TA2 or TB. Our findings suggest that more aggressive treat-

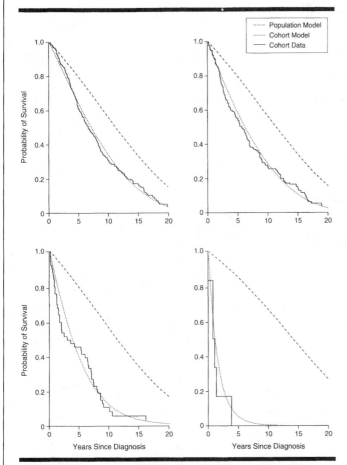

--- Population Model
..... Cohort Model
— Cohort Data

Figure 3.—Age-adjusted survival curves for levels of comorbidity indexed by the Index of Co-Existent Disease (ICED). Observed cohort data are shown as Kaplan-Meier curves. Smooth curves are age-adjusted survival predicted for each group by the bivariate hazard model and by the general population model. Top left graph is for ICED classification 0 (n=245); top right, ICED classification 1 (n=150); bottom left, ICED classification 2 (n=50); and bottom right, ICED classification 3 (n=6).

ment is unwarranted.

Men with moderate-grade (Gleason score 5 to 7) and high-grade (Gleason score 8 to 10) tumors face a progressively greater loss of life expectancy compared with the general population. We estimate that for men aged 65 to 75 years at the time of diagnosis, this loss of life is probably no greater than 4 to 5 years for moderate-grade tumors and 6 to 8 years for high-grade tumors. Because the goal of aggressive treatments, such as radical surgery or radiation therapy, is to cure affected men, our data provide quantitative upper-bound estimates of the potential years of life to be saved. Whether aggressive treatment is able to achieve these potential savings can be judged only by prospective randomized trials.

In the absence of trials with sufficient power to determine treatment efficacy among men with localized prostate cancer, clinicians and patients are forced to make inferences from results reported for case series of men treated with surgery or radiation therapy. Accordingly, our second finding, that patient comorbidities are nearly as potent a predictor of survival as are tumor histologic findings, carries particular relevance. Because men selected to undergo aggressive treatment may differ substantially from the general population, especially with regard to comorbidi-

ties, failure to adjust for this potential bias can result in inappropriate conclusions. For example, if men selected to undergo surgery generally have fewer comorbidities than men treated with radiation or conservative therapy, the survival among men treated with radiation or conservative therapy may appear to be inferior relative to surgery but is confounded by the effects of competing disease hazards.

A recent structured literature review of prostate cancer treatment case series revealed that 98% failed to stratify patients by comorbidity.[5] Adjusting case series data for expected survival given tumor histologic findings and comorbidity is not difficult (computational formulas are available from the authors on request). Our findings clearly demonstrate that age adjustment alone is an inadequate statistical control for the potential biases associated with case series results.

Two differences between incident cases of localized prostate cancer found today compared with those found during the 1970s act to ensure that the estimated loss in life expectancy owing to conservative management inferred from our analysis is a maximal estimate.

First, tumor staging was incomplete for many patients identified in our population-based study. Most patients lacked bone scans (80%), metastatic surveys (81%), or serum acid phosphatase levels (47%). No patient underwent prostate-specific antigen (PSA) testing, as this assay was unavailable in the 1970s. We attempted to exclude patients from our series who had more advanced disease at the time of diagnosis; however, some patients are likely to have had regional or distant disease, as judged by contemporary standards with use of PSA testing. Had we been able to exclude all patients with regional or metastatic disease using modern staging techniques, the reported cumulative mortality rates shown in Figures 1 through 3 would undoubtedly have been lower and the estimated loss in life expectancy compared with the male population would be smaller.

Second, because the current case finding for localized prostate cancer is largely driven by PSA testing, our results potentially differ owing to lead time advantage and length bias for contemporary cases identified by aggressive screening relative to those in our cohort.[16] The widespread availability of PSA testing and the ease of performing prostate biopsies has led to a dramatic rise in incident cases of localized prostate cancer.[17] These incremental cases carry a smaller tumor burden than many of the incident cases found during the 1970s, and the patients therefore would be expected on average to have a longer life expectancy. These biases as-

Table 2.—Estimated Hazard Ratios and Life Expectancies According to Gleason Scores for Men With Conservatively Treated, Clinically Localized Prostate Cancer*

		Life Expectancy†		
	Hazard Ratio‡	Age 65 y	Age 70 y	Age 75 y
All subjects	2.06 (1.87-2.27)	10.6 (10.0-11.2)	8.2 (7.7-8.7)	6.2 (5.8-6.6)
Gleason scores				
2-4	0.96 (0.68-1.36)	16.1 (13.4-19.0)	13.0 (10.6-15.6)	10.2 (8.2-12.5)
5-7	1.84 (1.56-2.17)	11.3 (10.3-12.4)	8.8 (7.9-9.8)	6.7 (6.0-7.5)
8-10	3.30 (2.78-3.93)	7.9 (7.0-8.8)	5.9 (5.2-6.7)	4.4 (3.8-5.0)

*Values in parentheses are 95% confidence intervals.
†Population life expectancies are 15.8, 12.7, and 10.0 years for ages 65, 70, and 75 years, respectively.
‡Relative to Connecticut men in 1986.

Table 3.—Estimated Hazard Ratios and Life Expectancies According to ICED Comorbidity Score for Men With Moderate-Grade, Conservatively Treated, Clinically Localized Prostate Cancer*

ICED Score for Gleason Score 5-7 Tumors		Life Expectancy†		
	Hazard Ratio‡	Age 65 y	Age 70 y	Age 75 y
0	1.55 (1.29-1.87)	12.5 (11.2-13.8)	9.8 (8.7-11.0)	7.5 (6.6-8.5)
1	2.02 (1.62-2.50)	10.7 (9.4-12.2)	8.3 (7.2-9.5)	6.3 (5.4-7.3)
2	3.81 (2.79-5.19)	7.1 (5.8-8.8)	5.4 (4.2-6.7)	3.9 (3.1-5.0)
3	16.8 (7.34-38.6)	2.3 (1.1-4.4)	1.6 (0.7-3.2)	1.1 (0.5-2.3)

*Values in parentheses are 95% confidence intervals. ICED indicates Index of Co-Existent Disease.
†Population life expectancies are 15.8, 12.7, and 10.0 years for ages 65, 70, and 75 years, respectively.
‡Relative to Connecticut men in 1986.

sociated with contemporary screening help to ensure that our computed loss of life expectancy associated with conservative management of localized disease is probably larger than can be expected in the 1990s, but this conclusion rests on the assumption that tumors identified by PSA testing progress in the same fashion as tumors identified previously.

Our findings carry implications for the interpretation of decision models of treatment outcomes for prostate cancer.[6,18-20] The accuracy of these models depends on estimates of long-term survival following alternative treatment strategies. Based on our analysis of the long-term survival of a population-based cohort of men who were diagnosed as having localized disease and treated conservatively, we present quantitative estimates of life expectancy for men aged 65 to 75 years and compare them to a relevant population life table. Tumor histologic findings and extant comorbidities are highly predictive of survival above and beyond patient age. Both of these factors must be controlled to allow for consistent and useful interpretations of case series survival data in men with localized prostate cancer.

Future studies must also include relevant information concerning treatment-associated morbidities.[21] We are currently participating in several efforts to assess patient quality of life following treatment of localized prostate cancer and will combine survival data from this study to construct decision algorithms that assist patients in this age group who face difficult treatment choices.

This project was supported by grant HS06770 from the Agency for Health Care Policy and Research, Rockville, Md.

The authors would like to thank Jonathan Epstein, MD, The Johns Hopkins School of Medicine, Baltimore, Md, for reading the histologic slides, Donald Gleason, MD, and David Bostwick, MD, for assisting with test-retest reliability of histologic readings, and the following Connecticut institutions, without whose assistance this research would not have been possible: Hartford Hospital; Yale–New Haven Hospital; St Francis Hospital and Medical Center, Hartford; Bridgeport Hospital; Waterbury Hospital; Hospital of St Raphael, New Haven; Danbury Hospital; New Britain General Hospital; Norwalk Hospital; St Vincent's Medical Center, Bridgeport; The Stamford Hospital; Middlesex Memorial Hospital, Middletown; Mt Sinai Hospital, Hartford; St Mary's Hospital, Waterbury; Lawrence and Memorial Hospital, New London; Manchester Memorial Hospital; Greenwich Hospital Association; Veterans Memorial Medical Center, Meriden; Griffin Hospital; Bristol Hospital; St Joseph Medical Center, Stamford; University of Connecticut Health Center/John Dempsey Hospital, Farmington; William W. Backus Hospital, Norwich; Park City Hospital, Bridgeport; Charlotte Hungerford Hospital, Torrington; Windham Community Memorial Hospital, Willimantic; Milford Hospital; Day Kimball Hospital, Putnam; Rockville General Hospital, Vernon-Rockville; Bradley Memorial Hospital, Southington; The Sharon Hospital; World War II Hospital, Meriden; New Milford Hospital; Johnson Memorial Hospital, Stafford Springs; Winsted Hospital, Uncas on Thames, Norwich; Veterans Home and Hospital, Rocky Hill; Veterans Affairs Medical Center–West Haven; and Veterans Administration Medical Center–Newington.

References

1. Kramer BS, Brown ML, Prorok PC, Potosky AL, Gohagan JK. Prostate cancer screening: what we know and what we need to know. *Ann Intern Med*. 1993;119:914-923.
2. Boring CC, Squires TS, Tong T, Montgomery S. Cancer statistics, 1994. *CA Cancer J Clin*. 1994;44:7-26.
3. Lu-Yao GL, Greenberg ER. Changes in prostate cancer incidence and treatment in USA. *Lancet*. 1994;343:251-254.
4. Lu-Yao GL, McLerran D, Wasson J, Wennberg JE, for the Prostate Patient Outcomes Research Team. An assessment of radical prostatectomy: time trends, geographic variation, and outcomes. *JAMA*. 1993;269:2633-2636.
5. Wasson JH, Cushman CC, Bruskewitz RC, Littenberg B, Mulley AG Jr, Wennberg JE, for the Prostate Patient Outcomes Research Team. A structured literature review of treatment for localized prostate cancer. *Arch Fam Med*. 1993;2:487-493.
6. Fleming C, Wasson JH, Albertsen PC, Barry MJ, Wennberg JE, for the Prostate Patient Outcomes Research Team. A decision analysis of alternative treatment strategies for clinically localized prostate cancer. *JAMA*. 1993;269:2650-2658.
7. Krahn MD, Mahoney JE, Eckman MH, Trachtenberg J, Pauker SG, Detsky AS. Screening for

prostate cancer: a decision analytic view. *JAMA*. 1994;272:773-780.
8. Johansson JE, Adami HO, Andersson SO, Bergstrom R, Holmberg L, Krusemo UB. High 10-year survival rate in patients with early, untreated prostatic cancer. *JAMA*. 1992;267:2191-2196.
9. Chodak GW, Thisted RA, Gerber GS, et al. Results of conservative management of clinically localized prostate cancer. *N Engl J Med*. 1994;330:242-248.
10. Greenfield S, Giovanni A, McNeil BJ, Cleary PD. The importance of co-existent disease in the occurrence of postoperative complications and one-year recovery in patients undergoing total hip replacement. *Med Care*. 1993;31:141-154.
11. Kaplan MH, Feinstein AR. The importance of classifying initial co-morbidity in evaluating the outcome of diabetes mellitus. *J Chronic Dis*. 1974;27:387-404.
12. Charlson ME, Pompei P, Alex KL, MacKenzi CR. A new method of classifying prognostic comorbidity in longitudinal studies: development and validation. *J Chronic Dis*. 1987;40:373-383.
13. Concato J, Horowitz RI, Feinstein AR, Elmore JG, Schiff SF. Problems of comorbidity in mortality after prostatectomy. *JAMA*. 1992;267:1077-1082.
14. Catalona WJ, Whitmore WF. New staging sys-

tems for prostate cancer. *J Urol*. 1989;142:1302-1304.
15. Elandt-Johnson RC, Johnson NL. *Survival Models and Data Analysis*. New York, NY: John Wiley & Sons Inc; 1980.
16. Black WC, Welch HG. Advances in diagnostic imaging and overestimations of disease prevalence and the benefits of therapy. *N Engl J Med*. 1993;328:1237-1243.
17. Potosky AL, Miller BA, Albertsen PC, Kramer BS. The role of increasing detection in the rising incidence of prostate cancer. *JAMA*. 1995;273:548-552.
18. Cowen ME, Chartrand M, Weitzel WF. A Markov model of the natural history of prostate cancer. *J Clin Epidemiol*. 1994;47:3-21.
19. Beck JR, Kattan MN, Miles BJ. Critique of decision analysis for clinically localized prostate cancer. *J Urol*. 1994;152:1894-1899.
20. Mold JW, Holtgrave DR, Bisonni RS, Marley DS, Wright RA, Spann SJ. The evaluation and treatment of men with asymptomatic prostate nodules in primary care: a decision analysis. *J Fam Pract*. 1992;34:561-568.
21. Litwin MS, Hays RD, Fink A, et al. Quality of life outcomes in men treated for localized prostate cancer. *JAMA*. 1995;273:129-135.

Conservatively Treated Prostate Cancer—Albertsen et al **631**

Printed and Published in the United States of America

10

EVALUATING INTEGRATIVE LITERATURE

Daniel J. Friedland, MD • Michael G. Shlipak MD, MPH •
Leslee L. Subak, MD • Stephen W. Bent, MD • Terrie Mendelson, MD

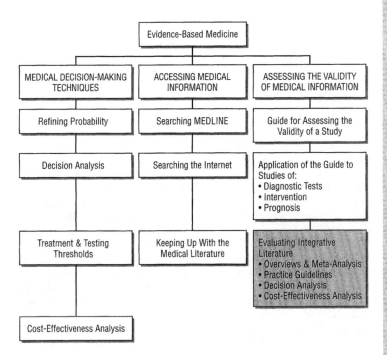

INTRODUCTION

In Chapter 8 we classified medical information as either *studies* or *integrative literature*. Recall that studies either describe individual variables (descriptive studies) or analyze the association between two or more variables (analytic studies). Integrative literature is distinct in that it "integrates" information reported in individual studies (and sometimes other integrative literature) within a particular framework. The individual frameworks that integrate information characterize the different types of integrative literature: overviews, meta-analyses, practice guidelines, decision analyses and cost-effectiveness analyses.

While the individual types of integrative literature may appear very different from each other, the process by which they are assembled is fairly uniform. Evidence-based integrative literature incorporates each component of evidence-based medicine (described in the introduction of this book), saving the clinician considerable time. In assembling *evidence-based* integrative literature the authors formulate an appropriate medical question, identify and retrieve all relevant studies, assess the validity of these studies and integrate this information within a particular framework to provide a summary finding or recommendation.

While saving the clinician time, the critical reader will want to consider the validity of the integrative literature (ie, whether the individual steps are optimally performed in the spirit of evidence-based medicine). If we determine that the summary finding or recommendation is valid, we then assess its applicability to the care of our patient (or patient population). Our general approach to evaluate integrative literature thus comprises five steps:

1. Is the problem framed in a clinically relevant manner?
2. Does the integrative framework incorporate all valid information?
3. Is the process of integrating information rigorous?
4. What is the finding or recommendation and is it presented appropriately?
5. Is the finding or recommendation applicable to the care of my patient?

In this chapter, we will apply this general approach to each type of integrative literature. Within each step, we will ask specific questions that pertain to the particular type of literature.

EVALUATING OVERVIEWS & META-ANALYSES

An **overview** is a summary of the medical literature on a focused clinical problem. The overview may address particular questions of incidence, prevalence, risk, diagnosis, treatment, or prognosis, or it may provide a summary of several of these factors with regard to a defined clinical problem. Many overviews are not comprehensive or balanced but represent the author's expert opinion on the basis of clinical experience and nonsystematic review of the literature. Reviews of this sort frequently propose diagnostic or treatment recommendations that are not substantiated in more rigorous, systematic analyses and cannot be relied on to provide evidence-based recommendations for clinical practice.

Some overviews do include a thorough literature search and critical appraisal of individual studies; the largest and most rigorously performed studies serve as the basis for the summary finding. These types of overviews are known as **systematic reviews.**[1] Although systematic reviews are evidence-based, the process by which the individual studies are integrated is *qualitative*. The summary finding thus does not demonstrate a magnitude of effect and may be biased by author opinion.

Meta-analysis is a type of systematic review that uses statistical techniques to *quantitatively* combine and summarize the results of previous research. By statistically combining the findings from many studies, meta-analyses are able to estimate the magnitude of the effect of an intervention or risk factor, as well as evaluate previously unanswered questions by performing subgroup analysis. If the methods of individual studies are similar, a meta-analysis may clarify the direction of effect when the findings of these individual studies are discrepant.[2,3]

The number of published meta-analyses in the English medical literature has increased dramatically, from only 13 between 1970 and 1980 to 416 between 1993 and 1996.[2,3] The role of meta-analysis has provoked some controversy, however. Some authors believe that meta-analysis may be as reliable as randomized controlled trials,[4] whereas others believe that the technique should be used only to generate rather than test hypotheses.[5] Although one recent study supported meta-analysis by finding results of smaller trials agreeing with larger trials in most cases (82–90%),[6] another study that compared the conclusions of meta-analyses with the results of subsequent large randomized controlled trials (generally considered to be the gold standard test of the efficacy of an intervention) found that meta-analysis did not accurately predict the results of the randomized controlled trials in 35% of the comparisons.[7] However, this study revealed that statistically significant differences in the results of the two study types occurred only 12% of the time. Controversy about the role and reliability of meta-analysis for medical decision making is likely to continue. Nevertheless, in the absence of a large randomized controlled trial, a meta-analysis of multiple smaller studies is probably the best source of information to answer a specific question as long as a rigorous meta-analytic technique is applied.

Many comprehensive guidelines and reviews discussing the technique of meta-analysis are available.[1–3,8] We will summarize the process of evaluating both meta-analyses and overviews using the aforementioned five-step approach. The evaluation of meta-analysis differs from that of overviews only in assessing the quantitative estimate of the finding. Use of this approach to evaluate overviews helps us determine whether they are truly systematic reviews that yield evidence-based findings which may enable us to better care for our patients.

Is the problem framed in a clinically relevant manner?

Are the population, predictor, and outcome clearly identified and relevant?

Overviews that summarize descriptive studies describe individual variables such as the demographic information about a population or the cause or natural history of a disease. Descriptive reviews usually provide background reading but not the type of information contained in summaries of analytic studies that are more likely to influence clinical practice. Analytic studies evaluate associations between variables so that one may identify risk factors and prognostic factors for a disease or determine the accuracy of a diagnostic test or the efficacy of an intervention. All meta-analyses summarize analytic studies.

You will recall from Chapter 8 (page 156) that a research question in an analytic study is composed of three components: the target population, the predictor, and the outcome. Thus, a review of analytic studies should clearly identify the spectrum of subjects and the predictor and outcome variables. The relevance of the review is partly dependent on the spectrum of subjects and conditions you treat in your clinical practice. Simply reading the question addressed by the overview should allow you to roughly determine whether the predictor (ie, the risk factor, prognostic factor, diagnostic test, or intervention) and type of subjects would be relevant to your practice.

If the subjects and predictor are relevant to our clinical practice, we then determine whether the outcome variable is clinically relevant. Outcome variables of morbidity and mortality are usually more useful than such intermediate variables as laboratory tests of risk factors for a particular disease. For example, a meta-analysis suggesting that the use of HMG-CoA reductase inhibitors reduces the incidence of stroke[9] is much more likely to change clinical practice than is a study indicating that soy protein intake reduces serum lipid levels.[10] Although both interventions may reduce morbidity, the study showing a clear risk reduction in the occurrence of stroke is much more meaningful than the study indicating a reduction in a laboratory value that may be a marker for increased risk of stroke.

Does the integrative framework incorporate all valid information?

Are prospective inclusion and exclusion criteria identified?
Is the search strategy comprehensive and explicitly described?
Is there an assessment of validity of the individual studies?
Is the process of study selection, searching, assessing validity and data abstraction reliable?

The validity of the summary finding is largely determined by the author's success in incorporating information from all relevant valid studies. This requires selection of studies using prospective inclusion and exclusion criteria, performing a comprehensive literature search, and assessment of the validity of individual studies. These processes and that of data abstraction should be reliable.

Prospective inclusion and exclusion criteria limit potential selection bias in the review that may occur if the authors primarily identify studies that support their own work or opinion. These prospective criteria should also ensure that the individual studies have the appropriate subjects and predictor and outcome variables to answer the particular research question, are sufficiently similar to be combined, and meet quality standards in study design and methodologic rigor.

The review should explicitly state the search strategy so that we can determine whether it is comprehensive. Comprehensive searches involve performing a thorough, up-to-date MEDLINE search that includes non-English language articles. Depending on the research question, other on-line databases (eg, AIDSLINE, CANCERLIT, EMBASE) should be included. Sources providing additional references include Index Medicus, the Science Citation Index, clinical trial registries (eg, Cochrane, NIH Inventory of Clinical Studies, VA Cooperative Studies Program Master List), granting agencies, governmental reports, bibliographies from textbooks and retrieved articles, and communication with experts.[1]

A thorough search may successfully identify all *published* articles, but it is more difficult to identify *unpublished* studies. Because studies with negative results are less likely to be published than studies with positive results,[11] inability to identify and retrieve unpublished studies may result in publication bias. However, while most meta-analysts believe that unpublished studies should be included in reviews, their inclusion is fraught with controversy.[12] Unpublished data may be less rigorous and more subject to bias. Furthermore, an adequate description of the methods may not be available to evaluate the validity of the study sufficiently. Indications of an author's effort to retrieve unpublished data include communication with experts and pharmaceutical companies and reviews of conference abstracts and repositories of unpublished data (eg, BRS Saunders, Clinical Trials Registry, Institutional Review Boards).[13] Although there are no perfect methods to estimate the effect of publication bias on the summary estimate, funnel plots or a number of other statistical tests may be used for this purpose.[13,14] If the authors are unable to sufficiently scrutinize the validity of unpublished studies, they may conduct a sensitivity analysis (see step 4), during which the summary estimate is calculated with unpublished studies both included and excluded.[12,13]

To assess whether each study retrieved is worthy of inclusion in the review, each study should be critically evaluated. It is essential that the authors assess the validity of each study to ensure the study design is rigorous, the subjects and variables are valid, and that the study findings are not attributable to the effect of chance, bias, or confounding. In meta-analyses, the quality of each study is sometimes graded using point scoring systems.[1] Incorporating quality assessment in the process of integrating information is discussed in the next section.

Because the thoroughness of a search, the inclusion and exclusion of studies, the assessment of study validity, and the process of data extraction may vary from individual to individual, a rigorous meta-analysis will involve many independent reviewers. We are assured of the reliability of these processes when multiple reviewers arrive at the same final study list and agree on the quality of the individual studies and data abstracted. A precise prospective definition of precise predictor and outcome variables further helps to improve reliability by limiting subjective interpretation when abstracting data. Particularly important is "blinding" the reviewer to the author, journal, year of publication, and study conclusion. This further limits bias in determining which studies should be included or excluded, in assessing a study's validity, and in performing data extraction.[2,3]

Is the process of integrating information rigorous?

Are the individual studies sufficiently similar that they can be combined?
Is the summary finding representative of the largest and most rigorously performed studies?

When the relevant information is integrated, the summary finding should reflect the most valid information. In **systematic reviews,** conclusions should be drawn from studies that address the same research question. However, simply comparing the number of studies with positive results with the number of studies with negative results is inadequate.[8] The author should assign greater qualitative weight to larger studies, as well as greater weight to randomized controlled trials than to observational studies (ie, cohort, case-control, and cross-sectional designs). However, even the most rigorous qualitative synthesis may be subject to the bias of author opinion, which may limit the ability to provide a truly accurate estimate of the magnitude of an effect. Nonetheless, there are times when it is best to discuss the finding in a qualitative review rather than presenting it quantitatively.

Meta-analysis quantitatively integrates results from individual studies and may provide an accurate estimate of effect size as long as quality studies are appropriately summarized. Most importantly, authors should combine studies that measure the same underlying effect. Thus, to ensure an accurate estimate of the magnitude of effect, the individual studies must be of good quality *and* have similar designs, methods, subjects, and predictor and outcome variables. If these factors are significantly different across studies, the summary finding may not be valid. In this situation, it is preferable for the finding to be summarized qualitatively rather than quantitatively. The next section discusses a statistical test of homogeneity that may also indicate the existence of important differences between studies.

Combining the results from individual studies by simple averaging of findings is not adequate primarily because such an approach does not account for differences in size of the individual studies. Of meta-analyses published between 1987 and 1990, only 78% were statistically adequate.[3] Many statistical methods are available to combine the findings from individual studies.[14–16] These methods calculate a summary estimate as a weighted mean of the individual study findings. The weight given to each study finding is typically the inverse of the variance of the finding (which itself is inversely proportional to the study sample size).

Adequate statistical integration of data from individual studies, however, does not necessarily ensure a reliable conclusion. The quality of the individual studies is critical but often inadequately addressed. In meta-analyses from 1955 to 1990, the issue was fully addressed in fewer than a quarter of reviews—and this number did not appear to increase with time. Quality was not assessed in almost half of the reviews.[3]

Inclusion of poor-quality studies leads to unreliable conclusions; this is otherwise known as the "garbage in, garbage out" phenomenon. Poor-quality studies may be excluded from the analysis using the aforementioned inclusion and exclusion criteria. If quality scores are used, studies with scores below a certain threshold may also be excluded.[1] When these criteria stipulate inclusion of the most rigorous study designs and methodology—for example, double-blind randomized controlled trials with at least 80% follow-up or, alternatively, studies designated high-quality scores—the summary finding will be most reliable. An interesting example of the use of quality scores is found in a meta-analysis by Warshafsky and colleagues,[17] which examined the effect of garlic intake on total serum cholesterol level. On the basis of the studies included in the meta-analysis, the authors concluded that ingestion of one half to one clove of garlic daily reduces total serum cholesterol levels by about 9%. The investigators appropriately performed a blinded, quality assessment of the individual studies using a quality scale ranging from 0 to 10. However, the five studies included in the meta-analysis received scores ranging only from 3.25 to 4.5, indicating the poor quality of *all* included studies. Because the summary estimate is based on poor-quality studies, the conclusion regarding efficacy of the intervention is undermined.

Some reviews may use the quality score to weight the relative contribution of individual study findings in calculating the summary estimate, although this approach is controversial.[18] If poor-quality studies are included in an analysis, their effect on the magnitude of the summary finding can be ascertained using sensitivity analysis, discussed next.

What is the finding and is it presented appropriately?

Are the key elements of each individual study clearly displayed?
What is the magnitude of the finding and is it statistically significant?
Is the finding homogeneous or heterogeneous?
Is a sensitivity analysis performed?

One of the most important benefits derived from reading a qualitative or quantitative overview is the time savings compared with evaluating the methods and findings of *all* the original literature. It is therefore very helpful when the author presents the key elements of the individual studies. Key elements, ideally presented in a table, include the study design, sample size, selection and characteristics of subjects, number of unreported or lost subjects, treatment dose and duration, outcome measures, and study result.[1] In qualitative overviews, such information enables the reader to judge whether the data are summarized fairly and whether discrepant findings are adequately discussed.

In meta-analysis, the summary effect may be described as a relative risk, odds ratio, effect size, relative or absolute risk reduction, or the numbers needed to treat to prevent a single event.[1] The magnitude of the summary effect should report its level of statistical significance using a p value or, better yet, a confidence interval (CI)[2,3] (see Chapter 8, pages 160–161). A p value of less than 0.05 indicates that the finding is statistically significant, which suggests that it is unlikely to have occurred by chance. Recall that the CI represents the range of values that are statistically compatible with the estimate of the study result, a 95% CI representing a range of values that would not differ from the estimate provided by the study at a statistical significance of 0.05. For example, if the 95% CI spans a relative risk or odds ratio of 1.0 or an effect size of zero, the result is statistically indistinguishable from no effect and is therefore not statistically significant. The width of the interval is determined by the number of study subjects and the precision of the measures. The narrower the CI, the more precise the result. If the finding is not significant and is imprecise even after many studies are summarized, we consider whether the finding may become significant in the future with the inclusion of additional studies (which would result in a larger number of subjects and a more precise result).

Meta-analyses use a statistical test of homogeneity to assess how different the individual study findings are from one another. Identification of heterogeneity suggests that the individual studies might have significant differences in methods, interventions, study populations, or overall quality. These differences between studies suggest that summarizing the data is akin to combining apples and oranges—and is therefore not meaningful. The test for heterogeneity is not very powerful for detecting differences across studies.[19] (This is the reason that important differences between studies are also considered qualitatively in step 3.) If heterogeneity is found, the authors should attempt to identify and account for important differences by redoing the analysis after exclusion of studies containing the difference or by stratifying the studies with respect to the difference. For example, in a meta-analysis by Sawaya and coworkers[20] that examined the efficacy of antibiotic prophylaxis at the time of induced abortion, significant heterogeneity was found between studies. There was no longer heterogeneity when the analysis was stratified according to low, mid-range, and high incidence of postabortion upper genital tract infection in the placebo group (reflecting an important difference in the propensity of these different populations to become infected). If heterogeneity cannot be explained and resolved, the summary estimate is less likely to be valid, and the finding should not be presented quantitatively but rather summarized in a qualitative overview.[8]

Meta-analyses should include sensitivity analyses, which recalculate the summary estimates for various inclusion criteria or other assumptions. For example, the summary finding may be calculated both including and excluding unpublished data, as well as studies of lesser quality or particular study populations. A recent meta-analysis by Saint and colleagues[21] evaluated the use of antibiotics in exacerbations of chronic obstructive pulmonary disease. The authors included studies of both inpatients and outpatients with exacerbations, assuming that the findings would be no different between these groups. They appropriately performed a sensitivity analysis to determine the impact on the summary estimate if inpatients were excluded and if outpatients were excluded. Since the summary estimate in each subgroup was similar, the authors concluded that the overall estimate represented both populations. In evaluating whether the summary estimate changes with varying assumptions, the authors demonstrate the robustness of the finding.

Is the finding applicable to the care of my patient?

Are the subjects adequately described and similar to my patient?
Is the predictor variable adequately described and applicable to my patient?
Will the finding result in an overall net benefit for my patient?

If the overview or meta-analysis has included all relevant studies and we believe the summary finding, we next determine whether the finding is applicable to our patient. Note that this step asks essentially the same question as that asked in step 5 of the study guide in Chapter 8—Will the study help me in caring for my patient?.

First, we ensure that the patients described in the overview are similar to our patient. The spectrum of subjects in the overview must be well enough described both in terms of demographic information and disease severity. If our patient is different from those in the review, the finding may not be applicable. (However, we may still find the review useful if it is applicable to other patients in our clinical practice). For example, it is now acknowledged that studies of prognosis and therapy of coronary artery disease (CAD) in men may not be generalizable to women.[22] We should thus exercise caution when applying the findings of most older reviews, which predominantly evaluated men, to a female patient in our practice. In addition, the impact of an intervention is often greater in patients with more advanced disease. For carotid endarterectomy, for example, the absolute risk reduction of stroke is greater in symptomatic patients than in asymptomatic patients.[23,24] If the overview does not explicitly state the severity of disease, the clinical setting where the patient received care may provide surrogate information. In general, patients treated in specialty clinics or referral centers have more advanced disease than do those treated in primary care clinics.[25]

Next we determine whether the predictor variable was well enough described and whether it is applicable to our patient. For reviews describing diagnosis or intervention, the diagnostic test and treatment should be sufficiently detailed and we will need the necessary resources and professional expertise to replicate them for our patient. Similarly for overviews of risk or prognosis, the risk factor and prognostic factor should be adequately described for us to assess if they apply to our patient.

Finally, it is important to weigh the costs (including all risks) and benefits associated with the findings to determine whether there is a net clinical benefit for your particular patient. The process for doing this is essentially the same as described in Chapter 8.

EVALUATING CLINICAL PRACTICE GUIDELINES

Clinical practice guidelines attempt to identify diagnostic and treatment strategies for common clinical problems, summarizing a vast quantity of medical knowledge into a readily usable format.[26] They have been defined by the Institute of Medicine as "systematically developed statements to assist practitioner and patient decisions about appropriate health care for specific clinical circumstances."[27]

More than 1600 clinical practice guidelines have been published by a variety of physician specialty organizations (eg, American College of Physicians, American College of Cardiology), volunteer health organizations (eg, American Heart Association, American Cancer Society), government agencies (eg, US Preventive Services Task Force, Agency for Health Care Policy and Research, Centers for Disease Control and Prevention), and independent research centers (eg, the RAND Corporation, Institute of Medicine). In addition, clinical practice guidelines are also developed by locally based medical organizations (eg, academic institutions, health maintenance organizations [HMOs]) and commercial organizations (eg, insurance agencies, consulting companies).[28]

Increasing pressure to provide more cost-effective medical care is fostering the development of an increasing number of clinical practice guidelines. Practice guidelines are in great demand by insurers: over 80% of HMOs encourage health care providers to follow specific guidelines,[29] and the National Committee for Quality Assurance, the major accreditation organization for managed care in the United States, requires practice guideline development, approval, and implementation as a condition of accreditation.[30]

The prescriptive nature of clinical practice guidelines is very seductive in an era in which clinicians are experiencing shrinking time for both the patient encounter and independent literature review. Furthermore, some clinicians may use particular clinical practice guidelines in the belief that they provide medicolegal protection. Practice guidelines, however, vary greatly in terms of their intended goals and perspectives, as well as in terms of the methodologic rigor with which they are assembled. Thus, before implementing a guideline, the critical reader will want to systematically assess its validity, as well as its applicability to the care of the individual patient. It is therefore very important that either the guidelines' policy statement or supporting article explicitly describe the process of assembly. Although it may seem like a lot of work to read a supporting article every time you evaluate a guideline, such organizations as the Agency for Health Care Policy and Research develop a host of guidelines that strictly comply with a uniform methodology. Thus, evaluating the one supporting article enables you to assess the validity of the entire series of guidelines.

Many approaches have been published to evaluate clinical practice guidelines.[31–33] We will employ the same five steps we used to evaluate overviews and meta-analyses.

Is the problem framed in a clinically relevant manner?

> Is the population, predictor and outcome clearly identified and relevant?
> What is the goal and perspective of the guideline?

As with overviews and meta-analyses, clinical practice guidelines should address an identifiable target population and predictors. The predictor should encompass all important diagnostic and therapeutic options for the management of a particular condition. In addition, the population and predictors should be clearly enough defined to allow the reader to determine the guideline's intended scope—the range of diagnostic tests and interventions administered by a defined group of providers for a specific group of patients. For example, the diagnostic and therapeutic strategies outlined by the Agency for Health Care Policy and Research guidelines for the management of depression[34] are intended to be used by primary care providers caring for their patients rather than for care delivered in psychiatric practice. The scope of patients is alluded to in the American College of Physicians' guidelines for using ambulatory electrocardiographic monitoring[35] by the statement that electrocardiographic ST-segment analysis is inaccurate in diagnosing coronary artery disease but may be useful in monitoring patients with known coronary disease.

The reader should also be able to identify the outcomes on which the recommendations are based to ensure they are clinically relevant. Recommendations based on studies that describe improvements in morbidity and mortality, rather than changes in laboratory values or risk factors, will be most relevant to the care of an individual patient.

Because clinical practice guidelines are prescriptive and biases in the recommendations may be difficult to detect, it is very important to identify the guideline's goal and perspective. Practice guidelines are developed to accomplish a variety of goals: to guide clinical practice in areas of uncertainty, decrease variation in practice style, increase quality of care, control escalating costs, and promote medical education through up-to-date literature synthesis. Furthermore, guidelines may be developed from the perspective of the patient, institution, or payer. For example, the American College of Physicians' guidelines for counseling postmenopausal women about preventive hormone therapy[36] are written from the perspective of the patient; the guidelines are intended to improve patient care through clinician counseling. On the other hand, a published practice guideline developed by a hospital to promote early hospital discharge of patients admitted with chest pain and low probability for myocardial infarction adopts an institutional perspective and is probably designed primarily to reduce hospital costs.

To facilitate our assessment of a guidelines' goal and perspective, as well as any potential biases favoring the author's supporting organization, the guideline developers should identify their source of funding, vocational titles, and professional, academic, or commercial affiliations. Identifying the guideline's goal and perspective helps us determine whether the guideline is consistent with our goals; a guideline intended to reduce costs may not necessarily improve the quality of patient care.

Does the integrative framework incorporate all valid information?

> Are prospective inclusion and exclusion criteria identified?
> Is the search strategy comprehensive and explicitly described?
> Has the validity of information incorporated been assessed?
> Has the guideline incorporated multidisciplinary input and patient preferences?
> Has the most up-to-date information been considered?

Clinical practice guidelines incorporate information from two main sources: published literature of differing methodologic rigor and expert opinion. It is often challenging to determine whether all valid information has been incorporated.

Because it is possible for guideline developers to find support for almost any recommendation if a very selective literature search is performed, prospective criteria for the inclusion and exclusion of studies should be formulated to limit potential bias. The literature search should be as comprehensive as that for overviews and meta-analyses, with efforts to retrieve all relevant published and unpublished material.

Once the relevant studies are identified, it is imperative that their validity be assessed. Unpublished material particularly deserves close scrutiny.

Although a variety of grading systems exist, they all consider the source of evidence; the more rigorous study designs receive the higher grades and expert opinion receives the lowest. The grading system used by the US Preventive Services Task Force[37] is provided in Table 10–1. (This grading system is a modification of the grading system originally developed by the Canadian Task Force on the Periodic Health Examination.[38])

Most diagnostic and therapeutic strategies involve a team approach to patient care. Multidisciplinary input is desirable to ensure the guideline recommendations are well balanced, as well as feasible, in considering all aspects of care. Generalist and subspecialty physicians, nurses, physical therapists, psychologists, social workers, public health officials, hospital administrators, and payers may all contribute. If the guidelines' intention is to improve patient care, the patient perspective is indispensable. The guideline should mention how patient preferences were assessed and incorporated; preferences derived from actual groups of patients are preferable to those assigned by providers.

Because "new and improved" diagnostic tests and interventions are continually becoming available, practice guidelines should be subject to an ongoing scheduled review process to ensure the incorporation of new data. To determine whether a guideline is outdated, search MEDLINE for relevant studies published after the cut-off date noted in the methods section, and compare the results of your search with the guideline's recommendations.

Is the process of integrating information rigorous?

Is the process by which the recommendations are formulated either evidence-based or explicit?

This step considers the process by which the information is individually weighted and synthesized to produce a recommendation. Woolf has divided the process of guideline assembly into four categories: informal consensus development, formal consensus development, evidence-based guideline development, and explicit guideline development.[39]

Informal consensus is the oldest process, and its legacy is the basis for an abundance of guidelines in use today. These guidelines are most often assembled using the BOGSAT principle—recommendations are formulated by a *b*unch *o*f *g*uys *s*itting *a*round *a* *t*able. These guidelines provide only recommendations and little background on the process by which they were synthesized. Even when evidence is cited in the discussion, there is little

TABLE 10–1. US PREVENTIVE SERVICES TASK FORCE SYSTEM FOR GRADING THE QUALITY OF EVIDENCE.[37]

Grade	Source of Evidence
I	Evidence obtained from at least one properly randomized controlled trial or a well-conducted meta-analyses based on properly randomized controlled trials
II-1	Evidence obtained from well-designed controlled trials without randomization
II-2	Evidence obtained from well-designed cohort or case-control analytic studies, preferably from more than one center or research group
II-3	Evidence obtained from multiple time series with or without the intervention
	Dramatic results in uncontrolled experiments (such as the results of the introduction of penicillin treatment in the 1940s) could also be regarded as this type of evidence
III	Opinions of respected authorities based on clinical experience, descriptive studies, and case reports, or reports of expert committees

documentation on how it was assessed and weighted to generate the recommendation. Guidelines developed in this manner are usually of poor quality because the recommendations are easily influenced by biased information and group dynamics.

Formal consensus was introduced in the 1970s. In 1977, the National Institutes of Health Consensus Development Program presented its structured approach to develop guidelines in a two-and-a-half-day conference.[40] Even though closed, plenary, and open sessions provided a more formal presentation of evidence than informal consensus, consensus was still the basis for reaching agreement on recommendations. Group dynamics—in which the most vocal may be most influential—potentially bias the recommendation. In the 1980s, the RAND Corporation introduced a more formal approach to assess expert opinion.[41] After receiving a package of relevant articles, individuals on the expert panel are asked to rate the appropriateness of a given procedure using a nine-point score (the Delphi technique). A score of 1 represents extreme inappropriateness and a score of 9 represents extreme appropriateness of the procedure. The scores are ultimately published as a distribution. Note, that these scores do not directly represent the strength of the individual evidence but rather the experts' overall impression of the merit of the procedure.

Evidence-based guidelines directly link recommendations to the strength of the underlying evidence. These guidelines weigh each source of information. The merits of studies that differ in methodological rigor and expert opinion are then factored together to produce a final graded recommendation. Examples of such guidelines are those produced by the Agency for Health Care Policy and Research, the Canadian Task Force, and the US Preventive Services Task Force. The US Preventive Services Task Force uses letter grades to denote whether the overall quality of evidence is "good," "fair," or "insufficient" (see Table 10–2).[37] This evidence-based guideline considers three criteria in assigning the grade: the burden of suffering from the target condition, the characteristics of the intervention, and the effectiveness of the intervention as demonstrated in published clinical research (refer to Table 10–1). Effectiveness of the intervention receives special emphasis.

Explicit guidelines were initially developed by Eddy to more explicitly weigh and present the specific information that generates the recommendation.[42,43] In this approach, the guideline developers specify the benefits, harms, and costs of the intervention. In addition, probability estimates for the most important outcomes and patient preferences for those outcomes are stated. Sometimes, the explicit guideline further incorporates the information into a decision or cost-effectiveness analysis.

Evidence-based and explicit guidelines represent the most rigorous processes for integrating information to generate recommendations. Thus, by identifying the process of guideline assembly we can ensure that we will be using the most evidence-based recommendations to care for our patients.

What is the recommendation and is it presented appropriately?

Are the recommendations graded according to the strength of the evidence?
Are the specific benefits, harms, costs, and patient preferences tabulated?

Evidence-based guidelines grade their recommendations according to the strength of the evidence (eg, Table 10–2).

Explicit guidelines tabulate the specific benefits, harms, and costs, as well as the probabilities and patient preferences for the most important outcomes. An excellent example of a

TABLE 10–2. MODIFIED SUMMARY OF THE US PREVENTIVE SERVICES TASK FORCE GRADING OF RECOMMENDATIONS.[37]

Grade	Summary of Strength of Evidence
A	There is good evidence to support the recommendation.
B	There is fair evidence to support the recommendation.
C	There is insufficient evidence for or against, but recommendations may be made on other grounds.
D	There is fair evidence to exclude the recommendation.
E	There is good evidence to exclude the recommendation.

balance sheet for this information, pertaining to colorectal cancer screening, is found in an article by Eddy.[44] The article contains a table that has column heads that read "No Screening" and "Fecal Occult Blood Testing/Endoscopy." Each column contains the probability of getting and dying of colorectal cancer; these differences between strategies reflect the net benefit of screening. Each column also lists the probability of a false-positive fecal occult blood test result, perforation from endoscopy, and measures of inconvenience, anxiety, and discomfort from testing; these differences represent the net harm of testing. In addition, costs of screening and cancer treatment are tabulated for each strategy.

If the explicit guideline includes a decision or cost-effectiveness analysis, sensitivity analysis should be performed to evaluate any change in recommendation that might result from any reasonable change in costs or the probability or preference for an outcome. Sensitivity analysis is further discussed in step 4 in the section on decision analysis.

Is the recommendation applicable to the care of my patient?

> Are the subjects adequately described and similar to my patient?
> Is the predictor variable adequately described and applicable to my patient?
> Will the recommendation result in an overall net benefit for my patient?

This step is similar to that in overviews and meta-analysis. After assessing whether the clinical practice guideline has included all of the valid information and whether formulation of the recommendation is rigorous, we determine whether the recommendation is applicable to our individual patient.

A sound guideline adequately describes the subjects for which it is intended so that we can determine if they are similar to our patients. The intended subjects should reflect the subjects in the primary studies on which the recommendation is based.

A sound guideline also adequately describes any diagnostic tests and interventions so we can duplicate them for our patient. If we have the necessary resources and local expertise, these predictors are considered applicable to our patient.

Finally, we weigh the costs and benefits of the diagnostic and therapeutic recommendations in the context of our patient's preferences to plan and implement an individualized strategy. If the guideline has been tested in a population representative of our patient, we may provide to our patient additional information regarding the likely outcome of the recommendation.

EVALUATING DECISION ANALYSES

In Chapter 2, we introduced the basic concepts of decision analysis and demonstrated how the technique can be useful in the treatment of an individual patient. This form of medical decision making is also applied to broad management dilemmas in public health. Although we prefer to base treatment strategies on evidence derived from randomized controlled clinical trials or meta-analyses of randomized controlled clinical trials, this level of evidence is frequently unavailable. Many clinical questions would take years of time, thousands of patients, and millions of dollars to answer through implementation of a randomized controlled clinical trial. As clinicians, we cannot delay all decisions until the best possible evidence is available. In these situations, a published decision analysis may be a helpful tool for making an evidence-based decision.

We will begin with a clinical situation in which decision analysis could be helpful. A published analysis will serve as an example for our approach to evaluate decision analysis.

> Suppose you are a primary care clinician with a practice including many women who are perimenopausal. You know that estrogen has been shown to reduce osteoporosis and the risk of hip fractures, and you have heard that hormone replacement therapy (HRT) reduces the incidence of CAD; however, you are concerned that the potential increase in endometrial and breast carcinomas may outweigh the benefits of HRT. Your patients depend on you to help them weigh these risks and benefits and to make a recommendation. Your initial inclination is to avoid HRT based on the principle of primum non nocere

(the first thing [is] to do no harm); you fear that your decision would result in cancer for some of your patients. On the other hand, if the evidence leans toward HRT providing a survival benefit by reducing the risk of fractures and CAD, your inaction is a poor decision that is costing your patients in potential survival time. Once again, you and each of your patients must make a decision.

Pondering the issue of HRT in postmenopausal women, you formulate the questions that you would like answered. Does HRT provide an overall survival benefit for those who receive it? Are there subgroups of patients who would benefit most, and are there subgroups who would be most harmed by HRT? If HRT is indicated, should you use estrogen alone or combinations of estrogen and progestin? Searching MEDLINE for answers, your initial attempt reveals no randomized controlled clinical trials that evaluate the potential survival benefit of HRT. Thinking that a decision analysis might be helpful, you combine a search of the subject headings "decision support techniques" and "hormone replacement," which yields six sources, including two decision analyses. You select one by Zubialde and coworkers entitled "Estimated Gains in Life Expectancy With Use of Postmenopausal Estrogen Therapy: A Decision Analysis,"[45] which seems to address the question you have. As the authors of this analysis note in their introduction, many nonexperimental studies have evaluated the impact of HRT on individual disease outcomes. Decision analysis is uniquely suited for the integration of these competing risks and benefits.

Unfortunately, decision analyses can be among the most difficult studies to read in the medical literature. Because the technique is highly quantitative and entirely dependent on the structure and data incorporated in the model, the published work tends to be lengthy and intimidating. Nonetheless, these articles can be evaluated with the same systematic method that you would apply to the other forms of integrative literature. In fact, both decision and cost-effectiveness analyses are easily evaluated using our five-step approach because the steps assembling the analyses (Chapters 2 and 4) almost perfectly parallel the steps we use to evaluate the analyses (see Table 10–3).

You will note that step 4 in evaluating analyses relates to both steps 4 and 5 used to assemble analyses. Step 5 in evaluating analyses then considers the applicability of the finding to the care of a specific patient.

You may also note that in order to maintain this parallel structure, it has been necessary to invert steps 2 and 3 relative to the approach used to evaluate overviews, meta-analyses, and clinical practice guidelines.

Reviewing Chapter 2 before reading this next section will facilitate your understanding regarding the importance of each specific question.

Is the problem framed in a clinically relevant manner?

Is the population, predictor, and outcome clearly identified and relevant?
Are the most reasonable strategies considered?
Is the time frame of the analysis appropriate?

As with other integrative literature, the research question should be important and have a clear focus with an identifiable target population, predictor, and outcome. If the subjects and predictor in the decision-analysis are relevant to our clinical practice, we then determine whether the outcome variable is clinically relevant. In Zubialde's article on HRT, we find the main question explicitly stated: "Is there a significant advantage in terms of life-expectancy benefit for women using postmenopausal estrogens?"

TABLE 10–3. STEPS FOR ASSEMBLING AND EVALUATING DECISION AND COST-EFFECTIVENESS ANALYSES.

Assembling Analyses	Evaluating Analyses
1. Formulate an explicit question	1. Is the problem framed in a clinically relevant manner?
2. Structure the decision	2. Is the process of integrating information rigorous?
3. Fill in the data	3. Does the integrative framework incorporate all valid information?
4. Determine the value of alternative strategies	4. What is the finding and is it presented appropriately?
5. Perform sensitivity analyses	5. Is the finding applicable to the care of my patient?

The importance of this clinical question is highlighted by the authors, who note the enormous number of women eligible for HRT. The subjects are postmenopausal women; the main predictor is a combination of estrogen and progestin. A secondary predictor is estrogen alone. Is this group of patients and type of intervention applicable to your practice? The main outcome is the clinically relevant variable life expectancy.

Next we evaluate the predictors in greater detail. We specifically determine whether the analysis considers the most reasonable strategies in the management of the particular condition. The three strategies compared in the analysis appear reasonable: no treatment, estrogen only, or estrogen and a progestin. Treatment is started after menopause and continued until death. Clinicians may wonder what impact the timing of HRT has on survival. Is there an age at which HRT should be discontinued? These more complex questions will not be answered by this decision analysis.

The time frame of the model should fit the natural history of the clinical situation. For example, a decision tree that compares treatments for dysuria should not rank different antibiotics based on their effect on survival, as patients rarely die of urinary tract infections. Conversely, a model that compares strategies for colorectal cancer screening should determine the overall effect on life-expectancy. The question of HRT can be settled only by weighing risks and benefits over decades of follow-up. The selected article addresses the long-term effects of HRT appropriately by choosing a time frame that extends from menopause until death.

Is the process of integrating information rigorous?

Is the type of analytic model appropriate?
Did the model account for all the relevant outcomes?

The type of model chosen should be appropriate for the patient and the clinical situation. A simple decision tree is appropriate for clinical scenarios that have all outcomes resolved in the near future (eg, treatment of dysuria) or that have a straightforward natural history over time (the ulcerative colitis example in Chapter 2). Alternatively, it is important to ensure that more sophisticated modeling techniques (such as the Markov model described in Chapter 2, pages 53–54, and Chapter 4, pages 87–88) have been used to adequately characterize more complex scenarios in which outcomes are projected over long periods of time and in which there are many intermediate health states through which patients transition.

Zubialde's analysis structures the decision using a Markov model, dividing women into HRT and no HRT cohorts. The Markov model cycles every year, with predetermined annual mortality rates in each cohort reflecting the effect of HRT over time. A standard decision tree could not have incorporated the complexity of the yearly cycles and annual mortality rates.

The structure of the model used in the decision analysis should be explicitly presented and preferably illustrated in the article. You should be able to determine whether the model accounts for all relevant outcomes that would be important to the patient. Life expectancy is important to both the patient and the physician, but intermediate outcomes of disease and disability may also need to be addressed in the decision analysis. Therapeutic strategies that involve the possibility of many levels of disease and disability are insufficiently evaluated by a model that classifies persons only as alive or dead. In fact, some states of health may involve such severe disability, such as a major stroke or profound dementia, that their utility may approach zero. On the other hand, life expectancy may be the right choice if no significant intermediate health states can be identified. The reader should feel comfortable that the published model reflects the natural history of the disease and all important outcomes of each strategy.

Because HRT may affect the risk of breast cancer, endometrial cancer, coronary artery disease, and osteoporosis, the model should include outcomes appropriate for each of these conditions. The outcomes chosen in Zubialde's analysis relate only to mortality. Each year, the patient has an age-specific probability of dying of endometrial carcinoma, breast carcinoma, coronary artery disease, or other causes. Intermediate outcomes related to the above diagnoses are excluded from the model. For example, if a woman needed to undergo mastectomy or hysterectomy because of a diagnosis of carcinoma, this model would not account for any related psychological and physical morbidity. Ignoring the decrement in quality of life that might be expected if HRT causes these "intermediate outcomes" biases the results of the study toward finding an overall benefit associated with HRT. Conversely, the model does not recognize the potentially beneficial effect of HRT on intermediate health states of CAD, such as nonfatal myocardial infarction or moderate angina pectoris. This could bias the results against finding a benefit from HRT.

The most significant outcome missing from this decision model relates to osteoporosis and the risk of fractures; the authors claim that the fact that HRT slows osteoporosis is already widely accepted. We expect that inclusion of osteoporosis and the prevention of fracture-associated mortality in the model would have increased the estimate of life expectancy in the HRT cohort. Its omission, therefore, represents a significant bias against finding an overall benefit from HRT in postmenopausal women. We will have to read further to determine whether this omission alters the conclusions of the study. On the other hand, omission of other outcomes—such as the potential increased risk of venous thromboembolism and gallbladder disease—may bias the finding toward demonstrating an overall benefit of HRT.

Does the integrative framework incorporate all valid information?

> Are the probabilities valid?
> Are the outcomes of effectiveness valid?
> Are the outcomes appropriately discounted?

In Chapter 2, the importance of incorporating valid data into a decision analytic model was discussed. After all, the results of the analysis are merely a reflection of the structure of the model and the data incorporated. Poor-quality information may lead to inappropriate conclusions and have a detrimental effect on patient care. Before scanning the results of the decision analysis, the reader should take care to evaluate the estimates selected by the authors.

It may be very difficult to determine the validity of the individual probabilities without retrieving and evaluating the primary data used in the model. Most readers, however, will not have time to directly review the primary studies and will rely on the credibility of the source. We can expect that probabilities extracted from studies are likely more reliable than numbers generated by modeling or expert opinion. Probabilities derived from experimental studies are usually more reliable than those derived from observational studies. Data obtained from large national databases and surveys may be more reliable and generalizable than data obtained from descriptive studies of relatively small populations. We may also feel a little more reassured when data are derived from studies published in highly respected peer reviewed journals. An analysis is most credible when it explicitly cites the source of all information incorporated in the model and comments on its validity.

In this HRT decision analysis, we find the value of each probability neatly tabulated and the source used to derive each is provided. The text also describes the authors' strategy for selecting these particular sources. The most important data incorporated in the model are the incidence and mortality rates of endometrial cancer, breast cancer, and coronary artery disease and the relative risk of each disease in HRT-treated compared with untreated women older than 50.

For **endometrial cancer,** the baseline incidence rates were obtained from population-based cohort data published in the *Journal of the National Cancer Institute* and the mortality rates are derived from cohort data published in *Cancer*. The relative risks of endometrial cancer for unopposed estrogen (5.7) and combined estrogen and progestins (1.6) compared with untreated women were estimated from a population-based case-control study published in *The Lancet*.

The incidence rates of **breast cancer** were derived from the National Cancer Institute's Epidemiology and End Results Study and the mortality rates were derived from a cohort study published in *The New England Journal of Medicine*. The authors incorporated only data for women at average risk for breast cancer. The relative risk of breast cancer for women receiving HRT, however, was less firmly known at the time of this study's publication. The authors cited two meta-analyses published in 1991 that addressed this question; one in *Archives of Internal Medicine* and another in *Journal of the American Medical Association*. The relative risks of breast cancer attributable to HRT was found to be 1.08 in the former study and 1.30 in the latter. Citing methodological questions with the latter study, Zubialde and colleagues chose the lower estimate as their "best estimate" and reserved the higher estimate for sensitivity analysis as the "worst-case scenario."

The incidence of **CAD** was derived from the large, well-known Framingham cohort. CAD mortality was estimated from a cohort study published in *Circulation* and from the medical treatment arms of three randomized control trials (Coronary Artery Surgery Study, European Collaborative Study, and Veterans Administration Cooperative Study). The protective effect of estrogen on coronary artery disease, a relative risk of 0.56, was derived from the Nurse's Health Study cohort. The variable unknown to the authors was a possible decrement in CAD survival benefit with the addition of a progestin to estrogen. They chose to model various degrees of declining benefit—from 0% to 40%—of combined therapy relative to the benefit of estrogen alone in sensitivity analysis.

The process ascribing the outcome measures of effectiveness should also be clearly described in the text of the article. Effectiveness may be measured in terms of life expectancy, quality-adjusted life expectancy (QALE), quality-adjusted life-years (QALYs), or utilities. As noted, this HRT analysis used only life expectancy as its outcome. Because HRT can influence many health outcomes—not just mortality (as discussed above in step 2)—QALE would have provided a better reflection of the overall impact of HRT.

If an analysis does incorporate utilities (either alone or, more commonly, as a component of QALE or QALYs, which adjust length of time for the utility of particular health states), the reader must carefully review the validity of the utilities. For the decision tree example in Chapter 2, the patient supplied the utilities using the standard gamble method for utility assessment. Other methods for deriving utilities are the time trade-off method and the visual analog scale. The visual analog scale may be less reliable as it generally underestimates utilities derived by the other methods (see Chapter 2, page 45). Optimally, utilities should be derived from persons who live with the outcome. If this approach is not feasible and published values are not available, a group of disease-free individuals can estimate utilities. Health care providers, doctors, and medical students frequently provide utilities because they are easily accessible to the medical researcher. However, these groups may systematically bias into the assignment of utilities, as they may be fundamentally different from the general public or your patient.

Discounting of outcomes has become the accepted method for reporting cumulative life expectancy or QALE. Most people value the present over the future. Because patients value outcomes in the present more than the same outcomes in the future, outcomes are discounted to their present value, as described in Chapters 2 and 4 (see pages 52–53 and 92, respectively).

The HRT analysis does not include a discount rate in its analysis of life expectancy. In analyses that use the outcome of life expectancy, discounting might be important if age-specific mortality, or the shape of the survival curve, differed among the three strategies. A "high discounter" might avoid a treatment strategy with a relatively high early mortality and late benefits, even if the average life-expectancy would be longer with the treatment. Typically, outcomes are discounted at an annual rate of 3–5%. Although early complications of HRT may be negligible, much of the assumed benefit of HRT accrues years after initiating therapy. Thus, omission of discounting probably overestimates the reported magnitude of efficacy of HRT.

What is the finding and is it presented appropriately?

What is the magnitude of difference between the different strategies?
Does a sensitivity analysis evaluate a reasonable range of uncertainty?

The purpose of a decision analysis is to give a definitive answer. The decision analytic process was developed to address the uncertainty surrounding the optimal management of a complex clinical situation. After reading the results of a decision analysis, we should know if there is a better option. In an analysis for an individual patient (as in Chapter 2), it may be sufficient to identify the best strategy. But, for decision analyses that address public health questions, the magnitude of the difference between the strategies should be clearly presented. A survival difference, for example, should quantitate the added life expectancy or QALYs of one strategy relative to the other. The exact difference in the average life expectancy or the quality-adjusted life expectancy per patient that is considered clinically significant is somewhat arbitrary. Some consider 2 months or more to be significant. On the other hand, if the difference between strategies is only a few days, the decision may be considered a "toss-up."

The authors of the decision analysis examining HRT and life expectancy presented the finding in a table that incorporates four levels of CAD risk. For all categories of CAD risk, combined HRT therapy confers a benefit in life expectancy ranging from 4 months in the lowest risk group to 2.3 years in the highest risk group. This baseline analysis assumes progestins do not decrease the benefit of estrogen on CAD mortality.

The baseline analysis incorporates the probabilities and utilities that the authors consider most valid. Because the findings depend on probabilities and utilities that are rarely based on perfect information and may not be appropriate for your patient, the authors should test the impact of uncertainty via sensitivity analysis (as described in Chapters 2 and 4, pages 48–52 and 96, respectively). The findings in the analysis may be recalculated over a range of the 95% CI of a point estimate, a range of values derived from different studies in the literature, or a clinically feasible range.[46] The less confidence there is in the accuracy of a probability value, the wider the range should be.[47] Thus, in addition to the baseline values of each estimate, the range of values over which sensitivity analyses are conducted should be explicitly stated.

One main benefit of sensitivity analyses is that they identify variables that deserve close scrutiny. The analysis is "sensitive" to changes in these variables because they cause relatively large changes in the magnitude of the finding. If the findings in an analysis show little change over a relatively broad range of values or a particular variable, the analysis is said to be "robust." An inaccuracy in the baseline value of a "sensitive" variable will more likely invalidate an analysis than a similar inaccuracy of a "robust" variable. Therefore, even though most clinicians who read a decision analysis will not have time to review the validity of all the primary data incorporated in an analysis, if the baseline value of a sensitive variable is of questionable validity, the reader should consider retrieving and evaluating the article from which the estimate was derived.

Sensitivity analysis in Zubialde's study focused on the two variables that the authors thought had the most uncertainty: the effect of HRT on the development of breast cancer and the effect of combined HRT on CAD-related mortality. The authors modeled the effect of added progestin on CAD risk reduction by decreasing the benefit shown with estrogen alone by 0–40%. As the reduction in HRT benefit rises from 0% to 40%, the benefit in life expectancy of combined HRT declines to 1.5 months in the lowest CAD risk group and to 1.2 years in the highest CAD risk group. The effect of HRT on the development of breast cancer was not presented in a table format. In the text of the results section of the paper, the authors note that increasing the relative risk of breast cancer to 1.3 in the HRT cohort decreases the life expectancy benefit of HRT by 70% in the low-risk CAD group, but only by 20%, 10%, and 7% in the average-, moderate-, and high-risk groups, respectively.

Note that while the authors decrease the benefit of estrogen therapy by up to 40% with the addition of progestin, they do not perform sensitivity analysis on the benefit of estrogen alone. Because all of the HRT benefit in this article derives from the reduction in risk of CAD and because the reported benefit of HRT is derived from observational data rather than from a randomized control trial, sensitivity analysis should have been performed over a relatively broad range of estrogen effect. Reducing the 0.56 relative risk of CAD by 40% with addition of a progestin still represents a 26% reduction in CAD risk with HRT. (This reduction in risk is especially impressive when compared with that described for other interventions reducing the risk of CAD, such as antihypertensive and lipid-lowering therapies.)

Is the finding applicable to the care of my patient?

Are the hypothetical subjects adequately described and similar to my patient?
Is the predictor variable adequately described and applicable to my patient?
Is the range of values for probabilities and outcomes applicable to my patient?
Will the finding result in an overall net benefit for my patient?

If we believe the finding, we may apply it to the care of our patient. Succinctly summarizing the above steps considering the rigor of the model's structure and the quality of data incorporated helps us crystallize the belief as to whether the finding is valid and therefore should be applied. If important biases are identified, we need to determine which strategy they favor. The quality of data incorporated in a decision analysis is often its Achilles' heel, because decision analysis is usually performed in the absence of a randomized control trial to resolve a clinical question.

A major bias in Zubialde's analysis is the omission of outcomes related to osteoporosis; such omission results in an underestimation of the magnitude of benefit of HRT. In addition, the omission of intermediate outcomes may also result in an underestimation of the benefit of HRT if one assumes that the reduction in morbidity associated with coronary artery disease and osteoporosis outweighs the expected increase in disability associated with endometrial and breast cancer.

Although the above biases support the article's conclusion of an overall HRT benefit, the reader should exercise caution. The conclusion finding a life expectancy benefit of HRT rests heavily on the incorporation of an impressive risk reduction of HRT on CAD that was derived from an observational study. While some clinicians might argue that the summary finding represents the best possible assessment of HRT efficacy based on the best available data, others may prefer to wait for the results of randomized control trials, particularly those elucidating the effect of HRT on CAD. (Such trials are in progress.) The latter-mentioned group of clinicians might argue that the application of results of decision analyses incorporating observational data should be reserved for situations in which one is compelled to make a therapeutic decision, as in the setting of life-threatening illness. They would assert that preventive strategies require experimental data before making universal recommendations. In this analysis of the preventive strategy of HRT, it would have been helpful if the authors had conducted sensitivity analysis over a reasonable range of estrogen benefit and reported a threshold at which estrogen would no longer be beneficial. Those who believe that the magnitude of estrogen benefit exceeds this threshold (and that the effect of omitting discounting and outcomes, such as venous thromboembolism is inconsequential) may accept the conclusion that the benefit of HRT outweighs its risks.

If one chooses to apply the finding to a particular patient, the hypothetical subjects in the analysis should be well enough described to determine whether they are similar to the patient. The hypothetical subjects should be similar to the populations of patients from which the data were derived. In the HRT analysis postmenopausal women are defined by an age 50 years and older; other demographic data are not provided. Because the finding is stratified by CAD risk groups, we need to determine to which risk group our patient belongs. Four CAD risk groups are defined in the methods section: "average" risk denotes the CAD risk of the general population of women; "low" risk is defined as the absence of five CAD risk factors (systolic hypertension, hypercholesterolemia, diabetes, cigarette smoking, and left ventricular hypertrophy); "high" risk is defined as the presence of all five CAD risk factors; and "moderate" risk is defined as a risk group intermediate between average- and high-risk groups. The authors do not specify the number of risk factors that characterize average- and moderate-risk groups.

It is also important for the analysis to sufficiently describe the diagnostic or therapeutic strategies; availability of sufficient local expertise and resources will enable us to reproduce the strategy for our patient. When a particular strategy uses an algorithmic approach, which involves a particular sequence of steps, we need to assess whether the steps are applicable to our practice. In Zubialde's study, the dose of each hormone is not specifically addressed. However, in this particular case, this omission may be appropriate since the ideal dose of HRT has not been determined in a clinical trial and the data incorporated in the analysis probably reflect a range of different dosages.

Finally, if the baseline probabilities and utilities in a valid analysis seem appropriate for our patient, the reported optimal strategy will result in an overall net benefit for our patient. Alternatively, if the baseline probabilities and utilities are different from our patient's, we turn to the sensitivity analysis to determine whether it indicates the best strategy for our patient. If our patient is at increased risk for CAD, for example, the sensitivity analysis indicates a greater magnitude of benefit with HRT. If the sensitivity analysis does not account for a different risk profile in our patient, however, the results should not be used. For example, this study applies only to women at average risk for breast cancer. If our patient has a family history of breast cancer, we cannot determine whether the reported CAD benefit outweighs the potentially increased risk of breast cancer.

EVALUATING COST-EFFECTIVENESS ANALYSES

In the previous section, we outlined a strategy for evaluating a decision analysis of hormone replacement therapy.

> While awaiting the results of a randomized control trial, you cautiously explain to individual women in your practice that the best available evidence suggests HRT offers a net health benefit. However, you are also a policy maker for an HMO that has a fixed budget. And although you currently believe that the benefits of HRT outweigh its risks, you need to know how much the HRT benefit will cost. Whereas **decision analysis** can help you determine the most effective strategy for a patient or patient population, **cost-effectiveness analysis** enables you to calculate how much the benefit costs.
>
> Realizing that implementing HRT in the entire postmenopausal population of your HMO will divert funds from other health care strategies, you would like to know how the costs and efficacy of HRT compare with other preventive strategies, such as mammographic screening for breast cancer, fecal occult blood testing for colon cancer, and use of Papanicolaou's smears for cervical cancer. You search MEDLINE, cross-referencing the terms cost-effectiveness analysis and hormone replacement and retrieve an article by Weinstein and Tosteson entitled "Cost-Effectiveness Analysis of Hormone Replacement."[48] Although it was published in 1990, you think it may be useful.

Since cost-effectiveness analysis is essentially a decision analysis that incorporates cost, the steps used to evaluate the validity of a cost-effectiveness analysis are almost identical to those used for decision analysis. We will use the same five-step approach to evaluate Weinstein and Tosteson's article and highlight the specific differences as they pertain to cost-effectiveness analysis. The main differences from decision analysis are the consideration of perspective in step 1 and costs in step 3, the presentation of the finding in step 4, and its application in step 5. Reviewing Chapter 4 before reading this section will make it easier for you to understand why each specific question is important.

Is the problem framed in a clinically relevant manner?

Is the population, predictor, and outcome clearly identified and relevant?
Are the most reasonable strategies considered?
Is the time frame of the analysis appropriate?
What is the perspective of the analysis?

The importance of this clinical question is highlighted by the authors who note the enormous number of women eligible for HRT and the very large annual cost (3.5 to 5.0 billion dollars) that is comparable to the annual cost of coronary artery revascularization or antihypertensive therapy.

Weinstein and Tosteson's analysis clearly identifies the subjects ("postmenopausal women") and predictor ("hormone replacement therapy"). If these subjects and the predictor are relevant to your practice, evaluate the outcome. All cost-effectiveness analyses, by definition, include cost as an outcome. The principal issue in determining the clinical relevance of the outcome lies in assessing the outcome measures of effectiveness. The most relevant outcomes of effectiveness for most preventive strategies are changes in life expectancy and changes in quality of life (measured as quality-adjusted life expectancy); both outcomes were used in the analysis.

The strategies are clearly outlined and represent commonly used HRT regimens: unopposed estrogen (0.625 mg/d conjugated estrogen) and combined estrogen-progestin therapy (25 days conjugated estrogen followed by 10 days of 10 mg/d medroxyprogesterone acetate). Treatment durations of 5 and 15 years are evaluated. Each regimen is compared with the strategy of no HRT. Commonly used regimens not considered are continuous progestin and estrogen therapy and the treatment duration of lifelong therapy.

The time frame of the model fits the natural history of the clinical scenario: beginning at the age of 50 years and continuing until death.

The perspective of the analysis principally refers to the viewpoint taken on costs. As discussed in Chapter 4 (see pages 86–87), costs may be viewed from the patient, program, payer, and societal perspectives. To facilitate comparability between cost-effectiveness analyses, the societal perspective should be taken. This is in accord with recent guidelines published by the Panel on Cost-Effectiveness in Health and Medicine.[49] Weinstein and Tosteson's analysis uses the societal perspective.

Is the process of integrating information rigorous?

Is the type of analytic model appropriate?
Did the model account for all the relevant outcomes?

As in decision analysis, the type of analytic model should be sophisticated enough to adequately characterize the complexity of the clinical scenario. While Weinstein and Tosteson's article did not explicitly describe the type of model used, the model does incorporate quality-adjusted life expectancy and discounting.

The clinical issues are the same as the previous decision analysis example: the potential benefits of the use of estrogen include reduced risk of CAD and osteoporosis and hip fractures, as well as relief of menopausal symptoms (eg, hot flashes and insomnia). Risks associated with HRT include potential increase in endometrial and breast carcinomas, gallbladder disease, and venous thromboembolism. The primary outcomes used in the model are life expectancy and QALYs. Although the structure of the model is not explicitly outlined, from the text we deduce that each strategy evaluated mortality from hip fracture, endometrial cancer, and breast cancer. Quality of life was evaluated in relation to menopausal symptoms and resumption of menstruation, level of disability with hip fracture, and diagnosis of endometrial cancer.

The main outcome omitted was the effect of HRT on coronary artery disease, although at the time the article was written, the authors cite evidence that the effect of HRT on CAD was inconclusive. If upcoming randomized controlled trials demonstrate a reduction in CAD with HRT, this analysis will underestimate the benefit of HRT and thus overestimate the cost-effectiveness ratio. By omitting a possible benefit of a reduction in other osteoporotic fractures, such as Colles' and vertebral fractures, the analysis may further underestimate the benefit of HRT. On the other hand, the model did not include a possible increase in the incidence of gallstones or venous thromboembolism with HRT and it did not account for a reduced quality of life associated with a diagnosis of breast cancer. These omissions probably overestimate the benefit of HRT and underestimate the cost-effectiveness ratio. If the reduction in CAD with HRT in experimental studies is shown to be as large as the observational data used in Zubialde's decision analysis[45] (which we evaluated in the previous section), the most likely overall effect of omitting the above-mentioned outcomes in Weinstein and Tosteson's analysis is an underestimate of the benefit of HRT.

Does the integrative framework incorporate all valid information?

Are the probabilities valid?
Are the outcomes of costs and effectiveness valid?
Are the outcomes discounted appropriately?

In the previous section on decision analysis, we discussed some tips for evaluating the validity of information incorporated in step 3. The probabilities in a cost-effectiveness study should be as rigorously evaluated as those in a decision analysis. In addition to evaluating the outcome measures of effectiveness, the reader of a cost-effectiveness analysis must assess whether all relevant costs are incorporated into the model and whether valid sources are used to estimate costs.

Weinstein and Tosteson's analysis cites the source of all data from which probability data are derived. Incidence rates for breast and endometrial cancer are based on the Third

National Cancer Survey. The relative risk for breast cancer associated with any estrogen was derived from a number of observational studies; the authors assumed a relative risk of 1.25 but acknowledged this value as controversial in the face of conflicting data. Survival after detection of breast cancer was based on unpublished data from the National Cancer Institute. Age-specific risks for endometrial cancer are derived from numerous epidemiologic studies. Women who receive unopposed estrogen are at increased risk for endometrial cancer: four-fold during the first 5 years of treatment, eight-fold from 5 years until treatment stopped, and four-fold for 5 years thereafter. Survival rates with estrogen-induced endometrial cancer assumed detection in stage 1, grade 1 as a result of annual monitoring and are derived from studies published in *Journal of the American Medical Association* and *Cancer.*

Age-specific incidence rates for hip fracture are estimated from a multiple regression model that incorporated age-specific bone mineral density of the hip. HRT was assumed to delay bone loss during the period of treatment. Age-specific probabilities of death after hip fracture are based on a study published in the *Journal of Bone & Joint Surgery.*

Death rates from other causes were obtained from *Vital Statistics of the United States* for women.

It thus appears that almost all data are derived from large national databases or studies published in reputable journals. The authors, however, do not comment on the reliability of the data incorporated. Ideally, the authors should test the robustness of all the key probabilities in the sensitivity analysis. If varying a particular probability causes large changes in cost-effectiveness, a policy maker should thoroughly evaluate the primary data to ensure that the baseline estimate in the model is valid.

Outcomes of cost are expressed in 1988 dollars. Cost estimates from before 1988 are appropriately adjusted to 1988 dollars using the medical component of the Consumer Price Index. It appears that all important direct costs associated for conditions included in the decision model have been considered: HRT and the associated physician visits; acute and long-term management of hip fracture; and management of endometrial cancer, endometrial hyperplasia, and breast cancer. In addition, the authors included the cost of an additional endometrial biopsy for the evaluation of unscheduled bleeding in the unopposed estrogen group. Costs of CAD, other osteoporotic fractures, gallbladder disease, and thromboembolism are not included. When possible, the authors use national cost estimates—Medicare prevailing charges or Medicare diagnosis-related group (DRG) reimbursements for specific procedures, both of which reflect the economic burden of care to society. The National Nursing Home Survey of reimbursement for nursing home residence is used to estimate annual nursing home costs. When national cost estimates were not available, the authors used Boston-area prevailing charges and adjusted for reimbursement. These costs are likely to be a reasonable representation of the direct societal costs of medical care. Drug charges were obtained from several pharmacies in the Boston area and averaged. The authors do not consider indirect cost (eg, lost wages) in the analysis. Perhaps they assumed that indirect costs would be similar for each strategy and would therefore not effect the incremental costs.

The outcome of effectiveness focused on the effect of HRT on quality of life. A number of assumptions are made. Weinstein and Tosteson assume that resumption of menses with HRT results in a loss of quality of life of 0.5% per year while relief of menopausal symptoms is assumed to result in a gain of quality of life of up to 2% per year. They also assume that the diagnosis of endometrial cancer causes a 20% reduction in quality of life for 5 years, that is, a loss of 1 quality-adjusted life year. The source or basis for these estimates is not mentioned. Utilities are incorporated for consequences of hip fracture: nursing home residence (0.4); disabled but living independently (0.8); acute, uncomplicated fracture (0.95 for 1 year only); and postfracture recovered (1.0). Although the method to derive these estimates is not explicitly described, a publication in the *American Journal of Medicine* is cited. Because the utilities appear relatively low, you retrieve the citation and find that the utilities were estimated by the article's authors and a panel of experts, not by patients. These estimates may or may not truly reflect the values your patients would place on these outcomes.

The authors appropriately discount all future costs at a commonly used rate of 5%. In addition, QALYs, which incorporate patient preferences, are discounted at the same rate.

What is the finding and is it presented appropriately?

What is the magnitude of difference between the different strategies?
Does a sensitivity analysis evaluate a reasonable range of uncertainty?

The relevant finding in a cost-effectiveness analysis is the incremental cost-effectiveness between one strategy and another. One strategy is often a regimen being considered for use and the other is usually the current acceptable regimen. For example, the relevant finding in evaluating screening mammography starting at age 40 years is determined by comparing this strategy with the current acceptable strategy of screening mammography starting at age 50 years. Comparing screening starting at age 40 years with a strategy of no screening at any age would not be meaningful.

The incremental cost-effectiveness ratio is the difference in costs between the two strategies divided by the difference in effectiveness between the two strategies (Δ costs/Δ effectiveness).

In Weinstein and Tosteson's analysis, each HRT strategy is compared with the reasonable alternative strategy of no HRT. The authors present the data in concise tables that show incremental costs and benefits and the incremental cost-effectiveness ratio of each HRT strategy.

The incremental lifetime discounted costs in 1988 dollars for each of the HRT strategies compared to no treatment are as follows: unopposed estrogen for 5 years (E-5), $1391; estrogen and progestin for 5 years (E-P-5), $1053; and estrogen and progestin for 15 years (E-P-15), $2514. E-P-5 costs the least of the three interventions because of the lower cost of uterine monitoring and treatment of uterine hyperplasia and cancer. While E-P-15 has the lowest cost for hip fracture, it is the most expensive intervention because of the increased cost of 10 additional years of HRT medication and the associated physician visits.

The effectiveness of each HRT strategy is presented as a net change in life expectancy and quality-adjusted life expectancy (QALE). This value represents the days of quality-adjusted life expectancy gained as a result of the net effects of HRT (ie, each HRT strategy is compared with no HRT) on hip fracture, endometrial and breast cancer, and mortality as a complication of uterine dilation and curettage. The net effect of each strategy on QALE (not discounted) is as follows: E-5, 55 days; E-P-5, 70 days; and E-P-15, 195 days. (Note that when QALE in days is divided by 365, it is equivalent to the more familiar QALY.)

Cost-effectiveness is calculated by dividing incremental costs by incremental effectiveness (in quality-adjusted life years and now discounted) of each HRT strategy compared with no treatment. The incremental cost-effectiveness is thus presented as cost per QALY; for E-5 it is $72,100; for E-P-5 it is $26,100; and for E-P-15 it is $24,000 per QALY. The authors also note the incremental cost-effectiveness of E-P-15 compared with E-P-5 is $22,650 per QALY.

Sensitivity analyses are performed in the article but only for the effect of menopausal symptoms and for the assumption made with respect to bone loss. The basis for assuming that resumption of menses with the addition of progestin results in a 0.5% per year decrement in quality of life and that relief of menopausal symptoms results in a 2% per year quality of life gain is not mentioned, and it is difficult to determine whether this represents a reasonable range of values. The results are particularly sensitive to these changes in quality of life. For example, for the E-P-5 strategy, the cost-effectiveness ratio more than doubles to $59,700 per QALY for a 0.5% per year loss in quality of life and is reduced more than two-thirds, to $8,000 per QALY for a quality of life gain of 2% per year.

The risk reduction for hip fracture is based on the "bone loss assumption," which assumes that HRT delays bone loss during treatment and that bone loss continues at the same rate it would have at age 50 without treatment. Sensitivity analysis evaluates the effect on the cost-effectiveness ratio of an alternative scenario suggested by several epidemiologic studies. The "epidemiologic assumption" assumes HRT reduces age-specific risk of hip fracture by 60%. The model is quite sensitive to this assumption, which more than doubles the cost-effectiveness of the E-P-15 strategy to $54,400 per QALY. If this strategy also results in a 0.5% loss in quality of life from resumption of menses, the cost-effectiveness ratio increases to $106,300 per QALY.

It would have been helpful if the authors presented sensitivity analyses on other probabilities incorporated in the model as well as on the utilities for hip fracture. By varying the baseline estimates of multiple variables, one may identify those variables that cause relatively large changes in the cost-effectiveness ratio. The identification of these "sensitive" variables invites particular close scrutiny of the primary data from which these baseline estimates were derived.

Because postmenopausal women have significant morbidity and mortality because of CAD, it would also have been helpful if the authors incorporated CAD as an outcome measure and performed a sensitivity analysis over a reasonable range of potentially protective or harmful effects of HRT. This would have allowed estimates of the effect of HRT on CAD using data published in the future.

Is the finding applicable to the care of my patient population?

Are the hypothetical subjects adequately described and similar to my patient population?
Is the predictor variable adequately described and applicable to my patient population?
Is the range of values for probabilities and outcomes applicable to my patient population?
Will the finding result in an overall net benefit for my patient population?

If we believe the finding on the basis of the structure and data incorporated within the model, we finally determine whether it can be applied to the care of our individual patient or patient population. A succinct summary of the rigor of the model and quality of data helps us assess whether we ultimately believe the finding (and thus whether it should be applied). The main omissions from the model are the effects of HRT on CAD, other osteoporotic events (other than hip fracture), gallbladder disease, and venous thromboembolism. If future experimental data demonstrate that HRT prevents CAD, HRT may be more cost-effective than presented here. On the other hand, if experimental data demonstrate little or no effect of HRT on CAD but rather increased venous thromboembolic events, HRT may be less cost-effective than presented here.

Most of the data incorporated in Weinstein and Tosteson's analysis are derived from observational data and assumptions made about quality of life. As with all types of integrative literature, we must be cautious. We may be tempted to place greater belief on the validity of the summary estimate than is warranted by the quality of the primary data. Our perceptions of the quality of primary data are easily buried in complex modeling, especially when modeling has been rigorous. As experimental studies and patient-derived data on utilities of menopausal symptoms and hysterectomy become available, an updated analysis on the cost-effectiveness of HRT will be more reliable. Nonetheless, at the time of its publication, we may cautiously accept the finding presented in Weinstein and Tosteson's analysis as a "best" estimate.

To apply the finding, the subjects and interventions should be well enough described that we may determine whether they are similar and applicable to our patient population. The individual study populations from which the data were derived represent the spectrum of subjects in the analysis. Although we know that the analysis refers to postmenopausal women (specifically, women 50 years and older), the demographics of women in the individual studies is not explicitly described. The dosage and duration of HRT is well enough described so that we can replicate the intervention for our patients.

Once we determine that the probabilities, costs, and utilities that characterize the risks and benefits of HRT are similar to our patient population, we can ultimately assess whether the finding benefits our patient or patient population. We may counsel individual patients using the finding from the effectiveness component of the analysis. For example, we might ask our patient if she would want to take cyclic estrogen and progestin therapy for 15 years for a potential 6-month gain in life expectancy (and possibly more if there is benefit on CAD) and decreased postmenopausal symptoms but with resumption in menses and possibly a 25% increased risk of breast cancer. In all cases, it is important to note that these estimates represent the average benefits to a population of women and may not reflect an individual's benefit.

When applied to a patient population, cost-effectiveness analysis may be used to determine the most efficient or productive use of limited resources, to maximize the aggregate health benefits, or to minimize the cost of achieving a given health goal. A strategy may be called cost-effective when, compared with its alternative, it is less costly or is cost saving with an equal or better outcome; it is more effective and more costly, with the added benefit worth the added cost; or it is less effective and less costly, with the added benefit of the alternative not worth the added cost. The determination of whether added benefit is worth the added cost is made by our society and depends on societal values and resource availability. "Worth" is a relative term that may change over time and with different perspectives (ie, patient, program, payor, societal). While the explicit quantification of acceptable cost for a given benefit is very difficult to define, useful benchmarks are medical interventions society chooses to implement or not implement. Many health care programs that are widely used and funded have incremental cost-effectiveness ratios in the range of $30,000–$50,000 per life year or per QALY, which therefore appears to represents a currently acceptable value.[49]

Weinstein and Tosteson's analysis reports a cost-effectiveness of $24,000 per QALY for 15 years of cyclic estrogen and progestin therapy, $26,100 per QALY for 5 years of cyclic estrogen and progestin therapy, and $72,100 per QALY for unopposed estrogen therapy; each HRT strategy is compared with the alternative strategy of no HRT (1988 dollars). For comparison, a cost-effectiveness analysis of annual fecal occult blood testing to detect colon cancer in the elderly (65–85 years) found the cost per life year gained to be about $35,000 versus no screening[50] (1989 dollars); annual screening mammography in women 50 years of age or older to be $21,400 per life year gained (and $21, 700 per QALY) versus no screening[51] (1995 dollars); and annual Papanicolaou testing for women (20–75 years) to be about $40,000 per life year gained versus no screening. The incremental cost per life year gained for decreasing the Papanicolaou testing interval from 2 years to 1 year was greater than $2,000,000 (article published 1990; we assumed 1989 dollars).[52]

Policy making is far more complex than implementing the most cost-effective strategies. It is very difficult to compare the cost-effectiveness ratios between analyses even if each respective analysis is rigorous and valid. Different analyses use different methodologies. Furthermore, cost estimates are usually obtained in different years; inflation will thus partly account for the magnitude of difference between estimates. For example, let's adjust the above-mentioned cost-effectiveness ratios to 1995 dollars using the medical component of the Consumer Price Index. The cost per QALY for 15 years of cyclic estrogen and progestin would be about $38,000, the cost per life year of annual fecal occult blood testing to detect colon cancer in the elderly (65–85 years) becomes about $52,000, and the cost per life year for annual Papanicolaou testing for women (20–75 years) would be about $59,000. In addition, the incremental cost per life year gained for decreasing the Papanicolaou testing interval from 2 years to 1 year becomes about $3,000,000. (We did not adjust the ratio for annual screening mammography for women 50 years of age and older because it is reported in 1995 dollars.)

To improve comparability between cost-effectiveness analyses, recent guidelines published by the Panel on Cost-Effectiveness in Health and Medicine[49] convened by the US Public Health Service have recommended the use of a reference case, a standard set of methodological practices for cost-effectiveness literature. The reference case is from the societal perspective and compares the intervention of interest to existing medical practice. All costs are evaluated in 1995 US dollars. The outcome should reflect incremental resources used compared with morbidity and mortality incorporated into a single measure, preferably quality-adjusted life years. Remember, when analyses are compared, the units of effectiveness should be similar (life years, quality-adjusted life years, lives saved, etc). In addition, outcomes of costs and effectiveness should be discounted and sensitivity analyses should be performed.

Even if analyses evaluating different types of strategies have similar methodologies and are comparable, other issues play an important role in policy making. When resources are limited, fundamental tensions may exist between the needs of the individual patient and the needs of the larger community or population.[53] Optimally, policy decision making considers principles of equity and ethics that incorporate the utilitarian perspective of doing the most amount of good for the most amount of people. The complex factors that guide the formulation of policy are, however, beyond the scope of this book.

SUMMARY

Table 10–4 provides a summary of the individual questions asked when evaluating overviews and meta-analyses, practice guidelines, and decision and cost-effectiveness analyses. Note that for decision and cost-effectiveness analyses, question 3 is asked before question 2.

TABLE 10–4. SUMMARY OF THE APPROACHES TO EVALUATING DIFFERENT TYPES OF INTEGRATIVE LITERATURE.

	Overviews and Meta-Analyses	Practice Guidelines	Decision and Cost-Effectiveness Analyses
1. Is the problem framed in a clinically relevant manner?	Is the population, predictor, and outcome clearly identified and relevant?	Is the population, predictor, and outcome clearly identified and relevant? What is the goal and perspective of the guideline?	Is the population, predictor, and outcome clearly identified and relevant? Are the most reasonable strategies considered? Is the time frame of the analysis appropriate? What is the perspective of the analysis?*
2. Does the integrative framework incorporate all valid information?	Are prospective inclusion and exclusion criteria identified? Is the search strategy comprehensive and explicitly described? Is there an assessment of validity of the individual studies? Is the process of study selection, searching, assessing validity, and data abstraction reliable?	Are prospective inclusion and exclusion criteria identified? Is the search strategy comprehensive and explicitly described? Has the validity of information incorporated been assessed? Has the guideline incorporated multidisciplinary input and patient preferences? Has the most up-to-date information been considered?	Are the probabilities valid? Are the outcomes of cost and effectiveness valid?† Are the outcomes discounted appropriately?
3. Is the process of integrating information rigorous?	Are the individual studies sufficiently similar that they can be combined? Is the summary finding representative of the largest and most rigorously performed studies?	Is the process by which the recommendations are formulated either evidence-based or explicit?	Is the type of analytic model appropriate? Did the model account for all the relevant outcomes?
4. What is the finding or recommendation and is it presented appropriately?	Are the key elements of each individual study clearly displayed? What is the magnitude of the finding and is it statistically significant? Is the finding homogeneous or heterogeneous? Is a sensitivity analysis performed?	Are the recommendations graded according to the strength of the evidence? Are the specific benefits, harms, costs, and patient preferences tabulated?	What is the magnitude of difference between the different strategies? Does a sensitivity analysis evaluate a reasonable range of uncertainty?
5. Is the finding or recommendation applicable to the care of my patient or patient population?	Are the subjects adequately described and similar to my patient? Is the predictor variable adequately described and applicable to my patient? Will the finding result in an overall net benefit for my patient?	Are the subjects adequately described and similar to my patient? Is the predictor variable adequately described and applicable to my patient? Will the recommendation result in an overall net benefit for my patient?	Are the hypothetical subjects adequately described and similar to my patient or patient population? Is the predictor variable adequately described and applicable to my patient or patient population? Is the range of values for probabilities and outcomes applicable to my patient or patient population? Will the finding result in an overall net benefit for my patient or patient population?

* This question applies only to cost-effectiveness analysis.

† For decision analysis, we consider only whether the outcomes of effectiveness are valid.

REFERENCES

1. Cook DJ et al: Methodologic guidelines for systematic reviews of randomized control trials in health care from the Potsdam consultation on meta-analysis. J Clin Epidemiol 1995;48:167.
2. Sacks HS et al: Meta-analyses of randomized controlled trials. N Engl J Med 1987;316:450.
3. Sacks HS et al: Meta-analysis: An update. Mount Sinai J Med 1996;63:216.
4. Olkin I: Statistical and theoretical considerations in meta-analysis. J Clin Epidemiol 1995;48:133.
5. Borzak S, Ridker PM: Discordance between meta-analyses and large-scale randomized controlled trials: Examples from the management of acute myocardial infarction. Ann Intern Med 1995;123:873.
6. Cappelleri JC et al: Large trials versus meta-analysis of smaller trials. JAMA 1996;276:1332.
7. LeLorier J et al: Discrepancies between meta-analyses and subsequent large randomized, controlled trials. N Engl J Med 1997;337:536.
8. Oxman AD et al: Users' guides to the medical literature. VI. How to use an overview. Evidence-Based Medicine Working Group. JAMA 1994;272:1367.
9. Blauw GJ et al: Stroke, statins, and cholesterol. A meta-analysis of randomized, placebo-controlled, double-blind trials with HMG-CoA reductase inhibitors. Stroke 1997;28:946.
10. Anderson JW et al: Meta-analysis of the effects of soy protein intake on serum lipids. N Engl J Med 1995;333:276.
11. Dickersin K et al: Publication bias and clinical trials. Controlled Clin Trials 1987;8:343.
12. Cook DJ et al: Should unpublished data be included in meta-analyses: Current convictions and controversies. JAMA 1993;269:2749.
13. L'abbe KA et al: Meta-Analysis in Clinical Research. Ann Intern Med 1987;107:224.
14. Petitti D: *Meta-Analysis, Decision Analysis and Cost-Effectiveness Analysis.* Oxford University Press, 1994.
15. Wolf FM: *Meta-Analysis: Quantitative Methods for Research Synthesis.* Sage Publications, 1986.
16 Greenland S: Quantitative methods in the review of epidemiologic literature. Epidemiol Rev 1987;9:1.
17. Warshafsky S et al: Effect of garlic on total serum cholesterol: A meta-analysis. Ann Intern Med 1993;119:599.
18. Moher D, Olkin I: Meta-analysis of randomized controlled trials: A concern for standards. JAMA 1995;274:1962.
19. Laird NM, Mosteller F: Some statistical methods for combining experimental results. Int J Technol Assess Health Care 1990;6:5.
20. Sawaya GF et al: Antibiotics at the time of induced abortion: The case for universal prophylaxis based on a meta-analysis. Obstet Gynecol 1996;87:884.
21. Saint S et al: Antibiotics in chronic obstructive pulmonary disease exacerbations: A meta-analysis. JAMA 1995;273:957.
22. Beery TA: Gender bias in the diagnosis and treatment of coronary artery disease. Heart Lung 1995;24:427.
23. North American Symptomatic Carotid Endarterectomy Trial Collaborators: Beneficial effect of carotid endarterectomy in symptomatic patients with high-grade carotid stenosis. N Engl J Med 1991;325:445.
24. Executive Committee for the Asymptomatic Carotid Atherosclerosis Study: Endarterectomy for asymptomatic carotid artery stenosis. JAMA 1995;273:1421.
25. Melton LJ: Selection bias in the referral of patients and the natural history of surgical conditions. Mayo Clin Proc 1985;60:880.
26. Eddy DM: The challenge. JAMA 1990;263:287.
27. Institute of Medicine: *Guidelines for Clinical Practice: From Development to Use.* National Academy Press, 1992.
28. Hong DW, Liang BA: The scope of clinical practice guidelines. Hosp Phys 1996;32:46.
29. Oberman L: HMOs pushing clinical guideline use by physician. Am Med News 1995;38:8.
30. Handley MR, Stuart ME: An evidence-based approach to evaluating and improving clinical practice: Guideline development. HMO Practice 1994;8:10.
31. Eddy DM: *A Manual for Assessing Health Practices and Designing Practice Policies.* American College of Physicians, 1992.
32. Hayward RSA et al: Users' guides to the medical literature. VIII. How to use clinical practice guidelines. Evidence-Based Medicine Working Group. A. Are the recommendations valid? JAMA 1996;274:570.
33. Hayward RSA et al: Users' guides to the medical literature. VIII. How to use clinical practice guidelines. Evidence-Based Medicine Working Group. B. What are the recommendations and will they help you in caring for your patients? JAMA 1996;27:1630.
34. Depression Guideline Panel: *Depression in Primary Care: Volume 1. Detection and Diagnosis.* Clinical Practice Guideline, Number 5. Rockville, MD. US Department of Health and Human

Services, Public Health Service, Agency for Health Care Policy and Research. AHCPR Publication No. 93–0550; April 1993.

35. American College of Physicians: Practice guideline: Ambulatory electrocardiographic monitoring. Ann Intern Med 1990;113:77.

36. American College of Physicians: Guidelines for counseling postmenopausal women about preventive hormone therapy. Ann Intern Med 1992;117:1038.

37. *Guide to Clinical Preventive Services: Report of the US Preventive Services Task Force,* 2nd ed. Williams & Wilkins, 1996.

38. Canadian Task Force on the Periodic Health Examination: The periodic health examination. Can Med Assoc J 1979;121:1193.

39. Woolf SH: Practice guidelines, a new reality in medicine. II. Methods of developing guidelines. Arch Intern Med 1992;152:946.

40. Institute of Medicine, Council on Health Care Technology: *Consensus Development at the NIH: Improving the Program.* National Academy Press, 1990.

41. Park RE et al: Physicians ratings of appropriate indications for six medical and surgical procedures. Am J Publ Health 1986;76:766.

42. Eddy DM: Practice policies: Guidelines for methods. JAMA 1990;263:1839.

43. Eddy DM: Guidelines for policy statements. JAMA 1990;263:2239.

44. Eddy DM: Comparing benefits and harms: The balance sheet. JAMA 1990;263:2493.

45. Zubialde JP et al: Estimated gains in life expectancy with use of postmenopausal estrogen therapy: A decision analysis. J Fam Pract 1993;36:271.

46. Drummond MF et al: User's Guides to the Medical Literature. XIII. How to Use an Article on Economic Analysis of Clinical Practice. A. Are the Results of the Study Valid? JAMA 1997;277:1552.

47. Krahn MD et al: Primer on medical decision analysis: 4. Analyzing the model and interpreting the results. Med Decis Making 1997;17:142.

48. Weinstein MC, Tosteson AN: Cost-effectiveness of hormone replacement. Ann N Y Acad Sci 1990;592:185.

49. Gold MR: *Cost-effectiveness in Health and Medicine.* Oxford University Press, 1996.

50. Wagner JL et al: Cost effectiveness of colorectal screening in the elderly. Ann Intern Med 1991;115:807.

51. Salzmann P et al: Cost-effectiveness of extending screening mammography guidelines to include women 40–49 years old. Ann Intern Med 1997;127:955.

52. Eddy DM: Screening for cervical cancer. Ann Intern Med 1990;113:214.

53. Bodenheimer TS, Grumbach K: *Understanding Health Policy: A Clinical Approach,* 2nd ed. Appleton & Lange, 1998.

APPENDIX
LIFE TABLE

TABLE A–1. EXPECTATION OF LIFE AT SINGLE YEARS OF AGE, BY RACE AND SEX: UNITED STATES, 1990.

Age	All races			White			All other					
							Total			Black		
	Both sexes	Male	Female	Both sexes	Male	Female	Both sexes	Male	Female	Both sexes	Male	Female
0	75.4	71.8	78.8	76.1	72.7	79.4	71.2	67.0	75.2	69.1	64.5	73.6
1	75.1	71.6	78.4	75.7	72.3	78.9	71.3	67.2	75.3	69.4	64.8	73.8
2	74.1	70.6	77.5	74.7	71.4	78.0	70.4	66.2	74.4	68.5	63.9	72.9
3	73.1	69.7	76.5	73.8	70.4	77.0	69.4	65.3	73.4	67.5	62.9	71.9
4	72.2	68.7	75.5	72.8	69.4	76.0	68.5	64.3	72.5	66.6	62.0	71.0
5	71.2	67.7	74.5	71.8	68.5	75.0	67.5	63.4	71.5	65.6	61.0	70.0
6	70.2	66.8	73.6	70.8	67.5	74.1	66.5	62.4	70.5	64.6	60.1	69.0
7	69.2	65.8	72.6	69.8	66.5	73.1	65.6	61.4	69.5	63.6	59.1	68.1
8	68.2	64.8	71.6	68.9	65.5	72.1	64.6	60.4	68.5	62.7	58.1	67.1
9	67.3	63.8	70.6	67.9	64.5	71.1	63.6	59.4	67.6	61.7	57.1	66.1
10	66.3	62.8	69.6	66.9	63.5	70.1	62.6	58.5	66.6	60.7	56.1	65.1
11	65.3	61.8	68.6	65.9	62.6	69.1	61.6	57.5	65.6	59.7	55.1	64.1
12	64.3	60.8	67.6	64.9	61.6	68.1	60.6	56.5	64.6	58.7	54.2	63.1
13	63.3	59.8	66.6	63.9	60.6	67.1	59.7	55.5	63.6	57.7	53.2	62.1
14	62.3	58.9	65.7	62.9	59.6	66.2	58.7	54.5	62.6	56.8	52.2	61.2
15	61.3	57.9	64.7	62.0	58.6	65.2	57.7	53.6	61.7	55.8	51.3	60.2
16	60.4	57.0	63.7	61.0	57.7	64.2	56.8	52.6	60.7	54.9	50.3	59.2
17	59.4	56.0	62.7	60.0	56.7	63.2	55.8	51.7	59.7	53.9	49.4	58.2
18	58.5	55.1	61.8	59.1	55.8	62.3	54.9	50.8	58.7	53.0	48.5	57.3
19	57.5	54.2	60.8	58.1	54.9	61.3	54.0	49.9	57.8	52.1	47.6	56.3
20	56.6	53.3	59.8	57.2	54.0	60.3	53.0	49.0	56.8	51.1	46.7	55.3
21	55.7	52.3	58.8	56.3	53.0	59.3	52.1	48.1	55.8	50.2	45.9	54.4
22	54.7	51.4	57.9	55.3	52.1	58.4	51.2	47.3	54.9	49.3	45.0	53.4
23	53.8	50.5	56.9	54.4	51.2	57.4	50.3	46.4	53.9	48.4	44.1	52.5
24	52.8	49.6	55.9	53.4	50.3	56.4	49.4	45.5	53.0	47.5	43.3	51.5
25	51.9	48.7	55.0	52.5	49.3	55.4	48.4	44.6	52.0	46.6	42.4	50.6
26	51.0	47.8	54.0	51.5	48.4	54.5	47.5	43.8	51.0	45.7	41.6	49.6
27	50.0	46.9	53.0	50.6	47.5	53.5	46.6	42.9	50.1	44.8	40.7	48.7
28	49.1	45.9	52.1	49.6	46.6	52.5	45.7	42.0	49.2	43.9	39.9	47.7
29	48.1	45.0	51.1	48.7	45.6	51.6	44.8	41.2	48.2	43.0	39.0	46.8

30	47.2	44.1	50.1	47.7	44.7	50.6	43.9	40.3	47.3	42.2	38.2	45.9
31	46.3	43.2	49.2	46.8	43.8	49.6	43.0	39.4	46.3	41.3	37.4	45.0
32	45.3	42.3	48.2	45.9	42.9	48.7	42.1	38.6	45.4	40.4	36.5	44.0
33	44.4	41.4	47.2	44.9	41.9	47.7	41.2	37.7	44.5	39.6	35.7	43.1
34	43.5	40.5	46.3	44.0	41.0	46.7	40.4	36.9	43.5	38.7	34.9	42.2
35	42.6	39.6	45.3	43.0	40.1	45.8	39.5	36.0	42.6	37.8	34.1	41.3
36	41.6	38.7	44.4	42.1	39.2	44.8	38.6	35.2	41.7	37.0	33.3	40.4
37	40.7	37.8	43.4	41.2	38.3	43.8	37.7	34.4	40.8	36.1	32.5	39.5
38	39.8	36.9	42.5	40.2	37.4	42.9	36.9	33.5	39.9	35.3	31.7	38.6
39	38.9	36.0	41.5	39.3	36.5	41.9	36.0	32.7	39.0	34.4	30.9	37.7
40	38.0	35.1	40.6	38.4	35.6	41.0	35.1	31.9	38.1	33.6	30.1	36.8
41	37.0	34.2	39.6	37.5	34.7	40.0	34.3	31.1	37.1	32.8	29.3	35.9
42	36.1	33.3	38.7	36.5	33.8	39.1	33.4	30.3	36.2	31.9	28.5	35.0
43	35.2	32.4	37.8	35.6	32.9	38.1	32.6	29.4	35.3	31.1	27.7	34.1
44	34.3	31.5	36.8	34.7	32.0	37.2	31.7	28.6	34.4	30.3	27.0	33.3
45	33.4	30.7	35.9	33.8	31.1	36.2	30.9	27.8	33.6	29.5	26.2	32.4
46	32.5	29.8	35.0	32.9	30.2	35.3	30.0	27.0	32.7	28.7	25.4	31.5
47	31.6	28.9	34.1	32.0	29.3	34.4	29.2	26.3	31.8	27.9	24.7	30.7
48	30.7	28.1	33.1	31.1	28.4	33.5	28.4	25.5	30.9	27.1	24.0	29.8
49	29.9	27.2	32.2	30.2	27.6	32.5	27.6	24.7	30.1	26.3	23.2	29.0
50	29.0	26.4	31.3	29.3	26.7	31.6	26.8	23.9	29.2	25.5	22.5	28.2
51	28.1	25.5	30.5	28.4	25.8	30.7	26.0	23.2	28.4	24.8	21.8	27.4
52	27.3	24.7	29.6	27.6	25.0	29.8	25.2	22.4	27.6	24.0	21.1	26.6
53	26.4	23.9	28.7	26.7	24.2	29.0	24.4	21.7	26.7	23.3	20.4	25.8
54	25.6	23.1	27.8	25.9	23.3	28.1	23.6	21.0	25.9	22.5	19.7	25.0
55	24.8	22.3	27.0	25.0	22.5	27.2	22.9	20.3	25.1	21.8	19.0	24.2
56	24.0	21.5	26.1	24.2	21.7	26.4	22.2	19.6	24.3	21.1	18.4	23.4
57	23.2	20.7	25.3	23.4	21.0	25.5	21.4	18.9	23.6	20.4	17.8	22.7
58	22.4	20.0	24.4	22.6	20.2	24.7	20.7	18.3	22.8	19.8	17.1	22.0
59	21.6	19.2	23.6	21.8	19.4	23.8	20.0	17.6	22.0	19.1	16.5	21.2
60	20.8	18.5	22.8	21.0	18.7	23.0	19.4	17.0	21.3	18.4	15.9	20.5
61	20.1	17.8	22.0	20.3	18.0	22.2	18.7	16.4	20.6	17.8	15.4	19.8
62	19.4	17.1	21.2	19.5	17.3	21.4	18.0	15.8	19.9	17.2	14.8	19.1
63	18.6	16.4	20.4	18.8	16.6	20.6	17.4	15.2	19.1	16.6	14.3	18.5
64	17.9	15.8	19.7	18.1	15.9	19.8	16.7	14.6	18.5	16.0	13.7	17.8

(continued)

TABLE A–1. EXPECTATION OF LIFE AT SINGLE YEARS OF AGE, BY RACE AND SEX: UNITED STATES, 1990. *(continued)*

Age	All races			White			All other Total			All other Black		
	Both sexes	Male	Female	Both sexes	Male	Female	Both sexes	Male	Female	Both sexes	Male	Female
65	17.2	15.1	18.9	17.3	15.2	19.1	16.1	14.0	17.8	15.4	13.2	17.2
66	16.5	14.5	18.2	16.6	14.6	18.3	15.5	13.5	17.1	14.8	12.7	16.5
67	15.9	13.8	17.4	16.0	13.9	17.5	14.9	12.9	16.4	14.3	12.2	15.9
68	15.2	13.2	16.7	15.3	13.3	16.8	14.3	12.4	15.8	13.7	11.7	15.3
69	14.5	12.6	16.0	14.6	12.7	16.1	13.8	11.9	15.2	13.2	11.2	14.7
70	13.9	12.0	15.3	14.0	12.1	15.4	13.2	11.4	14.5	12.7	10.7	14.1
71	13.3	11.5	14.6	13.3	11.5	14.7	12.7	10.9	13.9	12.2	10.3	13.5
72	12.7	10.9	13.9	12.7	11.0	14.0	12.1	10.5	13.3	11.7	9.9	12.9
73	12.1	10.4	13.3	12.1	10.4	13.3	11.6	10.0	12.7	11.2	9.4	12.3
74	11.5	9.9	12.6	11.5	9.9	12.6	11.1	9.5	12.1	10.7	9.0	11.8
75	10.9	9.4	12.0	11.0	9.4	12.0	10.5	9.1	11.5	10.2	8.6	11.2
76	10.4	8.9	11.3	10.4	8.9	11.4	10.0	8.7	10.9	9.7	8.2	10.7
77	9.8	8.4	10.7	9.9	8.4	10.8	9.5	8.3	10.4	9.2	7.8	10.1
78	9.3	7.9	10.1	9.3	7.9	10.2	9.1	7.8	9.8	8.8	7.4	9.6
79	8.8	7.5	9.5	8.8	7.5	9.6	8.6	7.4	9.3	8.3	7.1	9.1
80	8.3	7.1	9.0	8.3	7.1	9.0	8.1	7.0	8.8	7.9	6.7	8.6
81	7.8	6.7	8.4	7.8	6.7	8.4	7.7	6.7	8.2	7.5	6.3	8.1
82	7.4	6.3	7.9	7.4	6.3	7.9	7.2	6.3	7.7	7.0	6.0	7.6
83	6.9	5.9	7.4	6.9	5.9	7.4	6.8	5.9	7.3	6.6	5.7	7.1
84	6.5	5.6	6.9	6.5	5.5	6.9	6.4	5.6	6.8	6.2	5.3	6.7
85	6.1	5.2	6.4	6.1	5.2	6.4	6.0	5.3	6.4	5.9	5.0	6.3

United States Department of Health and Human Services. Vital Statistics of the United States. Hyatsville, 1990. Life Tables, Part IIA, Table 6–3.

INDEX